Measuring and Improving Patient Satisfaction

Patrick J. Shelton, DPM, MBA
Former Director of Education
Med Partners—Friendly Hills HealthCare Network
Managing Partner
France-Shelton Foot Health Centre
United Kingdom
Visiting Lecturer
University of Central England
West Midlands
United Kingdom

AN ASPEN PUBLICATION®
Aspen Publishers, Inc.
Gaithersburg, Maryland
2000

The author has made every effort to ensure the accuracy of the information herein. However, appropriate information sources should be consulted, especially for new or unfamiliar procedures. It is the responsibility of every practitioner to evaluate the appropriateness of a particular opinion in the context of actual clinical situations and with due considerations to new developments. The author, editors, and the publisher cannot be held responsible for any typographical or other errors found in this book.

Library of Congress Cataloging-in-Publication Data

Shelton, Patrick J.
Measuring and improving patient satisfaction/Patrick J. Shelton
p. ; cm.
Includes bibliographical references and index.
ISBN 0-8342-1074-6
1. Patient satisfaction.   I. Title.
[DNLM: 1. Patient Satisfaction.   2. Data Collection—methods.   3.
Organizational Innovation.   4. Quality Assurance, Health Care—organization &
administration.   5. Staff Development.   W 85 S545m 2000]
RA399.A1 S47 2000
362.1'068'5—dc21
00-020622

Orders: (800) 638-8437
Customer Service: (800) 234-1660

About Aspen Publishers • For more than 40 years, Aspen has been a leading professional publisher in a variety of disciplines. Aspen's vast information resources are available in both print and electronic formats. We are committed to providing the highest quality information available in the most appropriate format for our customers. Visit Aspen's Internet site for more information resources, directories, articles, and a searchable version of Aspen's full catalog, including the most recent publications: www.aspenpublishers.com

Aspen Publishers, Inc. • The hallmark of quality in publishing
Member of the worldwide Wolters Kluwer group.

Editorial Services: Kathy Litzenberg
Library of Congress Catalog Card Number: 00-020622
ISBN: 0-8342-1074-6

Printed in the United States of America

1   2   3   4   5

To Geraldine—my wife, soul mate, and colleague—
for her endless encouragement, support, and assistance
throughout the book development process.

Table of Contents

Preface

WHO THIS BOOK IS FOR . . . AND HOW TO USE IT

Everyone involved in health care necessarily has either a direct or an indirect interest in patient satisfaction. Therefore, this book is designed to benefit a diverse audience that includes, but is not limited to, the following:

- health care executives (chief executive officers, presidents, vice-presidents)
- health care management (directors, supervisors, managers)
- medical directors
- health care administrators in large health care organizations
- health care administrators in solo or group practices
- health care marketing or marketing research personnel
- health care customer relations/member services managers and staff
- health care training and development personnel
- health care organization information systems/technology personnel
- health care providers*—large health care organizations
- health care providers*—solo or group practices
- nursing personnel (RNs, LVNs/LPNs)
- medical assistants or nurse assistants

Because of the inherent individual and organizational background differences among readers, recommendations for the initial reading

---

*These include medical doctors (MDs), doctors of osteopathy (DOs), doctors of podiatric medicine (DPMs), doctors of chiropractic (DCs), optometric doctors (ODs), nurse practitioners (NPs), and physician's assistants (PAs).

sequence and emphasis are provided for each of the above reader categories. In each case, five chapters are listed in the order that I believe to be most relevant and meaningful to start with. After this, I suggest that you review the Table of Contents and then select and read those remaining chapters that appear most interesting to you. Ultimately, the entire book should be read in order to gain an overview of all aspects of understanding, measuring, and improving patient satisfaction. Above all, you should use the information to build on your existing patient satisfaction improvement efforts. Socrates was credited with saying that "knowledge is power." In an industry as dynamic and competitive as health care, the real power lies with applied knowledge. As you read each chapter, highlight or make a note of action steps you might take to measure and improve patient satisfaction in your organization.

HEALTH CARE EXECUTIVES (CEOs, PRESIDENTS, VICE-PRESIDENTS)

- Chapter 11: Addressing Administration-Based Improvement Priorities
- Chapter 13: Building and Sustaining a Service-Oriented Organizational Culture
- Chapter 5: The Patient's Mental Report Card: A Model of How Patients Judge Their Health Care Experiences
- Chapter 8: Identifying and Prioritizing Service Quality Improvement Needs
- Chapter 3: The Elements of Patient Satisfaction: What Patients Value in Health Care

HEALTH CARE MANAGEMENT (DIRECTORS, SUPERVISORS, MANAGERS)

- Chapter 1: The Importance of Patient Satisfaction (and Loyalty)
- Chapter 3: The Elements of Patient Satisfaction: What Patients Value in Health Care
- Chapter 5: The Patient's Mental Report Card: A Model of How Patients Judge Their Health Care Experiences
- Chapter 4: The Relative Importance Index: Determining the Relative Importance of Each Patient Satisfaction Element
- Chapter 8: Identifying and Prioritizing Service Quality Improvement Needs

MEDICAL DIRECTORS

- Chapter 1: The Importance of Patient Satisfaction (and Loyalty)
- Chapter 3: The Elements of Patient Satisfaction: What Patients Value in Health Care
- Chapter 4: The Relative Importance Index: Determining the Relative Importance of Each Patient Satisfaction Element
- Chapter 5: The Patient's Mental Report Card: A Model of How Patients Judge Their Health Care Experiences
- Chapter 8: Identifying and Prioritizing Service Quality Improvement Needs

HEALTH CARE ADMINISTRATORS IN LARGE HEALTH CARE ORGANIZATIONS

- Chapter 1: The Importance of Patient Satisfaction (and Loyalty)
- Chapter 5: The Patient's Mental Report Card: A Model of How Patients Judge Their Health Care Experiences
- Chapter 8: Identifying and Prioritizing Service Quality Improvement Needs
- Chapter 12: The "Bottom Line": Measuring and Reporting the Value of a Patient Satisfaction Improvement Program
- Chapter 13: Building and Sustaining a Service-Oriented Organizational Culture

HEALTH CARE ADMINISTRATORS IN SOLO OR GROUP PRACTICES

- Chapter 1: The Importance of Patient Satisfaction (and Loyalty)
- Chapter 2: The Definition and Dimensions of Service Quality
- Chapter 3: The Elements of Patient Satisfaction: What Patients Value in Health Care
- Chapter 5: The Patient's Mental Report Card: A Model of How Patients Judge Their Health Care Experiences
- Chapter 8: Identifying and Prioritizing Service Quality Improvement Needs

HEALTH CARE MARKETING OR MARKETING RESEARCH PERSONNEL

- Chapter 1: The Importance of Patient Satisfaction (and Loyalty)
- Chapter 4: The Relative Importance Index: Determining the Relative Importance of Each Patient Satisfaction Element

- Chapter 5: The Patient's Mental Report Card: A Model of How Patients Judge Their Health Care Experiences
- Chapter 6: Measuring Patient Satisfaction: Determining an Organization's Grades on the Patient's Mental Report Card
- Chapter 7: Patient Satisfaction Data Collection, Processing, and Communication

HEALTH CARE CUSTOMER RELATIONS/MEMBER SERVICES MANAGERS AND STAFF

- Chapter 1: The Importance of Patient Satisfaction (and Loyalty)
- Chapter 2: The Definition and Dimensions of Service Quality
- Chapter 3: The Elements of Patient Satisfaction: What Patients Value in Health Care
- Chapter 5: The Patient's Mental Report Card: A Model of How Patients Judge Their Health Care Experiences
- Chapter 13: Building and Sustaining a Service-Oriented Organizational Culture

HEALTH CARE TRAINING AND DEVELOPMENT PERSONNEL

- Chapter 1: The Importance of Patient Satisfaction (and Loyalty)
- Chapter 2: The Definition and Dimensions of Service Quality
- Chapter 3: The Elements of Patient Satisfaction: What Patients Value in Health Care
- Chapter 5: The Patient's Mental Report Card: A Model of How Patients Judge Their Health Care Experiences
- Chapter 9: Addressing Behavior-Based Improvement Priorities

HEALTH CARE ORGANIZATION INFORMATION SYSTEMS/ TECHNOLOGY PERSONNEL

- Chapter 1: The Importance of Patient Satisfaction (and Loyalty)
- Chapter 3: The Elements of Patient Satisfaction: What Patients Value in Health Care
- Chapter 4: The Relative Importance Index: Determining the Relative Importance of Each Patient Satisfaction Element
- Chapter 7: Patient Satisfaction Data Collection, Processing, and Communication
- Chapter 6: Measuring Patient Satisfaction: Determining an Organization's Grades on the Patient's Mental Report Card

HEALTH CARE PROVIDERS—LARGE HEALTH CARE ORGANIZATIONS

- Chapter 1: The Importance of Patient Satisfaction (and Loyalty)
- Chapter 3: The Elements of Patient Satisfaction: What Patients Value in Health Care
- Chapter 5: The Patient's Mental Report Card: A Model of How Patients Judge Their Health Care Experiences
- Chapter 4: The Relative Importance Index: Determining the Relative Importance of Each Patient Satisfaction Element
- Chapter 8: Identifying and Prioritizing Service Quality Improvement Needs

HEALTH CARE PROVIDERS—SOLO OR GROUP PRACTICES

- Chapter 1: The Importance of Patient Satisfaction (and Loyalty)
- Chapter 3: The Elements of Patient Satisfaction: What Patients Value in Health Care
- Chapter 5: The Patient's Mental Report Card: A Model of How Patients Judge Their Health Care Experiences
- Chapter 4: The Relative Importance Index: Determining the Relative Importance of Each Patient Satisfaction Element
- Chapter 6: Measuring Patient Satisfaction: Determining an Organization's Grades on the Patient's Mental Report Card

NURSING PERSONNEL (RNs, LVNs/LPNs)

- Chapter 1: The Importance of Patient Satisfaction (and Loyalty)
- Chapter 3: The Elements of Patient Satisfaction: What Patients Value in Health Care
- Chapter 5: The Patient's Mental Report Card: A Model of How Patients Judge Their Health Care Experiences
- Chapter 8: Identifying and Prioritizing Service Quality Improvement Needs
- Chapter 13: Building and Sustaining a Service-Oriented Organizational Culture

MEDICAL ASSISTANTS OR NURSE ASSISTANTS

- Chapter 1: The Importance of Patient Satisfaction (and Loyalty)
- Chapter 2: The Definition and Dimensions of Service Quality

- Chapter 3: The Elements of Patient Satisfaction: What Patients Value in Health Care
- Chapter 5: The Patient's Mental Report Card: A Model of How Patients Judge Their Health Care Experiences
- Chapter 8: Identifying and Prioritizing Service Quality Improvement Needs

Introduction

The topic of patient satisfaction has been a focus of my life for the past twenty five years. During more than twenty years of private clinical practice, I have devoted considerable attention to understanding how to identify, meet, and exceed patient expectations. While presenting practice enhancement seminars to thousands of participants nationwide over an eight year period, I had the opportunity to gather many creative ideas from providers and ancillary personnel for better serving patients.

Then, in the early 1990's, my course work involved in earning an MBA degree provided me with the foundation needed to formalize my patient's mental report card model. Five years of teaching the principles of marketing and management at the undergraduate university level helped me place this model in an organizational context. In 1996, Friendly Hills HealthCare Network (which was located in southern California and served about 400,000 patients at the time) gave me the opportunity to put this model to work in the form of The Straight-A's program. This program was designed to systematically measure and incrementally improve patient satisfaction and loyalty at each of the 42 Friendly Hills health care centers. While presenting this program as part of a Friendly Hills national Beyond Strategy conference in Chicago, Aspen Publishers encouraged me to consider publishing the principles presented. In this book, I have attempted to provide the reader with a practical overview of the principles and techniques essential for understanding, measuring, and improving patient satisfaction in a health care organization of any size.

In Chapter 1, the importance of improving patient satisfaction is emphasized by focusing the reader's attention on the variety of possible organizational benefits. Satisfied patients are more likely to remain loyal, to refer others to you, and to comply with instructions. Meanwhile, they are less likely to complain or, worse yet, initiate a malpractice suit. Furthermore, accrediting agencies, such as the Joint Commission for Accreditation of Healthcare Organizations (Joint Commission) and the National Committee for Quality Assurance (NCQA) increasingly scrutinize issues of patient satisfaction when conducting accreditation assessments. Large employers often make health care contracting decisions based on, along with cost, employee satisfaction with health care benefits. Competitive advantage is an inevitable consequence of combining the internal and external marketing benefits of high levels of patient satisfaction. This advantage, when linked with sound management, will most assuredly result in increased profitability.

Chapter 2 discusses the evaluative dimensions of service quality that apply to all service industries. Research conducted by Berry, Parasuramen and Ziethaml, revealed the following five dimensions: tangibles, reliability, responsiveness, assurance and empathy. Martin described a model wherein consumers view relative organizational emphasis on personal and/or procedural dimensions. Based upon this model, Disend identified four service types: "airhead service," "indifferent service," "by-the-book service," and "superior service." We have all experienced service of each type in a variety of settings. Most patients who have received health care on multiple occasions have observed each service quality type in the process.

Chapter 3 provides a comprehensive overview of the elements of patient satisfaction. These fall into one of six main categories: access, convenience, communication, perceived quality of health care received, personal caring, and health care facilities/equipment. Each of the elements within each of these categories can be observed by patients in terms of specific health care provider/organization behaviors or conditions. For example, the category of access includes ease of scheduling appointments by telephone, ease of scheduling appointments in person, waiting time between the preferred day and the visit, waiting time in the reception room, access to emergency medical care and ease of seeing provider of choice. Then, carrying the example one step further, the component behaviors or conditions that patients observe in conjunction with ease of scheduling appointments by telephone include: number of telephone rings before being answered, ability to speak with a "live" person, length of time spent on hold, staff helpfulness on the telephone, multiple day and time offers for the appointment and total time required to make the appointment. This level of detail is maintained throughout the chapter.

Chapter 4 introduces the relative importance index (RII). This allows for a relative quantification of the importance of various service indicators within each element of patient satisfaction. This is extremely important, since a patient's ultimate satisfaction perceptions are determined by attributes he or she considers the most important. The RII is typically measured in the setting of focus groups (for different targeted groups) where the higher the numerical "rating," the more important the service indicator is in driving satisfaction/dissatisfaction. Later, during patient satisfaction measurement, the RII can be multiplied by the percentage of patients who are dissatisfied to help prioritize improvement needs. This assures that you will focus your initial improvement efforts on those areas that the patients consider important <u>and</u> they are dissatisfied with. Other methodologies for determining the RII are discussed in this chapter as well.

Chapter 5 introduces the reader to The Patient's Mental Report Card (PMRC). This is a model of how patients judge their health care experiences. This judgement, in turn, drives patient perceptions of satisfaction/dissatisfaction and behaviors of loyalty/disloyalty. The PMRC is made up of "moments of truth" (MOTs) and surrogate perceptions (SPs). An MOT is an impression of the organization based on any interpersonal contact between any representative of the health care organization and the patient. Patients retain a sort of "cerebral videotape" of each MOT they experience, weighing it on the basis of it's contribution to your organization's failing, meeting or exceeding their expectations. An SP is an impression of your health care organization based upon the patient's observation of an inanimate object or condition. These are recorded in the mind of patients as "cerebral snapshots." In this chapter, you will get a detailed sequential look at a typical PMRC.

Chapter 6 carries the reader's understanding of the PMRC forward to the point of actually measuring the grades patients give your organization. Seeking and responding to patients' perceptions of service quality is one of the most essential non-clinical endeavors a health care organization can undertake. There are a variety of mechanisms available for obtaining feedback that reflects patient satisfaction. These include such things as: post-appointment telephone surveys, open-ended questionnaires, objective survey questionnaires, an internet web-site, dedicated computer kiosks, lay advisory panels, patient focus groups, complaint/grievance analysis and "mystery shoppers." A survey is the most commonly used method of gathering patient satisfaction data. Whether you choose to build your own survey instrument, purchase an off-the-shelf version, or have a consultant develop one, the more you know about the overall development, sampling, administration, and data collection processes, the better equipped you will be to make educated choices along the way.

Chapter 7 addresses the collection, processing and communication of patient satisfaction data. The collection of this data begins with the sequential handling of completed questionnaires and, after a series of steps, ends with tabulation, which provides summary figures. These figures then need to be described and summarized using tables, graphics and statistics. This process is extremely important because the manner in which you display data affects the ease of highlighting your organization's service quality strengths and weaknesses. The objective is to convert a complex set of data to a form that can be read and understood quickly by executives, managers, and others who will make improvement decisions based on the research. Then analysis of this data is aimed at making the data "actionable" rather than "dust-collecting." Once the data meaning is appreciated, it needs to be communicated throughout the organization in a timely fashion using the appropriate media for the various audiences.

Chapter 8 shifts the reader's attention away from the patient satisfaction measurement and data collection processes to the actions needed to appropriately respond to the data. Identifying improvement needs is based on input obtained from both internal and external organizational customers. The external customers include patients, family members of patients, third-party payers, employers contracting for employee health care benefits, accrediting agencies and regulatory agencies. Internal customers include health care providers, nursing staff, medical assistants, specialty services, frontline personnel and all levels of management. Most organizations have limited resources to allocate to the overall patient satisfaction improvement process. Therefore, it is essential that the most critical issues—those that have the biggest impact on patient satisfaction/dissatisfaction—be approached first.

The quantitative component of prioritizing improvement needs involves combining patient dissatisfaction survey data with the RII. The dissatisfaction index (DI) is the term given to the percentage of patient satisfaction survey respondents rating a given survey item as "fair" or "poor." When the RII is multiplied by the DI, the result is the improvement priority index (IPI). It is important to combine the IPI with input gathered from internal and external current and past customers. The identified priorities are then divided into three categories based on the change mechanism involved: behavior-based, systems/process-based, and administration-based. In the next three chapters, methods for responding to each of these improvement priority categories are presented in detail.

Chapter 9 provides the reader with the information needed to address behavior-based improvement priorities. Special attention must be given to those employee behaviors associated with the management of each MOT. Specific, concise and measurable performance standards need to be focused on behaviors and actions that are very important to patients, can actually be improved and are challenging but realistic. Training is a means by which we attempt to close the gap between an individual's present performance level and his or her desired performance level. This equips employees with the attitudes, skills and knowledge needed to carry our their responsibilities in a manner that is pleasing to patients. The effectiveness of patient satisfaction improvement (PSI) training needs to be evaluated on the basis of trainee reaction, trainee learning, trainee behavior (i.e. transfer to the job) and business results (improved patient satisfaction scores). Furthermore, any health care organization needs to carefully design consequences in such a way so that behaviors that produce desirable outcomes (i.e., favorably contribute to patient satisfaction) are positively reinforced.

Chapter 10 provides the reader with the information needed to address systems- and process-based improvement priorities. A well-trained and motivated staff can only contribute to improving patient satisfaction continuously to the extent that organizational procedures, processes, and systems are designed to support the delivery of quality service to patients. While a process is a sequential grouping of tasks, a system consists of a group of related processes. Continuous process improvement (CPI) is the term applied when an existing process requires incremental improvement; a radical redesign of the entire process is referred to as process reengineering. The key is to focus on those processes that produce favorable outcomes in areas that are important to patients. In this chapter, the FOCUS-PDCA process improvement model (as applied in health care) is discussed. Furthermore, several standard CQI tools and techniques are presented for use in conjunction with your organization's PSI efforts.

Chapter 11 is focused on facilitating administration-based improvement priorities. For our purposes, we use the term *administration* to refer to such common descriptors as senior or upper management, organizational executives, or simply organizational leaders. This chapter presents several ingredients that are considered essential for ensuring administration's commitment and support of your organization's patient satisfaction improvement efforts. These ingredients include: effective and credible leadership, a compelling vision, change as the foundation for continuous improvement (changing management paradigms, reengineering management and administration's role in managing organizational change), administration's obligation to "walk the talk" and communicating patient satisfaction data to administration.

Chapter 12 prepares the reader for answering the inevitable bottom line question. You will be provided with a systematic approach to documenting the overall organizational value of your patient satisfaction improvement program using both tangible and intangible measures. Tangible benefits can be appreciated in terms of cost/benefit ratios, returns-on-investment, increased market-share, decreased patient defection and so forth. Intangible benefits are directly linked to improvement efforts that cannot accurately be converted to monetary values. These would include such items as: increased job satisfaction for providers and/or staff, increased organizational commitment of providers and/or staff, improved teamwork, improved patient service quality, reduced patient complaints and reduced conflict.

In this chapter, a model is presented that attempts to simplify and systematize this process by using clearly defined sequential steps. This involves: gathering data from a variety of sources, isolating the effects of PSI training on performance improvements, converting appropriate data to monetary organizational value, itemizing PSI program costs and finally calculating the ROI for you PSI program.

Chapter 13 is concerned with the influences of organizational culture on PSI-related employee behaviors. In this context, we are using the term *culture* to mean the pervasive norms and values of the health care organization. World-class organizations have six cultural elements in common: passionate customer focus, urgent obsession with quality, continuous improvement, high levels of employee participation, teamwork and ethics/integrity. If improving patient satisfaction and loyalty is to be truly continuous, with all of the associated long-term organizational benefits, then a service culture—one based on a passion for service excellence—must be established and maintained.

The vision, values, and mission of your health care organization serve to unify the efforts of all levels of management and employees. The vision is a concise word picture of the organization at some future (preferred) time in a future (preferred) state, which sets the overall direction of the organization. Organizational values are the building blocks of your health care organization's culture. They are the collective principles and ideals that guide the thoughts and actions of an individual, or a group of individuals—the maps of the way things should be. Finally, your organization's mission should be summarized in a statement that specifies its purpose or "reason for being." It represents the primary objective toward which the organization's plans and programs should be aimed. A mission is something to be accomplished, whereas a vision is something to be pursued. To implement the vision, values and mission of your health care organization, it is recommended that potential service employees be screened for two complementary capacities: service competencies and service inclination.

Chapter 14 provides the reader with a framework for converting the information presented throughout the book into positive organizational action that will improve patient satisfaction. A PSI planning model is presented; this is designed to be used generally as an overall approach to your PSI program and individually for each of your behavior-based and systems-based improvement efforts. Keep in mind that each health care organization is somewhat different—serving different numbers and types of patients, functioning in different marketplaces, offering slightly different services, and operating in differing internal cultures. Therefore, it is important to recognize that you will need to adapt the approach recommended in the PSI planning model to meet your organization's specific needs. Once each PSI strategy has been implemented, it is important to periodically evaluate the effectiveness of the change with the intention of further improvement. This must, of course, always be aligned with changing patient expectations.

CHAPTER 1

The Importance of Patient Satisfaction (and Loyalty)

Patient satisfaction has always been and will, to a greater extent, continue to be, a fundamental requirement for the clinical and financial success of any sized organization providing health care, regardless of specialty. The monumental changes in health care delivery systems have focused attention on more affordable, more available, more efficient, and higher quality health care. When the federal government attempted to impose greater controls in the form of the proposed Health Reform Act, the American people refused to support it. Public opinion shifted in favor of having the marketplace, via "managed competition," create the needed cost, access, and quality changes. This has resulted in the rapid growth of managed care over the past decade.

Arguably, managed care can produce an increase in efficiency, resulting in decreased costs and greater access. However, Harvard University researchers recently found that 51% of Americans believed that managed care was eroding the quality of health care in America ("Lessons for HMOs," 1997). So, what exactly does "quality" mean to consumers today?

Traditionally, the process of managing quality in health care entails such activities as measuring outcomes (Do the patients get better?), checking the credentials of providers (Are the providers well qualified?), auditing clinical activities (Are clinical guidelines and protocols being followed?), and auditing medical records. But, quality care is more than good outcomes and cost-effective processes; it must also give rise to satisfied patients who are loyal to the health care organization.

DISTINGUISHING PATIENT LOYALTY FROM PATIENT SATISFACTION

The distinction between patient "satisfaction" and patient "loyalty" is an important one with significant economic implications. Simply put, satisfaction is an *attitude* based on a myriad of service quality perceptions, whereas loyalty is a *behavior*. It is the behavior of remaining a patient year after year that truly adds value to an organization's combined efforts to measure and continuously improve satisfaction. Reichheld (1996) underscored the economic implications of loyalty: "Raising customer retention rates by five percentage points could increase the value of an average customer by 25 to 100 percent" (p. 13). Managed care organizations (MCOs) therefore direct a substantial amount of their internal marketing efforts toward patient retention.

Although patient satisfaction may not be sufficient to ensure loyalty, it is a necessary antecedent. One can predict with reasonable certainty that dissatisfied patients will exercise the ability to "vote with their feet" and defect to any available competitor. Therefore, scores reported in patient satisfaction research have become increasingly important in today's health care marketplace. Physicians want to show MCOs that they can provide cost-effective care in a manner that doesn't compromise patient satisfaction. Hospitals want to demonstrate high patient satisfaction scores to MCOs, particularly during the bargaining process. And, of course, MCOs want to report high satisfaction scores (both inpatient and ambulatory) to major employers when they are negotiating contracts.

STAKEHOLDER PERCEPTIONS, BEHAVIORS, AND BENEFITS

The mandate for intensifying efforts to achieve and sustain patient satisfaction is unquestionable. The National Committee for Quality Assurance (NCQA) measures patient satisfaction as part of the accreditation process for MCOs. Most anyone directly involved in the health care industry could readily provide some rationale for this mandate. However, in order to motivate individuals (and therefore organizations) sufficiently to intensify patient satisfaction efforts, a brief overview of stakeholder perceptions, behaviors, and benefits is in order. Table 1–1 summarizes this overview.

Table 1–1 The Impact of Patient Satisfaction

Category of Patient Satisfaction Importance	Impact on Health Care Provider Organization
Patient perceptions	Higher consumer service quality expectations
	Negative media representation of managed care
	Technical similarity of health care processes
Patient behaviors	Greater patient compliance
	Fewer patient complaints
	Increased patient referrals—powerful "grapevine"
	Greater patient loyalty
	Lower medical malpractice claim likelihood
Stakeholder benefits	Third-party payer incentives and mandates

Meeting the Service Quality Demands of a Changing Environment

Today's consumers have higher expectations for service quality than ever before. This is the age of consumerism—the consumer dictates what is, and what is not, acceptable or exceptional. Understanding and managing patient expectations must form the foundation on which all satisfaction enhancement efforts proceed. After all, it is the patients' ongoing process of comparing what was expected to what was received that drives their perceptions of service quality and value received. When the service received meets their expectations, they feel satisfied; when their expectations are exceeded, they become enthusiastic. Satisfied patients feel that they got what they paid for; enthusiastic patients perceive remarkable value for their investment...and tell others about this perception!

An even greater challenge in a changing environment is constantly escalating patient expectations. Familiarity with a satisfactory service breeds complacency. What was previously considered a unique "extra mile" service dimension may now be viewed as ordinary. The service strategies that created a "Wow" response last year may well be received with a yawn this year. Although incapable of judging the technical quality of health care accurately, most folks recognize good service when they see it, hear it, feel it, and touch it. Typically, people have experienced exceptional service quality somewhere; this unconsciously becomes their benchmark on which comparisons to other services (including health care) are based.

In health care, the challenge becomes more complex when we consider that patient expectations may, in certain instances, be unrealistic, such as expecting to see a specialist for routine health problems, demanding sophisticated diagnostic or therapeutic procedures when simpler approaches are equally effective, and so forth. Through the processes of education and judicious demand management, health care providers/organizations can retain the capacity to deliver patient satisfaction by meeting realistic expectations.

Most major metropolitan marketplaces are now heavily penetrated by managed care, the dominant force in the health care industry. Russell Coile, Jr., president of Health Forecasting Group, stated that "managed care will be the dominant scenario for healthcare in the future" (1990, p. 133). This brings reduced premiums or expanded coverage, which would reward enrollees with healthy lifestyles. Peter Boland, president of Boland Healthcare Consultants, summarized managed care as follows:

> It entails different financial incentives and management controls intended to direct patients to efficient providers who are responsible for giving appropriate medical care in cost-effective treatment settings. It seeks to maximize value to healthcare purchasers by channeling volume to high quality providers participating in health maintenance organizations (HMOs), preferred provider organizations (PPOs) or other "point-of-purchase" arrangements. Managed care alters decision-making of physicians and hospitals by interjecting a complex system of financial incentives, penalties, and administrative procedures into the doctor-patient relationship. (1993, p. 3)

Negative Media Representation

Negative media representation of the managed health care industry has become commonplace. Allegations of inaccessibility to specialists, impersonalization, long waiting times, rushed visits with physician or nonphysician providers, care withholding, wrongful deaths, and so forth receive priority attention by investigative reporters. Whenever an adverse outcome occurs, the entire managed care delivery system is scrutinized as the culprit, spawning further investigations. This, in turn, heightens consumer skepticism that quality service is even possible in a managed care system. As a result, health care providers/organizations that focus attention on the details of achieving and sustaining patient satisfaction have a clear opportunity to differentiate themselves (demonstrate how they are different and better) from competitors.

Technical Similarity

Although typically incapable of judging the technical aspects of medical care, patients determine satisfaction based on service quality elements they are familiar with—communication, personal caring, responsiveness, and so forth. Many service-based organizations have gained competitive advantage by providing excellent service, resulting in heightened expectations and long-term customer retention. When consumer expectations are not met, whether they are realistic or not, dissatisfaction is the natural outcome. In a competitive marketplace, dissatisfied customers will switch to a competitor when they have an alternative available at a comparable cost.

It is interesting to note that parallel but dissimilar competitive forces are in place in Great Britain. Approximately 85% of the health care in Great Britain is provided by the National Health Service. Although access to a general practitioner is readily available, long delays for specialist care or sophisticated diagnostic testing is the norm. Then, long reception room waits typically precede the visit. If nonemergency surgery or specialized treatment is recommended, an additional long delay (months or years) may be anticipated. The remaining 15% of the population receive their health care through private, fee-for-service providers. By minimizing or eliminating the access and delay concerns present within the National Health Service, private practitioners are able to differentiate themselves in the minds of consumers. Consequently, they deliver higher levels of satisfaction to a population of patients who are comparatively price insensitive.

Improved Patient Compliance

When patients are happy with the communication and rapport the provider has established with them, there is a much greater likelihood that they will comply with instructions. Granted, there are a number of reasons for noncompliance that are out of the physician's control—such as financial, time, or transportation problems. However, the process of clearly communicating those recommendations that you determine to be in the patient's best interest is controllable.

All communication begins with a thought in the mind of the sender. The communication process is successful (therefore clear) when the same thought ends up in the mind of the receiver. The sender is charged with the responsibility of encoding the message in such a way that it can be accurately "decoded" by the receiver. A blatant "miscoding" of the message occurs if the sender encodes it in a language the receiver does not understand. Interpreters are commonly used to reencode the message into a language known to the receiver.

As health care providers, it is imperative that the messages we convey to patients are not encoded in the "foreign language" of technical or medical jargon. Initially, we need to assess the general intellectual level on which a particular explanation should be formed. A highly educated patient working in a technical field will appreciate an elaborate and detailed discussion. On the other hand, a less educated person working in a nontechnical environment would probably benefit from a more basic explanation of the same information. But, how do we ensure that the patients understand our explanations and/or instructions? Is it by asking them, "Do you understand?" Not at all! Clearly, the vast majority of people who are asked this question (following some sort of explanation by someone they respect) will respond "yes" even if they truly have little or no understanding. This is because we all possess an innate desire not to appear "stupid." It is much less intrusive to reframe the question so as to claim responsibility for message clarity. Try saying, "It is my responsibility to make sure this makes sense to you. Am I doing my job? Are there any aspects of what we have just discussed that you'd like me to clarify for you?" Or, you might ask patients to tell you how they would explain this information to friends or family. This is much less intimidating and sets the tone for patients to ask clarifying questions and for you to correct any misinformation contained in their mock explanation. In yet another approach, other providers prefer a tactic of probing to clarify the patients' understanding following the initial interview and instructions. For example: "Patients should check their blood glucose daily. Why is it important for you to check your blood glucose levels daily? And how would you explain what blood glucose is?"

Compliance with instructions can be further improved by discussing the reasoning behind any recommendations. We are all, by nature, rational beings; we will be much more inclined to cooperate if we understand why something is important. This is evident when we discuss the consequences of the recommended action or inaction.

Also, whenever appropriate, patients should be given options so they can participate in decisions related to their care. Patients are much more likely to cooperate with a regimen they themselves co-created. Finally, carefully explained step-by-step instructions should be accompanied by written take-home instructions to serve as a memory jogger once the patient leaves the office.

Applying techniques to ensure the comprehension of instructions or having consultants that specialize in writing instructions and patient education materials and/or coaching physicians on enhancing patient–physician communication is sometimes advisable to ensure compliance. After all, compliance is very difficult to achieve if patients do not comprehend the message being conveyed, or if barriers to compliance are not being dealt with.

Fewer Causes for Patient Complaints

Any size health care organization must have a clearly defined, easily accessible mechanism in place for patients to register a complaint about any aspect of their experience with the organization. Furthermore, this mechanism needs to be supported by a well-designed system for investigating and resolving any and all complaints. Ironically, patients are more sensitive to their perceptions of how you respond to their complaint than they are to the original cause of that complaint. Therefore, the first priority must be to have the complaint registration and resolution processes implemented and publicized. Next, carefully monitor the complaint types so as to focus patient satisfaction improvement efforts toward eradicating the root causes of common complaints. These will typically fall within one or more of the following patient satisfaction categories:

- access: arranging for and getting health care
- convenience
- communication
- quality of health care received
- personal caring

- health care facilities (both clinical and nonclinical)
- increased patient referrals—the powerful "grapevine"

Increased Patient Referrals and Greater Patient Loyalty

The process of selecting a health care organization is becoming increasingly complex in competitive marketplaces. When confronted with the marketing materials of each plan, the "consumer report card" reports issued by accrediting agencies, and media-based comparisons, consumers can understandably be confused. Should they look primarily at cost? Does an adverse outcome reported in the newspaper necessarily eliminate that health care organization from their choices? Confounded by classic "information overload," it is much easier for prospective patients to rely on anecdotal information provided by a current patient. If Aunt Ellen relates how caring and friendly everyone (provider and staff) was during her recent health care visit, coupled with how efficiently her medical problem was resolved, that's convincing!

Furthermore, if she encountered some problem during the process of getting care, many more people will hear about it—not just about the problem, but about all of the circumstances surrounding the problem, as well as how it was resolved by the organization. The Technology Assistance Research Program (TARP) study conducted by Gallup for the White House indicated that 87% of the people who encounter a problem with an organization will tell 13 other people about the experience; the remaining 13% will spread the story to 20 or more others (Zemke & Schaaf, 1990).

When coupled with TARP's findings that 96% of people who encounter a problem with a service organization never bother to complain, the mathematics of the complaint management grapevine are astonishing. Assume that your health care facility receives two complaints per month. "Not bad," you might say. However, this means that 50 people actually encountered a problem. Continuing the grapevine formula, 87% of these 50, or approximately 44, will tell 13 others—totaling 572, and 6 will tell at least 20 others—totaling 120. With such a seemingly acceptable number of complaints, 692 people will be given potentially unfavorable information about your organization. Keep in mind, though, that grapevine power can work in your favor if you actively solicit complaints so that more than 4% speak up and you consistently resolve problems in a manner that exceeds patient expectations. All in all, satisfied patients—especially ones whose expectations have been exceeded—will spread the word to others while remaining loyal themselves.

Lower Medical Malpractice Claim Likelihood

Medical malpractice defense attorneys indicate that deficient patient rapport is commonly the proverbial "straw that breaks the camel's back" when a patient initiates a malpractice lawsuit. Fredonia Jacques (1983) emphasized the role of good patient rapport, stating that patients are far less likely to sue when their physician is friendly and caring. Impersonal patient treatment precludes the establishment of good patient rapport. Critics point to uncaring physician attitudes, a breakdown in doctor–patient relations, and the absence of bedside manner as the primary blockades to establishing rapport. Poor patient communication adds fuel to the malpractice flame of eroding rapport.

Recall that two of the primary categories of patient satisfaction are communication and personal caring. When organizationwide attention is systematically directed toward enhancing patient satisfaction in these two categories, improved patient rapport is a natural result. Specifically, attention should be directed toward the following issues:

- telephone techniques
- accurate scheduling
- interpersonal skills
- communication skills

Third-Party Payer Incentives and Mandates

Third-party payers recognize that patient satisfaction represents a critical success factor for the competitive strength of their organization. Therefore, they insist on doing the following:

- Regularly measure and monitor patient satisfaction levels among their insureds.
- Contract with providers who sustain minimum "industry standard" levels of patient satisfaction.
- Contract with providers who develop and implement a systematic approach to improving patient satisfaction, with special emphasis on those improvement needs identified by the survey process.
- Compensate contracted providers or provider organizations in a manner that includes incremental financial rewards for exemplary patient satisfaction scores, as demonstrated on the insured's survey findings.

Large Employer Insistence

Employers who pay the bill for all or a portion of the health care benefit costs for their employees are particularly concerned about getting value for their investment. Of course, this means the highest perceived quality of employee health care for the lowest possible cost. However, there is more to the equation than that. Part of the "return on investment" employers seek is an increase in employee satisfaction that is commensurate with the magnitude of the investment. The employees' perceived quality of the compensation or benefit package is connected to a myriad of financial and nonfinancial issues. Receiving good health care for themselves and their dependents is of paramount importance to them. When they are highly satisfied with all aspects of their health care coverage, they perceive this benefit to be of greater value.

Employers typically measure and monitor employee satisfaction on a regular basis. If patients are dissatisfied with their health benefits, benefits managers will shop elsewhere for health care. Patricia Nazemetz, director, Corporate Benefits for Xerox Corporation, emphasized this very well: "One objective of Xerox' healthcare purchasing strategy is to move from being a mere payer of the bills to being an intelligent purchaser of healthcare needs of employees and their dependents. To meet this objective, Xerox is defining its purchaser requirements and will limit the suppliers from which it purchases healthcare programs and services" (Boland, 1993, p. 118).

Accrediting Agency Demands

Accrediting agencies such as the NCQA have used the Health Employer Data Information Set (HEDIS) program to provide employers with "apples-to-apples" comparisons among MCOs. Although HEDIS measures a host of attributes aside from satisfaction, such as preventive and clinical performance factors, patient satisfaction measurement is part of the assessment and is considered in the accreditation process. These requirements focus on overall levels of satisfaction that provide a general indication of whether a health plan is meeting enrollee expectations (i.e., level of acceptability). The NCQA requirements include reporting the percentage of surveyed members who indicated that they are "satisfied with the health plan." Xerox and many other employers support HEDIS and base their selection of providers on the plan's performance on HEDIS measures as compared to goals. As you design a new or renewed organizational commitment to improving patient satisfaction continuously, logic mandates that you dovetail each of your improvement initiatives with accrediting and regulatory agency requirements.

Internal Marketing Benefits

Marketing consists of the "ongoing process of identifying the needs and perceived needs of the a given target audience and matching your products/services to those needs" (Shelton, 1988). Typically, when individuals think of marketing, there is an overwhelming emphasis placed on "advertising." This is very much like confusing penicillin with antibiotics; a part is misunderstood as representing the whole. In reality, advertising is but one strategy in the large category of external marketing. This combined group of strategies serves to project a particular organizational image to the targeted consumer population at large. These strategies include such familiar tactics as print and electronic media advertising, promotional campaigns, and so forth.

Internal marketing, on the other hand, takes place once the consumer is in the process of doing, or has done, business with your organization. In marketing terms, it is external marketing that "makes the promises," whereas internal marketing is responsible for "keeping the promises." In fact, the majority of efforts directed toward enhancing patient satisfaction are best classified as internal marketing activities. In future chapters, detailed information will be presented about various internal marketing elements of patient satisfaction, including

- communication
- education on how to avoid illness
- communication about health care education programs
- reminders to use preventive services
- thoroughness of the provider's examination
- amount of time provider spent with the patient
- thoroughness of the medical treatment received
- personal caring
- facility and equipment cleanliness

Efforts to meet, and preferably exceed, patient expectations in these areas should occur within an organization and will determine whether patients will be satisfied or dissatisfied, be loyal or disloyal, and refer others or badmouth you.

All in all, it makes the greatest marketing sense to focus first on internal marketing, then to use external marketing to increase the number of consumers whose expectations can be exceeded. Organizations that take the opposite approach, choosing to begin with external marketing before they have their internal marketing act together, can actually accelerate their own demise. That's right! Marketing can actually drive an organization out of the marketplace by increasing the rate at which you dissatisfy consumers.

Increased Profitability

The number one objective of all marketing efforts in any industry is product/service differentiation—to develop and substantiate the claim that your offering is different and better than the same or similar offerings that are made available to the consumer by competitors. When a health care organization consistently focuses on enhancing patient satisfaction, the net result is a clearly differentiated position in the health care marketplace. The natural result, assuming competent management, is increased profitability.

LOOKING FORWARD

Over the past decade, many organizations have placed a great deal of emphasis on the process of achieving customer satisfaction. As a result, a myriad of techniques for measuring and, therefore, monitoring consumer perceptions of service quality have been devised. Unfortunately, the information garnered by survey research all too often ends up "collecting dust" on the desks of a few select members of the organization's senior management team. Consequently, there is little in the way of systematic service quality improvement. When this is the case, employees view the entire process as "spinning their wheels." Worse yet, patients are insulted when they take the time to provide feedback and realize that "nobody is listening" because improvements are not forthcoming.

Several of these measurement techniques will be explored in future chapters, with the objective of guiding you through the process of making the data "actionable." This ultimately leads to continuous incremental improvements implemented in areas that align patients' experiences with their expectations. When consumers experience the quality of service they expect, the perception of "satisfied" is the result. Furthermore, when that experience far exceeds expectations, sheer enthusiasm and delight are the result.

CONCLUSION

Patient satisfaction is a fundamental requirement for the clinical and financial success of anyone or any organization that provides health care. Although patient *satisfaction*, the process of meeting or exceeding patient expectations, is an *attitude*, it serves as an antecedent to patient *loyalty*, which is the *behavior* of remaining a patient year after year. One of the major challenges of the dynamic health care environment is keeping up with constantly escalating patient expectations. This requires having various mechanisms in place for remaining in touch with, and responding to, those changing expectations—an essential organizational commitment in today's competitive health care marketplace. The remainder of this book is dedicated to enabling the reader to make this commitment actionable.

There are a variety of benefits awaiting any prudently managed health care organization that makes and sustains this service quality commitment. Satisfied patients are more likely to remain loyal, to refer others to you, and to comply more with instructions, and less likely to complain or, worse yet, initiate a malpractice suit. Accrediting agencies such as the Joint Commission on Accreditation of Healthcare Organizations (Joint Commission) and NCQA (using HEDIS) increasingly scrutinize issues of patient satisfaction when conducting accreditation assessments. This must be borne in mind when designing all patient satisfaction improvement initiatives. Large employers use employee satisfaction with provided health care benefits as a determinant, along with cost, when making health care contracting decisions. When all of this is combined with the inherent internal and external marketing benefits of high levels of patient satisfaction, the inevitable result is a competitive advantage that is tantamount to increased profitability.

ACTION STEPS

1. Develop a method of measuring patient loyalty to your health care organization.
2. Review your current mechanism of recording/tracking patient complaints and grievances for accuracy.
3. Identify your organization's most common sources of new patients.

4. Review your current third-party payer incentives for increasing patient satisfaction levels.
5. Develop a method of tracking and monitoring patient compliance.
6. List current NCQA/Joint Commission requirements for measuring and improving patient satisfaction. Next to each item, indicate what your organization is (or will be) doing to align improvement efforts with these requirements.

REFERENCES

Boland, P. (1993). *Making managed healthcare work: A practical guide to strategies and solutions*. Gaithersburg, MD: Aspen.

Coile, R.C., Jr. (1990). *The new medicine: Reshaping medical practice and health care management*. Gaithersburg, MD: Aspen.

Jacques, F. (1983). *Verdict pending: A patient representative's intervention*. San Juan Capistrano, CA: Capistrano Press.

Lessons for HMOs: Time with patients is profitable [Editorial]. (1997, December 8). *Los Angeles Times*, B1.

Reichheld, F.F. (1996). *The loyalty effect: The hidden force behind growth, profits, and lasting value*. Boston: Harvard Business School Press.

Shelton, P.J. (1988). *ABC'S of practice prosperity, tape 1, The Medical Marketing Process, tape 2, Internal Practice Marketing*. [Audiotapes]. Anaheim, CA: Innovative Management Systems.

Zemke, R., & Schaaf, D. (1990). *The service edge: 101 companies that profit from customer care*. New York: NAL Books, p. 8.

SUGGESTED READING

Baum, N. (1997). Giving our patients a Federal Express experience. *American Medical News, 40*(8), 22.

Bendall, D., & Powers, T.L. (1995). Cultivating loyal patients. *Journal of Health Care Marketing, 15*(4), 50.

Brown, S.A. (1992). *Total quality service: How organizations use it to create a competitive advantage*. Scarborough, Ontario: Prentice Hall Canada.

Carlzon, J. (1987). *Moments of truth*. New York: Harper & Row.

Chang, R.Y., & Kelly, P.K. (1994). *Satisfy internal customers first!: A practical guide to improving internal and external customer satisfaction*. Irvine, CA: Richard Chang Associates.

Denton, D.K. (1989). *Quality service: How America's top companies are competing in the customer-service revolution...and how you can too*. Houston, TX: Gulf.

Disend, J.E. (1991). *How to provide excellent service in any organization: A blueprint for making all the theories work.* Radnor, PA: Chilton Book.

Fleming, P., & Geiger, S. (1997, February, unpublished manuscript). Proven connections: BI loyalty model. *BI Performance Services.*

Gabbott, M., & Hogg, G. (1998). *Consumers and services.* West Sussex, England: John Wiley & Sons.

Goodman, J., & Ward, D. (1994, June 2–3). *Giving world class customer service.* Seminar presented for M D Buyline, Technical Assistance Research Programs, Arlington, VA.

Heskett, J.L., Sasser, W.E., & Sclesinger, L.A. (1997). *The service profit chain: How leading companies link profit and growth to loyalty, satisfaction, and value.* New York: The Free Press.

How good is your health plan? (1996, August). *Consumer Reports,* pp. 28–30.

Leebov, W., Vergare, M., & Scott, G. (1990). *Patient satisfaction: A guide to practice enhancement.* Oradell, NJ: Medical Economics Books.

MacStravic, S. (1994). Patient loyalty to physicians. *Journal of Healthcare Marketing, 14*(4), 53.

Milakovich, M.E. (1995). *Improving service quality: Achieving high performance in the public and private sectors.* Delray Beach, FL: St. Lucie Press.

Nelson, A.M., Wood, S.D., Brown, S.W., & Bronkesh, S.Z. (1997). *Improving patient satisfaction now: How to earn patient and payer loyalty.* Gaithersburg, MD: Aspen.

Page, L. (1996, March 18). Federal study to standardize patient satisfaction data. *American Medical News,* p. 17.

Prager, L.O. (1996). Latest *Consumer Reports* rates managed care plans. *American Medical News, 39*(30), 4.

Rummler, G.A., & Brache, A.P. (1995). *Improving performance: How to manage the white space on the organization chart* (2nd ed.). San Francisco: Jossey-Bass.

Sachs, L. (1991). *The professional practice problem solver: Do it-yourself strategies that really work.* Englewood Cliffs, NJ: Prentice Hall.

Sutherland, S.F., & O'Connor, R.E. (1996). Why should physicians worry about patient satisfaction? *Delaware Medical Journal, 68*(1), 19–22.

Tate, P. (1997). *The doctor's communication handbook* (2nd ed.). Oxon, UK: Radcliffe Medical Press.

Taylor, S.A., & Cronin, J.J. (1994). Modeling patient satisfaction and service quality. *Journal of Health Care Marketing, 14*(1), 34.

Woodruff, R.B., & Gardial, S.F. (1996). *Know your customer: New approaches to understanding customer value and satisfaction.* Oxford, England: Blackwell.

Zeithaml, V.A., & Bitner, M.J. (1996). *Services marketing.* London: McGraw-Hill.

Zeithaml, V.A., Parasuraman, A., & Berry, L.L. (1990). *Delivering quality service: Balancing customer perceptions and expectations.* New York: The Free Press.

CHAPTER 2

The Definition and Dimensions of Service Quality

In the arena of health care, it is helpful to keep in mind the theoretical distinction between the medical and nonmedical dimensions of perceived service quality. Although consumers are limited in their capability to judge the technical (medical) quality of a health care experience, they are ready and willing to base their service quality perceptions on nonmedical components of receiving health care. These perceptions, in turn, function as primary determinants of overall patient satisfaction. This chapter will serve as an introduction to the "science" of service quality, highlighting research conducted throughout a variety of service industries. The information in this chapter, then, functions as a foundation for Chapters 3 and 5, wherein this information is translated into a detailed model for analysis of the determinants of patient satisfaction throughout all components of the health care environment.

Zeithaml, Parasuraman, and Berry (1990) conducted 12 focus groups nationwide in search of a definition of service quality. They concluded that "service quality, as perceived by customers, can be defined as the extent of discrepancy between customers' expectations or desires and their perceptions" (p. 18). This supports the notion that the key to ensuring good service quality is meeting or exceeding what customers expect from the service. Therefore, a thorough understanding of customer expectations is the critical foundation on which perceived high-quality service must rest. In health care, of course, the term customer usually refers to the patient. In a health care organizational setting, the patient is, in fact, the primary external customer.

THE SHAPING OF PATIENT EXPECTATIONS

A number of factors appear to shape patient expectations. Word-of-mouth communication, or what patients hear from other patients, is a strong determinant of patient expectations. When one patient shares the details of how efficient the office was run, or how friendly the staff was, the potential patient then expects similar treatment. Also, the personal needs of a patient, in terms of time sensitivity, specialized care, preventive advice, or just plain empathy, all influence the patient's expectations for an upcoming health care experience.

Next, there is the patient's past experience(s) in using the same or similar services. When difficulty obtaining appointments and long waiting times have typically marked a patient's experiences with health care, he or she is delighted when this expectation is "exceeded" by easy appointment scheduling and/or minimal waiting time. Conversely, when a patient has become accustomed to efficiency and punctuality, anything short of this leads to dissatisfaction.

Finally, external marketing communications from health care providers/organizations play a key role in shaping patient expectations. Upscale, full-color brochures with photographs depicting a caring, unrushed physician interacting with a patient may lead the patient to choose that provider based on the expectation that this is how he or she will be treated. Marketing claims made in print or electronic media used to differentiate one health care organization from another also establish clear expectations on the part of the patient. When the patient's actual experience differs from that which was promised (in ways important to the patient), overall satisfaction is either positively or negatively impacted.

HOW PATIENTS MEASURE SERVICE QUALITY

Management guru Tom Peters (1994) indicated that "customers perceive service in their own unique, idiosyncratic, emotional, irrational, end-of-the-day, and totally human terms. Perception is all there is!" Several themes seem to emerge repeatedly in the literature about service quality.

- Service quality is more difficult for customers to evaluate than goods quality. A patient's assessment of the quality of health care services is more complex and difficult than his or her assessment of the quality of automobiles.
- Patients do not evaluate service quality solely on the outcome of a service; they also consider the process of service delivery. The antibiotics may have resolved the throat infection, but if discourtesy and an uncaring attitude marked the patient's interaction with the provider, the perception may well be "poor service quality."
- The patient defines the only criteria that count in evaluating service quality. Only patients can judge service quality; all other judgments are irrelevant.

THE EVALUATIVE DIMENSIONS OF SERVICE QUALITY

The SERVQUAL instrument for measuring service quality was developed by Zeithaml, Parasuraman, and Berry in 1985. It was derived by combining 10 evaluative dimensions (see below) obtained through exploratory research with their conceptual definition of service quality (above). This unique approach to quantifying service quality is, without a doubt, the most popular model in perceived service quality literature. It was designed to be applicable across a broad spectrum of services and can be adapted or supplemented to fit the characteristics or specific research needs of a health care organization.

The 10 evaluative dimensions of service quality that form the foundation for the SERVQUAL survey instrument, as adapted for health care, are as follows:

1. *Tangibles:* the appearance of physical facilities, equipment, personnel, and communication materials. Typical patient questions: "Does the facility look clean, neat, and free of infection?" "Does the equipment used here appear up-to-date and well maintained?"

2. *Reliability:* the ability to perform the promised service dependably and accurately. Typical patient questions: "Will the doctor/provider really return my phone call as the staff promised?" "Are my laboratory results going to be available to me in 3 days as promised?"

3. *Responsiveness:* the willingness to help customers and to provide prompt service. Typical patient question: "If I have a question about my treatment, will they take the time to thoroughly explain it to me?"

4. *Competence:* possession of the required skills and knowledge to perform the service. Typical patient question: "Can my health problem really be managed by my GP?...or should I be referred to a specialist?"

5. *Courtesy:* politeness, respect, consideration, and friendliness of contact personnel. Typical patient questions: "Will the receptionist greet me in a friendly, personal manner?" "Will the nurse in the back office respect my privacy when I am disrobing for my examination?

6. *Credibility:* trustworthiness, believability, and honesty of the service provider. Typical patient questions: "Does this health care organization have a good reputation?" "What are the credentials of the doctor/provider I will be seeing?"

7. *Security:* freedom from danger, risk, or doubt. Typical patient questions: "Will the parking lot be well lit and safe for me when I arrive for my evening appointment?" "Will the doctor/provider explain any possible risks or potential complications associated with the treatment he or she recommends?"

8. *Access:* approachability and ease of contact. Typical patient questions: "Will I be able to get an appointment for care when I really need it?" "Will I have to wait much longer than I'd like?" "Can I see a specialist right away or do I have to let the general practitioner try to treat me first?"

9. *Communication:* keeping customers informed in language they can understand. Listening to them is equally important. Typical patient questions: "Will the staff take the time to clearly explain what I am supposed to do before and after my upcoming surgery?" "Will the doctor/provider explain my condition using words I understand instead of a lot of medical jargon?"

10. *Understanding of the customer:* making the effort to know customers and their needs. Typical patient questions: "Will I be treated as a human being, rather than a case number or clinical condition?" "Will anyone remember who I am?...and greet me by name?"

These 10 dimensions were then ultimately subjected to rigorous statistical analysis, resulting in a SERVQUAL instrument that contained 5 distinct dimensions that captured facets of all of the 10 originally conceptualized dimensions. The items making up the consolidated dimensions and the required concise definitions are as follows:

1. *tangibles:* the appearance of physical facilities, equipment, personnel, and communication materials
2. *reliability:* the ability to perform the promised service dependably and accurately
3. *responsiveness:* a willingness to help customers and provide prompt service
4. *assurance:* knowledge and courtesy of employees and their ability to convey trust and confidence
5. *empathy:* caring, individualized attention the firm provides its customer

William B. Martin (1989) indicated that there are essentially two dimensions to service quality: procedural and personal (Figure 2–1).

The *procedural* dimension of service quality refers to all of the systems, processes, and mechanisms an organization uses to accomplish its work and meet customers' needs. This includes such things as the appointment scheduling process, special services referral process, rules, standard operating procedures, forms, decision-making and complaint-handling processes, and so forth. Patients would evaluate the procedural dimension in terms of the health care organization's efficiency, responsiveness, convenience, flexibility, and similar traits. The *personal* dimension represents the human side of service. This interpersonal component encompasses the health care organization's attitudes, friendliness, training, ability, willingness, and similar traits.

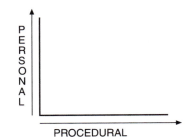

Figure 2–1 The Dimensions of Service Quality. *Source:* Reprinted with permission. *Managing Quality Customer Service,* William B. Martin, PhD, Crisp Publications, Inc. 1200 Hamilton Court, Menlo Park, California 94025.

THE PROCEDURAL DIMENSION OF SERVICE QUALITY*

The procedural dimension of service quality adapted for health care is made up of seven areas around which service standards should be developed.

1. *Timing:* Patients who feel constrained by time are sensitive to a variety of timing issues such as how quickly the telephone is answered, how long they are left on "hold," the length of time from the appointment scheduling phone call until the actual appointment date, how long it takes a receptionist to greet the patient on arrival at the office/clinic, the amount of waiting time in the reception room and again in the actual treatment room, time waiting for tests and test results, and so forth.
2. *Flow logic:* Patients who are being asked to perform a sequence of tasks (fill out and return forms, get weighed, attend health education classes, etc.) while under a health care provider's care prefer to do so in a logical order that avoids redundancy of their efforts and general inefficiency.
3. *Accommodation:* Patients need to feel that the health care organization's service systems are designed around their needs

---

Source: Reprinted with permission. *Managing Quality Customer Service,* William B. Martin, PhD, Crisp Publications, Inc. 1200 Hamilton Court, Menlo Park, California 94025.

and that health care providers are willing to be flexible enough to adapt to their special needs and/or requests, even if it means "bending the rules" somewhat.

4. *Anticipation:* Providing for patient needs (assisting an elderly patient out of a reception room chair or onto a treatment table, comforting an anxious child prior to a vaccination, etc.) without patients having to ask demonstrates your empathy for their circumstances.

5. *Communication:* All members of the health care team are expected to communicate with one another about matters pertaining to the patients' health care experience. Patients become frustrated when they tell their whole symptom history to a nurse or medical assistant (who is taking copious notes) followed by a rushed physician entering the treatment room asking, "What seems to be the problem?" Additionally, patients wish to receive clear communication from health care providers in their explanations, recommendations, verbal and written instructions, and so forth.

6. *Patient feedback:* Recall that 96% of people who experience a service problem with an organization do not bother to complain, meaning that the provider or organization misses out on valuable service quality information. Therefore, patients are interested in knowing that you actively welcome and solicit their input on a regular basis and that you are ready and willing to listen to and resolve their service concerns. Measuring and monitoring patient satisfaction is the only way to "keep score" in the service quality game—taking definitive steps to respond to the data is the only way to win that game.

7. *Organization and supervision:* W. Edwards Deming emphasized that the biggest enemy to quality is variation; this applies to services as well as products—patients must receive the same high quality of service from all members of the health care team and from the same people throughout time (Al-Assaf & Scmele, 1993). This takes time-consuming training and careful supervision. The way in which the various components of the health care service delivery process are organized and coordinated is important as well.

THE PERSONAL DIMENSION OF SERVICE QUALITY*

The personal dimension of service quality adapted for health care is made up of six areas around which service standards should be developed.

1. *Appearance:* Patients' positive or negative reaction to what they see strongly impacts the perception of their experiences. This perception begins with the physical appearance (cleanliness, neatness, maintenance, etc.) of the health care facility, both externally and internally; it continues with the physical appearance of the health care team.
2. *Attitude, body language, and tone of voice:* Patients begin forming their impression of this dimension on the telephone. An abrupt, impatient, rude, or hurried voice on the other end of a telephone sets the stage for a negative experience for the patient; then, when the patient is welcomed (or not welcomed) into the health care facility by staff, body language determines the "real message" whereby the patient feels like he or she is either welcome or an interruption in the staff members' day.
3. *Attentiveness:* Patients want to feel as though you are interested in them as individuals with unique needs, wants, and sensitivities; furthermore, they wish to be recognized as individual people (with names) instead of as clinic conditions or numbers.
4. *Tact:* Patients often seek health care for conditions that are related to the consequences of their own lifestyles. In many instances, they are aware that they don't eat a healthy diet, get enough rest, or exercise regularly, or that they smoke or drink too much. Tact involves the right choice of words to get the message across in a meaningful but respectful way. An insensitive choice of words will only create hurt feelings, hostility, and defensiveness in the patient.
5. *Guidance:* Patients often experience difficulties in navigating through the various components of modern health care facilities. The anxiety of seeking and receiving health care is worsened when patients are unsure of how to find the radiology depart-

---

Source: Reprinted with permission. *Managing Quality Customer Service,* William B. Martin, PhD, Crisp Publications, Inc. 1200 Hamilton Court, Menlo Park, California 94025.

ment, clinical laboratory, or other facilities. When clear written directions accompany verbal directions, along with easily readable signage, way-finding is perceived as much less troublesome. This, in turn, enhances the overall service quality perception.

6. *Gracious problem solving:* Given the nature and complexity of health care delivery, it is no wonder that problems tend to occur. Patients generally don't mind encountering a problem provided it is resolved to their satisfaction in a timely manner. If it is not, a complaint may result. A convenient and nonintimidating mechanism should be in place to both solicit and process this complaint. Barlow and Moller (1996) indicated that

in simplest terms, a complaint is a statement about expectations that have not been met. It is also, and perhaps more importantly, an opportunity for an organization to satisfy a dissatisfied customer by fixing a...service breakdown. In this way, a complaint is a gift that customers give to a business. The company will benefit from opening this package carefully and seeing what is inside. (p. 11)

THE FOUR TYPES OF SERVICE QUALITY

Based on Martin's model of service quality, Disend (1991) described four distinct types of service quality.

1. *Airhead service* places high emphasis on the personal or people dimension of service quality, with low emphasis on the procedural or systems and processes dimension. On the personal dimension, people smile a lot, they are friendly and well-meaning, and they appear concerned. However, they are also poorly trained, inept, and uncertain of what to do. On the procedural dimension, staff behavior is haphazard, confusing, disjointed, and inconsistent. The message sent to patients receiving this type of service is: "We've been to smile school, we'll try to please you, but we really don't know what we're doing." In any health care organization that lacks an infrastructure of systems and processes

to best serve patients, or that fails to provide training for staff, this sort of behavior may be typical among new employees. This is particularly disturbing to patients who are often feeling less than optimum and generally have a variety of needs and wants that require the help of competent staff.

2. *Indifferent service* places low emphasis on both the personal and the procedural dimensions of service quality. On the personal dimension, people are disinterested, impersonal, inattentive, and distant. It is clear that they are untrained or poorly trained and they are definitely unmotivated. On the procedural dimension, staff is unresponsive, slow-moving, and inconsistent. Everything seems to be complicated and confusing for them, and the appearance of a patient requesting any type of assistance or information is viewed as an interruption or inconvenience. Cavett Robert, a past president of the National Speakers Association, once stated that "people don't care what you know until they know that you care." This is especially true in health care. Imagine a patient who is anxious about his or her health problem arriving at the reception counter only to be completely ignored by a receptionist who is on a personal phone call discussing social plans for the upcoming weekend! Then, when the receptionist finally acknowledges the patient's presence, there's not even a hint of empathy or concern for the patient's problem. This sends the clear message to patients: "You are an interruption in my routine.... Don't bother me.... I've got more important things to do than take care of your needs."

   Well over a decade ago, *Consumer Reports* published the results of a study entitled "Why Customers Quit." This study revealed that a small percentage of customers left because of moving, dying, or switching to a competitor. However, 68% of them stopped doing business with an organization because of an attitude of indifference that was displayed to customers by staff.

3. *By-the-book service* places little emphasis on the personal dimension of service quality, focusing the greatest efforts on the procedural or systems/processes dimension. On the personal dimension, people are apathetic, insensitive, impersonal, disinterested, and unresponsive. When dealing with this type of staff member,

patients get the feeling they are talking to a walking rule book! On the procedural dimension, interactions with patients are precise, efficient, consistent, and unwavering. The highest priority is adhering rigidly to "sacred rules" that allow no room for flexibility or adaptation to special patient needs. This communicates to patients the all-too-common phrase we all loathe to hear: "That's not our policy."

4. *Superior service* places equally high emphasis on both the personal and procedural dimensions of service quality. On the personal dimension, people are friendly, caring, attentive, energetic, and well trained. As a result of their training, they are knowledgeable, confident, flexible, and responsive. On the procedural dimension, patients experience service that is prompt, efficient, convenient, and uncomplicated. The message that is sent to patients receiving superior service quality is, "We're here to help and we know what we're doing.... What else can we do for you?"

Everyone has, at one time or another, experienced superior service quality—perhaps even when obtaining health care. Those who have frequently received superior service probably have a higher level of expectations than those who have not. Nevertheless, in a competitive marketplace, health care organizations of all sizes and forms should take proactive measures to improve the level of perceived service quality for patients continuously.

CONCLUSION

Research demonstrates that service quality, as applied to any service industry, is perceived by customers along 10 evaluative dimensions. These are: tangibles, reliability, responsiveness, competence, courtesy, credibility, security, access, communication, and an understanding of the customer. Further research consolidated these dimensions down to five: tangibles, reliability, responsiveness, assurance, and empathy.

Another general view of service quality is based on a two-dimensional model, dividing behavioral attributes into personal and procedural segments. The procedural dimension is made up of seven attributes: timing, flow logic, accommodation, anticipation, communication, patient feedback, and organization and supervision. The personal dimension consists of six attributes: appearance, attitude/body language/tone of voice, attentiveness, tact, guidance, and gracious problem solving. This model then defines four distinct types of service quality: "airhead" (high personal/low procedural), "indifferent" (low personal/low procedural), "by-the-book" (low personal/high procedural), and "superior" (high personal/high procedural).

This introduction to the "science" of service quality serves as a foundation for Chapters 3 and 5, wherein this information is translated into a detailed model for analysis of the determinants of patient satisfaction with all aspects of health care.

ACTION STEPS

1. Prepare a grid containing the original 10 SERVQUAL evaluative dimensions. Based on your current understanding, do a "gut feeling" assessment of your organization along each dimension.
2. Prepare a similar grid using the personal and procedural dimensions of service quality. Do another "gut feeling" assessment of your organization.
3. Using Figure 2–2 as a guide, visit various direct-patient-contact areas of your health care organization to get an impression of where each department/facility would fit on this grid.
4. Based on the findings in steps 1–3 above, form a list of current service quality strengths and weaknesses.

REFERENCES

Al-Assaf, A.F., & Scmele, J.A. (1993). *The textbook of total quality in health care.* Delray Beach, FL: St. Lucie Press.

Barlow, J., & Moller, C. (1996). *A complaint is a gift: Using customer feedback as a strategic tool.* San Francisco: Berrett-Koehler.

Disend, J.E. (1991). *How to provide excellent service in any organization: A blueprint for making all the theories work.* Radnor, PA: Chilton Book.

Martin, W.B. (1989). *Managing quality customer service: A practical guide for establishing a service operation.* Menlo Park, CA: Crisp.

Peters, T. (1994). *The pursuit of wow.* New York: Vintage Books.

Zeithaml, V.A., Parasuraman, A., & Berry, L.L. (1990). *Delivering quality service: Balancing customer perceptions and expectations.* New York: The Free Press.

SUGGESTED READING

Anderson, K., & Zemke, R. (1991). *Delivering knock your socks off service.* New York: AMACOM.

Bell, C.R., & Zemke, R. (1992). *Managing knock your socks off service.* New York: AMACOM.

Delene, L.M., & Lee, H. (1994). The importance of various healthcare quality dimensions from the physician's viewpoint. *Journal of Ambulatory Care Marketing, 5*(2), 47–56.

Deming, W.E. (1982). *Out of the crisis.* Cambridge, MA: Massachusetts Institute of Technology, Center for Advanced Engineering Study.

Gabbott, M., & Hogg, G. (1998). *Consumers and services.* West Sussex, England: John Wiley & Sons.

Katz, J.M., & Green, E. (1997). *Managing quality: A guide to system-wide performance management in health care* (2nd ed.). St. Louis, MO: Mosby-Year Book.

Taylor, S.A. (1994). Distinguishing service quality from patient satisfaction in developing health care marketing strategies. *Hospital and Health Services Administration, 39*(2), 221.

Taylor, S.A., & Cronin, J.J. (1994). Modeling patient satisfaction and service quality. *Journal of Health Care Marketing, 14*(1), 34.

Zeithaml, V.A., & Bitner, M.J. (1996). *Services marketing.* London: McGraw-Hill.

CHAPTER 3

The Elements of Patient Satisfaction: What Patients Value in Health Care

Patient satisfaction or dissatisfaction is determined by a variety of closely linked elements that, when combined, drive each patient's perceptions of the overall health care experience. In order to appreciate the complexity of patient experiences with health care fully, it is helpful to place each component process figuratively under a microscope. In this chapter, we will discuss six general categories of satisfaction elements: access, convenience, communication, perceived quality of health care received, personal caring, and health care facilities/equipment. Within each satisfaction element, we will also consider specific health care provider/organization behaviors or conditions that lead to patient satisfaction/dissatisfaction. Later, in Chapter 5, we will explore these issues as patients experience them.

ACCESS

Access, in this context, refers to those processes that involve patients arranging for and obtaining health care. The elements and corresponding behaviors that, when combined, lead to satisfaction or dissatisfaction within each element in the category of access are presented in the following paragraphs.

Ease of Scheduling Appointments by Telephone

Frequently, a patient's first impression of the operational aspect of a health care office/organization is made when he or she calls to make an appointment. Depending on the patient's time sensitivity, efficiency expectations, and overall patience level, this could be perceived as either a pleasant or an unpleasant experience.

Service indicators that patients observe in conjunction with this element include the following:

- *Number of telephone rings before being answered:* This may vary regionally; however, most people expect the telephone to be picked up within three rings. Nothing is quite as frustrating for a patient—especially if there is a sense of urgency—than to wait 10 or 12 rings before a response is heard.
- *Ability to speak with a "live" person:* Although patients are becoming increasingly accustomed to automated telephone systems, they are only considered tolerable to the extent that they expedite the call. If, in fact, the patient can get through to the appointment scheduler directly by pressing a telephone button, this is viewed with greater favor than waiting for an operator to transfer the call. On the other hand, when there is an elaborate "tree" of multiple keypunch response options, or there are confusing instructions, it is difficult for anxious patients to remain calm.
- *Length of time spent "on hold":* Next to numerous rings prior to answering, enduring long periods of time left "on hold" ranks high among frustrating telephone experiences. This is especially true when the on-hold period begins without the caller's consent. Guidelines for managing the "on-hold" process will be discussed in Chapter 5.
- *Staff helpfulness on the telephone:* Having appropriately trained people projecting the desired positive impression of your health care facility/organization is critically important. Patients who experience "airhead" service quality on the telephone—with a smiling tone of voice but multiple incorrect call transfers, inaccurate messages taken, and so forth—will probably switch to a competitor at first opportunity. People don't expect their first telephone contact person to know everything, but they do expect telephone staff to be knowledgeable enough to put them in touch with the right person to help them.
- *Multiple day and time offers:* The majority of patients have many priorities, each of which imposes its own time management challenges. Therefore, patients need to be given options of dates and times available for their appointment. This allows them to take control and responsibility for scheduling a realistic appointment time, thereby decreasing the chance of a "no show."

- *Total time required to make an appointment:* Patients are usually very time-conscious for a variety of reasons. A working person may be calling during his or her coffee or lunch break and cannot afford any long daytime segments of time on the telephone.

Ease of Scheduling Appointments in Person

When patients are already present in your office or clinic, they expect to be able to schedule their next appointment conveniently and efficiently. Clear procedures and a consistently accurate scheduling system are essential to preventing bottlenecks from occurring during the process.

Component behaviors or conditions that patients observe in conjunction with this element include the following:

- *Convenient and functional position of the scheduler:* Often, the person scheduling appointments is the same person (and sitting at the same in-office location) responsible for answering telephones as well as for checking patients in prior to treatment. Thus, patients wishing to make another appointment are expected to wait in line as a "third priority" behind checking-in patients and telephone answering. Patients facing this scenario may well think that "making me wait in a line to schedule a follow-up appointment just doesn't make sense!" More importantly, they are right to think this. Providing a well-marked, distinct area for exiting patients to schedule appointments can eliminate confusion and increase efficiency. Of course, if true efficiency is what you seek, there's always computer-based scheduling that is positioned right in the treatment room! Then, exiting patients bypass the front desk on their way out with an appointment in hand.
- *Minimal wait to speak with the scheduler:* For the same reasons cited above, this may present a challenge. Appropriately cross-trained staff covering a separate exiting patient appointment desk can help to minimize this wait unless there are multiple doctors producing multiple patients exiting simultaneously. Then you're back to a bottleneck situation, which requires reengineering of the appointment scheduling process. All the staff training in the world will not rectify the inherent inefficiencies of a "sick" scheduling process or system.
- *Total time spent with the scheduler:* The fundamental information required to manage the reappointment process efficiently includes: (1) access to the schedule of all providers, (2) a thorough

understanding of the average length of time it takes each physician/provider to complete the most common different treatment types, and (3) the type of visit for which the patient is being scheduled. If any of this information is unavailable at the time the patient is attempting to schedule the appointment, some delay will result in longer total time spent with the scheduler.

• *Written verification of the appointment time received:* All health care facilities experience the challenge of managing "no shows" appropriately. Although some go so far as to charge patients a percentage of the normal fee, others simply juggle the schedule using short-notice lists of patients waiting to get an appointment. In fact, the best way to manage the problem is to prevent it. Written verification of the appointment, in the form of either an appointment card or a mailed follow-up note, serves as the first-line reminder of the scheduled visit. Subsequent to the first missed appointment, patients should be placed on a list to receive an appointment reminder, either by mail or via telephone call, 24 hours prior to the scheduled date.

Waiting Time between the Preferred Day and the Visit

Clearly, this is one of the primary concerns for patients when they consider how accessible their health care provider is. At one time, patients typically measured how good a doctor was by how difficult it was to get an appointment with him or her. Now, patients expect to be able to get in within a "reasonable" time period, especially if they perceive their problem to be urgent. An appointment system should be designed to be flexible enough to allow for patients' specific time constraints.

Component behaviors or conditions that patients observe in conjunction with this element include the following:

• *Availability of the preferred day:* If Wednesdays are the only days a patient can get off of work for a nonurgent doctor visit, then that patient expects to be able to get in on a Wednesday within the next several weeks. Consistent inability of a health care provider/ organization to offer appointments on preferred days should raise a "red flag" of procedural concern. It may be that capacity needs to be expanded in terms of longer hours, more treatment rooms, more support staff, or more providers. If patients can never seem to get in when they wish to, negative satisfaction survey responses will surely reflect this.

- *Availability of the preferred time:* For whatever lifestyle or work reasons, patients typically have a preference whether to be seen in the morning or in the afternoon. Within that framework, patients appear to be satisfied to accept specific appointment times other than those initially requested. The key issue appears to be that patients are offered a choice.
- *Nature (urgency) of the visit and provider's responsiveness to the expressed urgency:* There is often a discrepancy between the way health care providers and patients define "urgent." Health care providers view urgency in terms of the adverse consequences that could occur if the patient is not seen immediately; patients link urgency to their desire for immediate management of their discomfort, concern, or anxiety. One of the major challenges of managed care consists of educating patients so that they take responsibility for their well-being and access the appropriate level of care. When a patient calls your telephone advice system at 2 AM and receives helpful advice about home care for a health problem, he or she perceives this as responsive. On the other hand, if patients cannot get advice or an appointment to resolve an "urgent" matter, dissatisfaction results.

Waiting Time in the Reception Room

Classically, the number one patient complaint is "waiting time"; this most often refers to time in the reception room. Although delays (beyond 15–20 minutes) are bound to occur, they should be the exception rather than the rule. Furthermore, the manner in which such delays are "managed" will determine how they are perceived by patients.

Component behaviors or conditions that patients observe in conjunction with this element include the following:

- *Explanation provided for an extended wait:* The key to sustaining patient satisfaction in the midst of delays is to provide updated, honest information in a timely manner. Guidelines for explaining delays will be discussed in Chapter 5.
- *Total wait time in the reception room:* This is the amount of time between the time the patient arrives in the reception room until he or she is escorted to the treatment room. It is easy for health care providers and staff to underestimate the amount of time patients spend

waiting in the reception room. Patients, on the other hand, are likely to overestimate this time, especially when they expect no delay. Also, when a patient arrives early for an appointment, he or she begins measuring waiting time from the moment of arrival instead of from the appointed visit time, as it should be measured. Patient perceptions of waiting time are definitely influenced by the manner in which they are treated by staff during the delay.

Waiting Time in the Treatment Room

This involves several time segments: waiting for the nurse or medical assistant to obtain and chart basic information about the patient's symptoms or condition, waiting for the health care provider to enter the room, waiting for staff to "set up" for any special diagnostic or therapeutic procedures ordered by the provider, waiting for the provider to reenter the room, and so forth.

Component behaviors or conditions that patients observe in conjunction with this element include the following:

- *Explanation provided for an extended wait:* The same principles for delays in the reception room (see Chapter 5) also apply to delays in the treatment room. Patients deserve to be kept informed about anticipated delays in any of the time segments described above. If it will take 15 minutes to set up for a special examination, let the patient know. When patients can see that you are truly preparing for their examination or treatment, delays become somewhat more tolerable because progress is observable.
- *Total wait time in the treatment room:* From the moment the patient is brought into the treatment room until he or she exits the room following the visit, the patient's mental clock is ticking away. Inordinately long waits for any of the time segments detract from overall satisfaction. This is particularly true with patients who have work-related time constraints.

Access to Emergency Medical Care

Nothing diminishes the perceived value of health care coverage in the mind of a patient more than the thought of not being able to get needed help in an emergency. Then, if an emergency is encountered, and care is difficult or impossible to get, the resulting dissatisfaction will likely send the patient to a competitor for future care.

Component behaviors or conditions that patients observe in conjunction with this element include the following:

- *Ease of reaching emergency care by telephone:* Aside from the physical factors of telephone management (prompt answering, minimal on-hold time, trained staff, etc.), patients want to know that help is just a telephone call away. This help may be in the form of telephone advice from a trained nurse specialist or other provider about what to do to handle a particular emergency at home prior to getting medical attention.
- *Directions provided for getting care:* Clear and precise instructions for a patient (or patient's family) who is experiencing the emotional strain of an emergency are critically important. This advice might entail straightforward information pertaining to interim management of a laceration or potential fracture, or just clear travel directions to the nearest emergency facility.
- *Transportation to emergency services:* Patients or their families are often not capable or not equipped to provide transportation on an emergency basis. Specially equipped ambulances driven by highly trained emergency medical technologists can literally make the difference between life and death in a variety of cardiovascular emergencies. Patients seek the security of knowing that this would be available to them should they experience a life-threatening problem.

Ease of Seeing the Provider of Choice

This may become an issue with a variety of managed care organizations, depending on their structure. In a preferred provider organization, the patient can see an out-of-network provider, but it is likely to cost more. In an exclusive provider organization, there is no covered option to see an out-of-network provider. In an integrated delivery system, member patients are often required to see their assigned general practitioner (GP) first before accessing the services of a specialist; then, this service may only be available through a contracted specialist functioning within the network.

Component behaviors or conditions that patients observe in conjunction with this element include the following:

- *Ability to see the preferred provider type:* Patients typically have experience(s) with and preferences for various provider types; for example, patients with chronic foot problems request the services of a podiatrist. Patients with chronic low back pain may wish to receive periodic adjustments by a chiropractor instead of seeing the GP or an orthopaedist. Additionally, society is somewhat conditioned to seek the services of specialists at the first sign of an ailment that appears to be within that field. Thus, the patient with a sore throat may insist on seeing an ear, nose, and throat specialist; the patient with gastric upset may wish to see a gastroenterologist; and the patient with simple acne may seek care by a dermatologist. Additionally, patients who expect to be seen by a physician may resist an appointment with a nurse practitioner for a routine health problem.

The best way to manage demands for specialist services when a GP could easily handle the problem involves educating patients as to the scope of GP care. Once patients have a positive experience with this approach, the GP may well become the "preferred provider type," thus improving patients' perceptions of availability.

- *Ability to see the specific provider requested:* The contribution of this perception to overall satisfaction varies with the age, health status, and health care experiences of each patient. Generally speaking, senior citizens who have grown up accustomed to seeing one particular physician (often a GP) all their lives consider it very important that they continue to see that physician. Younger patients, however, have typically experienced the constraints imposed by an evolving health care delivery system. Therefore, they may be quite happy to see whatever provider can help their problem, without the demand to see the same one each visit.

Ease of Using the Telephone Advice System

Telephone advice systems enable patients to call to discuss their health-related problems by telephone with a licensed nurse. Consistent information and direction are then given by the nurse through the use of approved pediatric and adult protocols. This process benefits the health care organization by encouraging the proper use of services by patients, who typically call to discuss whether a visit to the physician is necessary. Through the use of physician-approved protocols, the nurse may be able to give patients self-care instructions in lieu of an office visit. This results in a decrease in the number of phone calls directly into the provider's office and a decrease in unnecessary office visits, freeing up appointment spaces for patients who really need them. Additionally, instruction for self-care and patient education increases overall patient satisfaction because it saves patients time and extends advice availability to after hours.

Component behaviors or conditions that patients observe in conjunction with this element include the following:

- *Immediate response to the patient's call*: Once this convenient service is implemented, patients expect to be able to get through to the telephone advice nurse without extensive delays. If the health-related matter is something the patient perceives as urgent, and he or she is unable to speak with the nurse quickly, the patient may revert back to going to the emergency room or physician's office instead of practicing self-care at home. The primary issue, from an organizational standpoint, is to have adequate staffing to manage the volume of phone calls received.
- *Clarity of instructions from the telephone advice nurse*: The patient-perceived value of a telephone advice system is based on trust that the system can meet the patient's individual health-related needs. The quality of communication that occurs in this setting will determine its true value. Therefore, the advising nurse must listen very carefully to the patient's "story" with empathy, asking relevant questions periodically and providing explanations and explicit instructions using laymen's terminology.

CONVENIENCE

In today's society, time is a precious commodity; people are "time-poor." Therefore, they are very sensitive to anything that appears to rob them of a disproportionate amount of their precious time. This could be in the form of travel time, waiting time, or just plain ease of accomplishing a simple health-related task, such as filling a prescription. Additionally, employed patients aren't always able to get time away from work during normal business hours to receive needed health care. Therefore, availability of services during nonbusiness hours becomes an important satisfaction issue.

The elements and corresponding behaviors that, when combined, lead to satisfaction or dissatisfaction within each element in the category of convenience are presented in the following paragraphs.

Location of the Health Care Center

This is primarily related to the anticipated travel time for patients to access the facility. This, in turn, is a function of distance from home or work, the ease of getting to the health care center by car or public transportation, and the amount of traffic congestion that is typically present.

Component behaviors or conditions that patients observe in conjunction with this element include the following:

- *Convenient location near home:* This is particularly important for home-based businesspeople, nonworking parents wishing to obtain their own health care or to bring children in for health care, and active retired people. The implication for health care organizations is to locate facilities based on current and projected future demographic data that align with targeted patient populations.
- *Convenient location near work*: This is particularly important for working people who prefer to get their health care during, immediately before, or directly after normal business hours.

Hours of the Health Care Center

Years ago, the phrase "bankers' hours" referred to the now-antiquated concept of businesses operating at times that were convenient to the business rather than to the customer. Now, people are accustomed to and expect services to be available at their convenience.

Component behaviors or conditions that patients observe in conjunction with this element include the following:

- *Convenient hours of the nonprovider staff:* Many services, such as routine laboratory tests, blood pressure checks, weighings, and so forth can be provided by the nonprovider staff. By making these available prior to or following normal business hours, patients can arrange to receive these services on shorter notice than would be needed for a provider appointment.
- *Convenient hours of the health care provider(s):* A thorough understanding (via market research) of the patient population being served by a health care facility/organization is needed to determine what patients consider to be most convenient. Access to health care providers during nontraditional hours can be very important to working patients, thereby giving a competitive advantage to those providers. The total number of working hours for providers may not need to be expanded.
- *Availability of early morning appointments:* Multiple-provider facilities may wisely choose to have some providers cover early morn-

ing hours, with their clinical day ending mid-afternoon, prior to rush-hour traffic.

- *Availability of evening appointments:* Other providers in a multiple-provider facility might prefer to start clinical hours mid-morning (after rush hour) and end in the evening (after rush hour). This arrangement may be particularly appealing to families with small children where both parents work during the day.

Parking Quality and Availability

Although in some locations public transportation is readily available, the prevalent mode of transportation for patients is likely to be by automobile. In congested metropolitan areas, parking is often at a premium and should be provided for patient convenience. After driving through traffic, the last thing a patient wants to encounter is difficulty or concern with any aspect of the parking process.

Component behaviors or conditions that patients observe in conjunction with this element include the following:

- *Ease of finding a parking space:* Appropriate planning should provide for ample parking spaces given the size of the patient population being served. This translates into less patient time wasted looking for a parking space—the absence of dissatisfaction, with moderate contribution to satisfaction.
- *Closeness of parking spaces to the building entrance:* If patients and staff share the same parking facilities, priority should be given to patients for spaces located closest to building entrances. Signs posted in front of conveniently located spaces such as "reserved for employee of the month" or "doctors' parking only" send the message that the patients are second priority.
- *Location and number of "disabled" parking spaces:* Our general population is aging, with a greater percentage of patients designated as disabled for purposes of parking. People have become accustomed to commercial stores providing ample, convenient disabled parking spaces. Thus, this is the expectation they bring with them to your health care facility.
- *Lighting in the parking lot during evening hours:* Aside from the family home, the family automobile tends to be one of the largest investments people make. A well-lit parking facility contributes to people's sense of security when parking or exiting or entering their vehicles. A poorly lit parking area invites would-be car thieves and vandals to "explore" the selection of desired items unnoticed.

- *Presence of security personnel in the parking area:* Female patients and elderly patients of both genders are constantly being warned about the dangers of being abducted in a parking lot. The presence of security personnel to guard against undesirables roaming the area and to escort patients to their vehicles during after-dark hours would undoubtedly be appreciated by patients.

Services Available for Filling Prescriptions

The required three-way cooperation between providers, pharmacists, and patients is best facilitated by physical proximity. Once the patient's health problem has been diagnosed and the appropriate prescription written, patient compliance begins with getting the prescription filled. When provisions are made for this to take place at the patient's convenience, his or her perceptions of overall efficiency will most likely improve satisfaction.

Component behaviors or conditions that patients observe in conjunction with this element include the following:

- *Convenient location of pharmacy services:* This is directly related to the convenient location of health care facilities in general. If the pharmacy is located within the health care facility, patients appreciate the "one-stop shopping" concept they have become so familiar with in their retail shopping experience. Additionally, a convenient location within the building, with minimal walking and elevator use required, is especially appreciated by mothers with young children and elderly patients with mobility limitations.

  When on-site services are not available, patients usually appreciate the offer to "call" the prescription in to their preferred pharmacy. Keeping that telephone number on file increases the convenience for staff to make the call. The end result is what patients truly appreciate—having the filled prescription waiting for them to pick up at the pharmacy.

- *Availability of prescribed medications in stock:* Efficient pharmaceutical inventory management must be based on current usage data so that commonly ordered medications are available to patients with little or no delay. In a managed care setting, there is often a "formulary" of approved medications that is categorized according to therapeutic action, relative clinical efficacy, and cost. Furthermore, arrangements should be made for rapid acquisition of less commonly prescribed medications that appear on the list but are not cost-effective to maintain in stock.

- *Written instructions provided regarding prescribed medication:* When patients are in the clinical setting, where a variety of "dos and don'ts" are being explained, instructions about how medications should be taken may not be heard clearly or understood. Therefore, this is the time to adhere to the old adage, "If it is worth saying, it is worth having in writing." Because the therapeutic value and effectiveness of any pharmaceutical agent is dependent on the delivery of adequate dosages at specific intervals via the proper route, it makes good sense to have all this information available to the patient for his or her reference following the clinical visit. Whether this information is provided by the health care provider or the pharmacist will vary based on the specific circumstances; what must remain consistent is the distribution of written instructions with each medication prescribed for patients. This is of particular significance to patients who are taking multiple medications (e.g., senior citizens who take an average of 5.6 medications at any given time), because the likelihood for confusion is much greater.
- *Total time spent waiting to fill a prescription:* It is important to conduct regular research about the time required for patients to get prescriptions filled. The efficiency of your internal or external pharmacy services will, in part, determine the amount of time patients need to wait for filled prescriptions. Actual waiting times should be kept to a minimum. However, the more important consideration is the comparison of actual waiting time to expected waiting time. If patients expect to wait 15–20 minutes, then a 10-minute turnaround is perfectly acceptable to them; on the other hand, if they expect the prescription to be ready within 5 minutes, the same 10-minute delivery time may be deemed "unacceptable." In this case, either the expectations need to be "corrected," or the speed of delivery increased, or both.

Services Available for Refilling Prescriptions

Many medications (antihypertensives, oral or injectable diabetic agents, etc.) require long-term, if not lifetime, continuation. This dependence becomes a habit for patients, yet the process of repeatedly refilling the prescription may be perceived as an inconvenience. If the process is efficiently managed, this minor inconvenience can be prevented from developing into a chronic nuisance.

Component behaviors or conditions that patients observe in conjunction with this element include the following:

- *Ability to request a refill by telephone:* This clearly requires coopera- tion between the physician/provider and the pharmacist. Typi- cally, the pharmacist is contacted by the patient or provider with a request for a refill. If this request is initiated by the patient, the provider must be contacted by the pharmacist to obtain refill per- mission, unless an original written prescription indicated a num- ber of refills. In some cases, of course, the patient needs to be ex- amined by the provider to determine and document whether continuation of the medication is medically indicated. This should be communicated to the patient, especially in a fee-for- service or co-pay-based managed care environment, where pa- tients may suspect that periodic "checkups" have more of a rev- enue generation basis than a therapeutic basis.
- *Refill ready when promised:* The rule of thumb is to "underpromise and overdeliver"; very simply, we are creating expectations when a promise is made. If the patient is informed that the prescription will be available in 20 minutes, that is when the patient expects to get it. Failing to meet those expectations will result in dissatisfac- tion, meeting them will lead to satisfaction, and consistently ex- ceeding them will produce an enthusiastic "raving fan."
- *Total time required to refill a prescription:* Systems and processes should be in place to keep this time to a minimum. The impor- tance of overall refill efficiency increases proportionately with the volume demand. Patients do not want their time to be wasted. Although a high volume demand on the pharmacy may provide an explanation for delays, time-pressured patients are reluctant to truly take this into consideration and reduce their expectations.

Completing Laboratory Work Ordered by the Provider

Often, the diagnosis associated with a particular set of symptoms is contingent on obtaining timely results from various laboratory tests. This requires patients to get to the laboratory soon after the provider visit, the laboratory personnel to perform the needed test efficiently, other laboratory personnel to "process" the specimen obtained, and clerical personnel to provide a report of test results. This report must then be communicated to the awaiting provider.

Component behaviors or conditions that patients observe in con- junction with this element include the following:

- *Convenient location of the laboratory:* In many cases, having the specimen obtained by nursing staff within the provider's office will obviate the necessity for patients to make their way to the lab. On the other hand, some tests are best performed completely by laboratory personnel. In this case, the more conveniently located the laboratory facility is, the sooner a patient can report for needed testing.

- *Convenient hours of the laboratory:* Working patients may find it difficult enough to get time off to see a health care provider, let alone additional time for getting laboratory work performed. Therefore, having the option to go to a conveniently located laboratory during work hours would be helpful.
- *Total wait time at the laboratory:* Testing that requires specialized personnel, procedures, or equipment is best performed on an appointment basis. Routine testing that is initiated by phlebotomy should be available on a walk-in basis because an experienced phlebotomist will typically take a very short time to obtain the needed blood specimen.
- *Prompt availability of results:* Patients are often anxious to know about the nature and/or progress of their condition. This means that if it is a new diagnosis, they wish to get on with the necessary treatment regimen as soon as possible. If a chronic condition is being monitored to measure the efficacy of an existing treatment approach, the provider is usually anxious to get needed information to guide future treatment.

Getting Radiographs, Sonograms, or Computed Tomography Scans Ordered by the Provider

For all of the same reasons that convenience and efficiency of clinical laboratory operations are important to the patient and health care provider alike, needed radiographic studies must be performed, interpreted, and reported as quickly as possible. The progress of a healing fracture or the nature and extent of a new orthopaedic injury carries particular urgency in the minds of both patients and providers.

Component behaviors or conditions that patients observe in conjunction with this element include the following:

- *Convenient location of radiography services:* This refers to convenient location within the health care organization. In practical terms, it needs to be located in relatively close proximity to where patients are seen by the provider.
- *Convenient hours of radiography services*
- *Total waiting time in radiography services*

- *Prompt availability of radiography results:* This is often directly related to how "realistic" the workload of the interpreting radiologist is. A huge backlog of radiographs waiting to be read by an
overworked radiologist can create a bottleneck. At some point,
consideration ought be given to increased staffing.

COMMUNICATION

In 1992, I asked health care providers to "take an honest look at how
you interact with patients" (Shelton, p. 64). The quality of any service
organization, health care included, is directly reflected in the emphasis
placed on quality communication. Think about the last time you received outstanding service. Then recall the critical role that communication played in your overall impression of that organization. Similarly, the perceived quality of your health care organization is, in part,
a byproduct of the quality of provider-to-patient, provider-to-staff,
staff-to-patient, and staff-to-provider communications. In his study of
more than 1,000 letters from dissatisfied patients at a Michigan health
maintenance organization, sociolinguist Richard Frankel (1992) found
that more than 90% of the letters were generated because of the way
members of the medical staff communicated with patients. A survey of
1,500 patients and doctors conducted by the Bayer Institute for Health
Care Communications suggested that patients regard communication
with their health provider as "very important." Patients who rated
their communication with their physician as excellent were more than
four times more likely to believe they receive excellent health care
than those who did not (Is Good Communication Synonymous with
High Patient Satisfaction?, 1996).*

Unfortunately, communication finesse is all too often neglected in
one or more important areas of health care delivery. This, in turn,
functionally impairs the health care provider/organization's incremental pursuit of service quality excellence.

"I know you believe you understood what you think I said, but I'm not
sure you realize that what you heard is not what I meant to say." Humor-
ous, yes, but, more important, this statement underscores the fact that
communication is indeed a complex process. First, a sender initiates the
communication by *encoding* the message in a way he or she believes is
meaningful to the intended receiver, either with symbols, words, gestures, physical contact, or body language. Next, the appropriate channel

---

Source: This and next four paragraphs reprinted from P.J. Shelton, Communication: A Mirror of Practice Quality, *Podiatry Today,* Vol. 4, No. 1, pp. 19–20,
© 1992.

or method of transmission is selected to get the message to the receiver who, in turn, *decodes* it into meaningful information. The accuracy of the receiver's interpretation is influenced by expectations (people hear what they want to hear), education and experience, personal assessments of symbols and gestures, and mutuality of meaning with the sender.

A fundamental understanding of the communication process is required, for example, in the explanation of a patient's diagnosis, treatment recommendation, or instructions. Equipped with a well-stocked "toolbox" of medical jargon, many physicians/providers feel compelled to encode the message (i.e., the explanation) to the patient using terminology intended to impress rather than inform the patient.

What happens when someone tries to tell you how to do something you've never done before? The verbal instructions can simply bewilder you. Imagine yourself in a patient's place. You might hear something like this: "Remove the outer gimbolo down to the level of the frambis. Insert the dolophisk into the baroon with either a gelspur or a plim…. Soak the twistuculus for 20 minutes and place a clean gimbolo over the gimphris." Sounds ridiculous, but this is a clear example of a common barrier to effective communication: *no mutuality of meaning*. Similarly, health care providers must consider the patient's education and background so that language or differing perceptions don't preclude understanding. A health care provider's explanation of a complex clinical condition to a college professor must necessarily differ from that presented to the average consumer. But in all instances, words must be chosen carefully because 500 of the most common (nonmedical) English words have an average of 28 meanings each.

The elements and corresponding behaviors that, when combined, lead to satisfaction or dissatisfaction within each element in the category of communication are presented in the following paragraphs.

Patient's First Impression of the Provider

The average clinician may perform 150,000 patient interviews during a medical career. A patient's first impression can be critical to his or her satisfaction level. As a society, we have come from conditioned-based care, to physician-based care, to patient-centered care, to relationship-centered care. Studies show that patients prefer to be involved in their care decisions.

Provider's Explanation of the Medical Problem

The challenge to the provider is to convert the complex intricacies of various clinical conditions into understandable and meaningful information in the minds of patients.

When speaking to patients, it should be kept in mind that people process information predominantly using one of three mechanisms: visual, auditory, or kinesthetic (feeling). In their research supporting the classic neurolinguistic programming, Grinder and Bandler discovered that individuals provide a host of verbal clues about which information processing mechanism they primarily use. For instance, a visual learner will use phrases such as "I see" and "I can see what you mean." Such individuals will benefit most from visual explanatory modalities such as models, diagrams, photographs, drawings, videos, and so forth.

On the other hand, auditory learners frequently use phrases like "I hear what you are saying" or "It sounds reasonable to me." Verbal explanations will be most meaningful to them. Finally, for the kinesthetic learner, you should communicate in terms of feelings, participative experience, and physical contact. Use phrases such as "How do you feel about having this corrected surgically?" or "I want you to experience the feeling of moving this joint the way I showed you." Simply initiating physical contact (handshake, examination) in a concerned empathetic way will set the stage for particularly effective communication with kinesthetic learners.

Component behaviors or conditions that patients observe in conjunction with this element include the following:

- *Understandable terminology used:* If the use of a particular medical term is included in the explanation, make sure the term is discussed in laymen's terms at a level that is reflective of the patient's education and background. The explanation may be best preceded by stating to the patient: "If any of the terms I mention during my explanation are unfamiliar to you, please stop me and ask for clarification. It's my job to have this information make sense to you." Remember, the objective is to inform, not impress, patients.
- *Visual aids used to aid in the explanation:* Although this is particularly important for visual learners, all patients can benefit from supplementing verbal explanations with visual aids. A simple anatomical model can put structural relationships into clear perspective. Similarly, a simplified diagram drawn in real time on a dry-erase board adjacent to the patient treatment table/chair can add to patient understanding. Additionally, patients consider this "customized" approach to add a personal touch that is unavailable with the use of standardized preprinted diagrams. Complex conditions can often be explained best with the assistance of a profes-

sionally produced videotape, supplemented with a diagram focusing on the unique aspects of the patient's condition, which may or may not have been emphasized on the videotape. Regardless of the modality used, patients deserve to have some visual component included in all clinical explanations.

- *Adequate amount of time spent on the explanation:* Nothing is more frustrating to patients than to sense that the provider simply can't or won't spend the time to explain his or her clinical condition. A rushed, cursory explanation of a complex condition may well leave a patient more confused than he or she was prior to the explanation. Supplementing the actual time spent in explanation with professionally prepared pamphlets, books, videos, or classes can lead patients to perceive that sufficient time has been spent on ensuring an understanding of their clinical condition.
- *Questions answered:* It can be very helpful to precede any explanation with an invitation for questions: "I will make every effort to explain this in a way that makes sense; however, if something is unclear or does not make sense to you, please don't hesitate to ask. Answering your questions is part of my job!" Additionally, it is well recognized that many times, a simple explanation makes perfect sense at the time, but the patient's attempt to explain the same information to a spouse or other family member causes unidentified confusion to surface. Therefore, make the following offer to patients: "If you think of any questions pertaining to your condition between now and your next visit, don't hesitate to call. If I can't come to the phone at the time, I'll make every effort to return your phone call the same day."

Provider's Explanation of Procedures and Tests

Just as patients wish (and deserve) to have a clear explanation of their medical condition, they should also be informed of the rationale and logistics associated with any necessary procedures or tests. This is particularly important in the case of invasive procedures or tests. Although the medical-legal requirements for informed consent document the fact that some form of explanation was provided, full understanding often requires further discussion. The greatest anxiety stems from facing the unknown. A patient's imagination may create a plethora of unfounded fears. Therefore, the more information you can give patients about exactly what they will experience, the more they can mentally prepare. For example, patients about to undergo elective surgery under general anesthesia should be told about everything that will occur leading up to their being brought into the operating room.

Component behaviors or conditions that patients observe in conjunction with this element are similar to those related to the provider's explanation of the medical condition, including the following:

- *Understandable terminology used*
- *Visual aids used to aid in the explanation*
- *Adequate amount of time spent on the explanation*
- *Questions answered:* Be prepared to answer questions that patients raise based on an article they read or publicity they saw surrounding a particular procedure or test. It is acceptable to admit that you are not familiar with "the article." Thank the patient for bringing it to your attention and state that you want to review the research before responding.

Provider's Explanation of the Prescribed Medication

Today's sophisticated consumer expects to be given an explanation of the rationale behind any prescribed medication. This explanation may go so far as to include why a particular medication was chosen over other alternatives, particularly if those options require less out-of-pocket expense to the patient.

Component behaviors or conditions that patients observe in conjunction with this element include the following:

- *Reason for taking the medication explained:* This reason should include a logical explanation of the anticipated outcome of taking the medication, such as, "Your infection is caused by xyz bacteria. This particular antibiotic is the most effective means of eliminating that bacteria and therefore clearing up your infection within approximately 7–10 days." Furthermore, patients should be advised of the potential adverse consequences of not taking the prescribed medication as directed.
- *Understandable terminology used*
- *Possible side effects or adverse reactions explained:* Patients should be warned about likely consequences associated with the ingestion of prescribed medications. Although this information is required to be present on pharmaceutical labels, it bears emphasizing by the provider and pharmacist alike. Patients should be instructed to contact their physician/provider if specified side effects or adverse

reactions occur. Even mild, but unexpected, reactions can cause considerable unnecessary anxiety on the part of patients. If patients are forewarned, they will usually weather such experiences in stride. More serious side effects, such as drowsiness associated with narcotic analgesics or antihistamines, require a modification of planned activities in the interest of safety.

- *Instructions for the medication provided:* Written instructions supplementing the administration details present on the medication label should clearly delineate route, dosage, and frequency, and any special instructions (i.e., "Take after meals," "Do not take on an empty stomach," or "Do not take with alcohol") should be distributed to patients at the time they receive their medication. This is also a good time to reinforce the importance of taking the medication as directed and what to do if they forget a dose.
- *Questions answered*

Communication between the Provider and Staff

Patients can readily sense when there is a lack of teamwork among those providing health care; this often boils down to poor communication.

Component behaviors or conditions that patients observe in conjunction with this element include the following:

- *Communication prior to the patient visit:* When patients offer information related to their chief complaint or clinical progress to nursing staff, this should be communicated to the provider prior to the office visit. Otherwise, patients become exasperated with the necessity to repeat their story from the beginning. Demonstration of this communication can be as simple as: "Nancy told me that your discomfort has decreased considerably. Have you discontinued the pain medication?"
- *Communication during the patient visit:* Patients often ask staff members a question that is best answered by the provider. If the issue in question is raised by the staff member on behalf of the patient during the visit, patients perceive a team approach to keeping them informed.
- *Communication following the patient visit:* Frequently, patients will raise a question or express an opinion to a staff member following the provider visit. Communicating this information to the provider can be helpful, particularly if it reveals a misunderstanding

or apprehension that could easily be cleared up by a brief phone call to the patient.

Willingness of the Provider To Listen

Of all the communication skills, the rarest and most vital is listening. This key skill elevates our communication from a one-way (monologue) process to the two-way (dialogue) process essential in the health care setting. Although we were given two ears and one mouth, seldom are they used proportionately! In his best-seller, *Seven Habits of Highly Effective People,* Stephen Covey (1989) emphasized the importance of listening (habit #5): "Seek first to understand, then to be understood" (p. 235). The author continues, "You've spent years learning how to read and write, years learning how to speak. But what about listening?...What training and education have you had that enables you to listen so that you really, deeply understand another human being from that individual's own frame of reference" (p. 237).

Listeners essentially fall into one of five basic categories: the "nonlistener" who ignores the speaker, the "marginal listener" who pretends to be listening, the "evaluative listener" who often parrots words back but makes no attempt to truly understand the speaker, the "active listener" who gives full attention to the speaker, and the "empathetic listener" who enters the speaker's frame of reference and seeks full emotional and intellectual understanding. The patient's perception of the quality of communication with the provider will, to a great extent, be based on the type of listener the provider is.

Component behaviors or conditions that patients observe in conjunction with this element include the following:

- *Eye contact maintained:* Little detracts more from rapport than a failure to maintain eye contact during communication. When a provider has his or her eyes glued to the patient's clinical chart while the patient is speaking, the patient perceives (perhaps rightfully so) that the chart is more important to the provider than the patient is.
- *Clarification of understanding:* It is important for providers to ask questions and use phrases that demonstrate interest, such as "go ahead" or "tell me more." Then, providers should paraphrase what the patient says, which achieves clarity by summarizing what has been covered. Finally, providers should empathize with patients, using phrases such as "I understand how you feel."

- *Unrushed appearance:* No matter how much time the provider allocates for listening to the patient, if one hand is on the doorknob of the treatment room toward the end of the visit, the patient will perceive that he or she is keeping the provider from getting on to "more important" things, such as the next patient or a telephone call.

Explanation of Required Consent

According to the American Medical Association (1990, p. 6),

> Informed consent is a legal doctrine that requires a physician to obtain consent for treatment rendered, an operation performed, or many diagnostic procedures.... In most states, the law makes it a nondelegable duty of the treating or performing physician.... It is essential that the patient fully understand the treatment to be rendered, the operation to be performed, or the diagnostic procedure to be undertaken.

There are two basic standards of informed consent. The "reasonable physician" standard is based on what is customary practice or what a reasonable practitioner in the medical community would disclose under the same or similar circumstances. The "patient viewpoint" standard is based on what a reasonable person in the patient's position would want to know in similar circumstances. This is based on the patient's perception rather than on a professional perception of what the patient should know.

The physician (provider) should discuss with the patient: (1) the risks and benefits of a proposed treatment or procedure, (2) alternatives to a proposed treatment or procedure, (3) the risks and benefits of the alternative treatments or procedures, and (4) the risks and benefits of doing nothing (commonly referred to as "watchful waiting").

The topic of thorough informed consent is discussed in greater detail in Chapter 5.

Component behaviors or conditions that patients observe in conjunction with this element include the following:

- *Understandable terminology:* It is prudent to describe the treatment or procedure using the appropriate medical terminology followed by an explanation of same using easily understood laymen's vocabulary. Thus, a "partial ostectomy of the proximal phalanx of the left hallux" is explained to the patient as "the removal of a small portion of bone from the first bone of the left big toe—see diagram below." Although laymen's terminology is helpful, a simple and clearly drawn diagram can contribute a great deal to a patient's true understanding of the nature of the planned treatment or procedure.

- *Alternative treatments explained:* Providing patients with the opportunity to make an informed decision about their well-being is appropriately aligned with the spirit of informed consent law. When all reasonable alternative approaches to treatment, coupled with the respective risks and benefits of each approach, are explained, patients rightfully feel as though they are making the informed choice. Patients should also be told about the consequences of doing nothing.
- *Questions answered:* Once the formality associated with the reading, explanation, and signing of the consent forms has been completed, patients should be given the opportunity to have their questions answered. This should be provided in such a fashion as to minimize intimidation. Do not ask, "Do you understand?" Rather, state that "it is my responsibility to have this all make sense to you. Am I doing my job? Are there any areas of our discussion you'd like clarified?"

Education To Manage the Health Problem

Health education for patients has emerged as a key factor in a managed care environment. This is due to the emphasis placed on preventive measures to maintain health and increase appropriate utilization of health care services. These measures also include the development of educational systems and processes that enhance the patient's health status, improve recovery in times of illness, and act as catalysts to healthy behavior change.

Component behaviors or conditions that patients observe in conjunction with this element include the following:

- *Availability of written educational material:* Patients want and need to have concise written information about the management of their health problem. Explanations and instructions only given orally are often misunderstood or confused. This sets the stage for noncompliance, and ultimately suboptimum treatment outcomes. Printed materials that enhance a patient's understanding of his or her condition are greatly appreciated by both patients and their family alike. Advanced testing of patient comprehension of the materials is advisable.

- *Availability of educational programs:* The management of certain complex chronic health problems, such as diabetes mellitus, requires detailed instruction and guidance over a period of time. By making classes available where patients can relate to others with the same clinical problem, appropriate lifestyle and dietary choices are encouraged. This, in turn, can prevent costly complications, reduce overall morbidity, and potentially improve the quality of life and even prolong life.
- *Availability of educational videos:* Many of today's patients recognize that they must share responsibility for understanding and managing their health problem. To this end, they appreciate having educational videos available on a loan basis for convenient home viewing. Many excellent illness prevention and health problem management videos are available on the market today. These are often accompanied by supplemental written materials or workbooks that allow the patient to actively participate in the learning process.

Schauffler and associates (Schauffler, Rodriguez, & Milstein, 1996), explored the relationship between health education provision and overall patient satisfaction. Their study conclusively demonstrated that

> patient satisfaction with the physician is positively and statistically significantly associated with patients' reports that their physician or other health professional discussed one or more health education topics with them in the last three years, regardless of the type of health plan in which the person was enrolled. Patients who reported having discussed any health education topics with a health care provider were more likely to be satisfied with their physician [provider] than patients who reported they did not. (p. 62)

Education on How To Avoid Illness

With lifespans ranging longer than ever before, a myriad of health problems related to lifestyle can be either minimized or prevented completely by taking relatively simple measures. By providing education in the form of written materials, classes, or take-home videos, health providers can visibly demonstrate their concern for patient well-being.

Communication about Health Care Education Programs

It can be quite discouraging to observe a well-qualified and prepared health educator present a class on diabetes management that is poorly attended, especially because many diabetics are very concerned about the implications of their disorder. Although some patients may have unexpected family matters preventing them from attending a class they signed up for, poor attendance may be more commonly related to a lack of publicity for the class. If the effort is being made to provide patients with appropriate classes, there needs to be a coordinated approach to making patients aware that the classes are available. In fact, patients may become more agitated knowing that there was a class they missed (because they were not informed about it) than if there were no class available at all!

Component behaviors or conditions that patients observe in conjunction with this element include the following:

- *Information supplied by the provider to the patient:* Patients who feel that they have a good rapport with their provider see him or her as their ultimate advisor about their health problem(s). As such, a recommendation for health education materials, videos, or classes coming from the provider is likely to be taken seriously and acted on. This is the ideal opportunity for patients to be made aware that these items are available.
- *Information supplied by the provider's staff to the patient:* In a managed care environment, the provider is frequently pressed for time and must rely on his or her staff to pass needed information on to patients. Patients particularly appreciate having staff refer them to or arrange for them to sign up for any classes recommended by the provider and/or to obtain any materials that may be helpful in the management of their health problem.
- *Program announcement sent by mail to patients:* Although the provider and his or her staff should be the primary source of information about, and referral for, health education resources, this is best supplemented by mailing information directly to the patient's home. This mailer should contain necessary telephone numbers and/or registration forms to stimulate patients to take immediate action in accessing health education resources.
- *Signs/posters visible to patients at health care centers:* Prior to the patient's visit with the provider, interest in health education can be stimulated by the presence of well-designed signs or posters focusing

on the benefits of such education. Then, when the provider and/or staff make a recommendation for accessing these resources, patients are likely to listen more intently and be more receptive to the idea.

Reminders To Use Preventive Services

Typical preventive services include immunizations, mammograms, routing physical examinations and health assessments, and counseling regarding behavior (smoking cessation, dietary counseling, stress reduction, etc.) that the patient can undertake to lower the risk of ill health. Providing reminders for patients to use these services is seen by patients as evidence of truly caring providers. These reminders could be in several forms.

- mailed written reminders
- telephone reminders
- health care provider recommendations
- health care center staff reminders
- notations referenced and charted during office visits

PERCEIVED QUALITY OF HEALTH CARE RECEIVED

The Joint Commission on Accreditation of Health Care Organizations (Joint Commission) defined quality as "the degree to which patient care services increase the probability of desired outcomes and reduce the probability of undesired outcomes given the current state of knowledge" (Katz & Green, 1997). The Joint Commission further outlined a number of factors that determine the quality of patient care and recently redefined these factors as dimensions of performance, including the following:

- *appropriateness:* the degree to which the care/intervention provided is relevant to the patient's clinical needs, given the current state of knowledge
- *availability:* the degree to which the appropriate care/intervention is available to meet the needs of the patient
- *continuity:* the degree to which the care/intervention for the patient is coordinated among practitioners, between organizations, and across time
- *effectiveness:* the degree to which the care/intervention is provided in the correct manner, given the current state of knowledge, in order to achieve the desired/projected outcome(s) for the patient

- *efficacy:* the degree to which the care/intervention used for the patient has been shown to accomplish the desired/projected outcome(s); the ratio of the outcomes (results of care/intervention) for a patient to the resources used to deliver the care
- *safety:* the degree to which the risk of an intervention and the risk in the care environment are reduced for the patient and others, including the health care provider
- *timeliness:* the degree to which the care/intervention is provided to the patient at the time it is most beneficial or necessary

Patients, on the other hand, are considerably more limited in their capacity to truly measure the quality of health care. Consequently, patients focus on certain observable components of the health care experience to derive their perception of quality. Although the outcome (improved health) is one important indicator, the process of obtaining care from the provider forms a patient's foundation for assessing the quality of care. In a 1997 survey with 43,771 respondents in 23,554 families residing in 12 randomly selected states, The Center for Studying Health System Change reported the number of families not satisfied with the quality of health care they received within the previous 12 months (Exhibit 3–1).

The elements and corresponding behaviors that, when combined, lead to satisfaction or dissatisfaction within each element in the category of perceived quality of health care received are presented in the following paragraphs.

Thoroughness of the Provider's Examination

Patients are aware that health care providers have undergone a tremendous amount of training and that the process of applying what they know to individual patients involves a bit of detective work. In the classic

Exhibit 3–1 The Number of Families Not Satisfied with the Quality of Health Care (Received within the Previous 12 Months)

Miami, FL	16%	Greenville, SC	11%
Phoenix, AZ	14%	Indianapolis, IN	11%
Orange County, CA	13%	Little Rock, AR	11%
Cleveland, OH	12%	Boston, MA	10%
Newark, NJ	12%	Lansing, MI	10%
Seattle, WA	12%	Syracuse, NY	8%

training video entitled "It's A Dog's World" (CRM films, 1994), a series of events leading up to and including an actual office visit with a physician (or veterinarian, in the case of the dog) is humorously portrayed. After the patient waits what seems to be an eternity in both the reception room and the treatment room, the physician enters the room only to perform a cursory 3-second "examination" followed by a directive, "You need an x-ray." No attention is given to the patient's history of the injury, nor could the quick look begin to assess the extent of the injury. The patient, rightfully so, is quite upset by this disinterested and uncaring approach; then, to add insult to injury, the physician quickly exits the treatment room with no explanation...to take a phone call! By the end of the video, the patient recalls each rude and discourteous encounter with staff and the physician as he rips the appointment card for follow-up "care" into pieces and throws it into the air.

Although a provisional diagnosis may be apparent to the provider within seconds of encountering a patient, patients expect their presenting complaint to be thoroughly evaluated.

Component behaviors or conditions that patients observe in conjunction with this element include the following:

- *Attention to total health indicators:* During the staff or provider's history-taking process and/or vital signs-checking, information related to the patient's general health should be obtained. If, for instance, significantly elevated blood pressure is noted as a finding unrelated to the chief complaint, then the patient should be made aware of it and given some guidance for future monitoring and/or treatment of the hypertension. Furthermore, patients become frustrated when history-based information is not addressed or at least taken into consideration when formulating the treatment plan for the presenting problem. After taking the time to complete a medical history form, a patient who has indicated a history of gastric ulcer is likely to be upset when the provider recommends a stomach-irritating medication (such as nonsteroidal anti-inflammatory agent).
- *Focused attention to the health problem area:* Careful examination with concerned questioning to ascertain the details of the chief complaint history demonstrates to patients that their problem is receiving all of the provider's attention.

Amount of Time the Provider Spends with the Patient

Perceived insufficient time with the provider is a potent dissatisfier for many patients. It is important, however, to distinguish between actual and perceived time spent. When the provider spends most of the visit fiddling with the chart and giving in to multiple distractions, listening only superficially, and generally communicates in a distant manner, patients may feel that an actual 15-minute visit lasted only 5 minutes. Conversely, when the provider's attention is 100% focused (undivided attention) on listening to, examining, and communicating with the patient in a caring manner, that same 15-minute visit may be perceived by patients as lasting 20 or 30 minutes. "My doctor always appears to be in a rush" and "He [my doctor] doesn't spend time with me" are typical comments from patients.

Patients' perceptions of how much actual time the provider spent with them are influenced by many things.

- *Friendliness:* Does the provider appear relaxed, concerned? Is eye contact sustained?
- *Questions asked:* Does the provider enable patients to ask the questions they want to ask?
- *Questions answered:* Do patients get the answers they need and want?
- *Hurriedness:* Does the provider show a desire to get rid of the patient (by putting hand on door, looking at watch, etc.)?

All of the above items suggest a need to focus on quality time, not just to increase the time spent with patients. The actual time spent may have little or no relationship with patients' perceptions.

Thoroughness of the Medical Treatment Received

Patients expect more than a "drive-through, fast-food" approach to the management of their health problem. They want to play an active role in determining the treatment approach, understand the rationale behind the recommended treatment as well as the expected outcome, and know what to do to prevent any potential recurrences of the current problem.

Component behaviors or conditions that patients observe in conjunction with this element include the following:

- *Alternative approaches outlined:* Providing patients with information about the alternative treatment options, with a clear indication of the pros and cons of each, allows them to play an active role in choices about their well-being.

- *Immediate treatment rendered*: Patients need to feel that the treatment is comprehensive enough, with the intention of eradicating the problem's cause, versus simply comforting the patient on a temporary or palliative basis.
- *Supplemental treatment measures provided*: Are there dietary or lifestyle changes that would help manage the chief complaint or prevent it from recurring? How about specific measures the patient can take to ensure the success of the main treatment regimen?
- *Directions for follow-up care provided*: Patients want to know what can be done to monitor the current problem in the future. Are future periodic visits recommended? Are there things they can do at home to help resolve the problem?

Teamwork of the Provider with the Nursing/Supporting Staff

All consumers have a keen ability to sense whether or not the employees and management of an organization are working together as a team to best serve customer needs. Patients can also readily observe the presence or absence of teamwork in the health care setting. In any health care facility, patients are better served and more satisfied when they are cared for by people who share common values and goals with others on their team. When they work together, members of a team can get things done efficiently and convey confidence and competence to patients.

Component behaviors or conditions that patients observe in conjunction with this element include the following:

- Provider and nursing staff exhibit a cooperative spirit.
- Staff assist the provider with medical treatment.
- Staff prepare the patient for the provider visit.
- Provider delegates to staff to increase overall efficiency.

PERSONAL CARING

Cavett Roberts, a past president of the National Speakers Association, was credited with the following statement: "People don't care what you know until they know that you care." This rings especially true in the health care environment. In a 1996 nationwide survey conducted by Roper Starch Worldwide (1996), 1,411 Americans with all types of health care coverage revealed that consumers place great importance on their physician's caring and concern. A "caring atmosphere" is somewhat difficult to define, but typical observable characteristics include friendliness, courtesy, respect, and personal concern. Because the delivery of health care is increasingly a cooperative team-oriented environment, this personal caring must be exhibited by all members of the team: providers, nursing/ancillary staff, and receptionists alike.

The elements and corresponding behaviors that, when combined, lead to satisfaction or dissatisfaction within each element in the category of personal caring are presented in the following paragraphs.

Friendliness Shown by the Provider, Nursing/Ancillary Staff, and Receptionists

The process of building rapport with patients is achieved as a result of many small understandings and micro-interactions. Each time a patient enters the health care facility, the health care team has a chance to display caring, friendliness, and recognition of the patient as an individual.

Patients enjoy being recognized as an individual with a life beyond their illness or physical well-being. They respond favorably when you recall something personal, like the fact that they went on vacation or that their daughter's wedding was last month. Just the mention of one of these relevant topics brightens people's days. Furthermore, it says to the patient, "This physician/nurse/receptionist actually cares enough about me to remember this. I'm not just a number here." Also, if the provider/nursing/ancillary staff/receptionist spends a few moments discussing something important to the patient, it sends a deeper message that you aren't concerned only with the patient's physical problems. Neil Baum, a New Orleans urologist, emphasized this point (Baum & Henkel, 1992): "One of the best ways to lay the groundwork and make your patients feel comfortable is to develop the habit of discussing nonmedical topics in the first 30–60 seconds of each patient visit. My rule of thumb for new patients is to spend at least two minutes talking about other subjects before launching into a discussion of what medical problem brought them into the office" (p. 27). Finally, these moments can serve to relax the patient and ready him or her for what may be a more anxiety-provoking discussion—the real reason they came in.

Component behaviors or conditions that patients observe in conjunction with this element include the following:

- *Greets the patient by name:* Many years ago, Dale Carnegie developed the concept that there is no sweeter sound to a person's ear than the sound of that person's own name being spoken. We know in health care that patients want to be treated as individuals, not as clinical conditions or chart numbers. Therefore, systems should be in place to facilitate each patient being greeted by name.
- *Smiles when greeting patients:* You can positively affect the inflection in your voice tone by smiling, especially when you first greet someone. The reason for doing so is not just psychological, but physiological. When you smile, the soft palate raises and makes the sound waves more fluid. Any voice teacher will tell you that the wider you open your mouth and the more teeth you show, the better tone you get. The same applies to speaking; smiling helps your voice sound friendly, warm, and receptive.
- *Treats the patient as a welcome visitor:* Consumers can readily detect whether they are perceived by an employee of a service organization as a welcome visitor or as an interruption in the person's day.
- *Goes the "extra mile" to treat the patient as a guest:* Patients expect to be acknowledged when they enter the office or clinic, but when they are greeted with warm enthusiasm, their expectations are exceeded. Making patients truly feel that you are glad to see them sets a positive tone for the remainder of the visit. Think in terms of how you are made to feel when you visit a welcoming friend.

Courtesy Shown by the Provider, Nursing/Ancillary Staff, and Receptionists

Component behaviors or conditions that patients observe in conjunction with this element include the following:

- *Pleasant tone of voice*
- *Professional attitude:* A friendly transaction is a clear and understandable goal in any business. Treating customers courteously, attentively, and professionally mimics the "transaction treatment" we would give to a close personal friend.
- *Attentive listener*

Respect Shown by the Provider, Nursing/Ancillary Staff, and Receptionists

Component behaviors or conditions that patients observe in conjunction with this element include the following:

- *Patient addressed by surname:* Our senior citizen population is rapidly approaching 15% of the American population. They are particularly sensitive to having "young folks" assume that they can be addressed by their first name. Quite simply, they resent it. It is much wiser to err on the side of conservative respect and address patients by "Mr., Miss, Ms. or Mrs. Surname," unless they request otherwise.
- *Privacy and confidentiality:* Patients feel very strongly about confidentiality. They don't want to go to a health care facility where personal information is made public. They feel that this violates privacy and shows disregard for the extremely private and precious nature of health and lifestyle information. Wendy Leebov, president of The Einstein Consulting Group, indicated the following:

  Three keys to confidentiality are particularly important to patients:
  - *Keep records confidential:* Patients need to know that their medical records are seen only by the provider and appropriate staff. In situations where patients are likely to be concerned about this, you should take initiative to state that the patient need not worry about confidentiality and to clarify your policy will ensure theirs.
  - *Discussing cases in the office:* Many patients don't like the idea that their physician would discuss their condition with the office staff. Because of this, care must be taken in public areas to keep all mention of patients strictly professional. If Mr. Harmon hears you discussing Mrs. Jones' mastectomy with the receptionist, he can't help but wonder what you will say when he leaves.
  - *Discussing patient cases with another patient:* This may seem extremely obvious, but patients state that doctors sometimes drop casual comments like: "I saw 'so and so' the other day." This information may seem harmless, but patients begin to wonder about the physician's discretion.

- *Tactful handling of financial matters:* Patients are typically sensitive about others hearing about delinquent payments, negotiating payment arrangements, or any other confidential financial information.
- *Cultural sensitivity:* Along with the diversity of the population comes a need for awareness—awareness that although patient expectations differ from one individual to another, the expectations of ethnic, religious, or cultural minorities have much greater variation than what health care providers are commonly familiar with.

Patients' expectations are influenced not only by what they see, hear, and experience, but also by the norms and values with which they live their lives and make everyday decisions.

Personal Concern Shown by the Provider, Nursing/ Ancillary Staff, and Receptionists

Component behaviors or conditions that patients observe in conjunction with this element include the following:

- *Empathy demonstrated:* Patients need to feel that their circumstances and feelings are appreciated and understood by the health care team member without criticism or judgment. This doesn't necessarily mean that the team member agrees with these feelings or the patient's point of view—patients are likely to get things wrong too. But, empathizing with patients shows them that they are being listened to and that somebody is willing to help them. If patients feel that the attention they receive is genuinely caring and tailored to meet their needs, it is far more likely that they will develop trust and confidence in the organization.

  Experiential learning can be used to help all who are involved in the delivery of health care to identify better with patients. For example, the best way for staff to understand what patients feel when they are in a cast is to place staff members in a cast for a prescribed period of time and ask them to perform normal functions. In the case of a leg cast, combined with crutches, the ability to anticipate patients' need to have assistance up and down stairs is heightened considerably.
- *Caring attitude displayed:* Caring shows that, indeed, you are very much interested in what the patient has to say. This may be in the form of spending a few extra minutes with the patient to determine what his or her real needs, wants, and expectations are. This information can be translated into action by taking a patient's special circumstances into consideration when providing instructions for home care, or simply by showing interest and concern above and beyond what would be expected by the patient.

Telephone Courtesy When Calling the Office or Health Care Center

Whether patients are calling a small medical office, a multispecialty group practice, or one of many health care centers that are owned and operated by a medical management corporation, the image of the organization is projected by the person(s) answering the telephone. For all intents and purposes from the patient's perspective, the person answering the telephone is the organization. If this encounter is routinely mismanaged, patients will soon get fed up and seek the services of a competitor who better meets their needs on the telephone. This was discussed in detail earlier in this chapter (under "access").

Component behaviors or conditions that patients observe in conjunction with this element include the following:

- *Prompt answering of the telephone:* The patience level of busy individuals will commonly accommodate 2–4 rings. If it takes much longer, a frustration-driven hang-up can be expected.
- *Length of time on "hold"*
- *Calls returned as promised:* Patients become understandably frustrated when they consent to waiting for a return call about their clinical condition or laboratory results only to be let down. There should be some form of tracking system to make sure patient calls are returned within the same day. In fact, many health care facilities provide a time range within which their calls will be answered—if an expectation is set, follow-through is essential.
- *Efficient transfer of calls to other parties:* Hayes and Dredge (1998) conducted research to determine what customers hate when they telephone organizations: "Being passed from pillar to post…. It can be difficult in a large organization to identify whom the customer should be speaking to but nobody likes being passed from department to department and having to tell their story all over again each time."

Strawberry Communications, a subsidiary of the Zig Ziglar Corporation, provides telephone etiquette training for better customer relations. This training recommends the following approach to transferring calls:

> Lead the customer from department to department. First, inform the client that he will be transferred and where. Ask his permission. Second, place the client on hold and begin the transfer. Third, stay on the phone until the called party answers. This protects your customer against busy signals or no answer. Fourth, when the called party answers: announce the party to be transferred and if possible give additional information re-

garding the client's problem etc. Fifth, successfully connect both parties and announce to each that the transfer has been completed (Strawberry Communications, 1987, p. 63).

- *Pleasant voice tone*: When dealing with patients face to face, building rapport often relies on visual signs such as eye contact and other body language, whereas on the telephone, the ability to strike up a comfortable bond with patients depends to a great extent on the voice. The pace, tone, pronunciation, and volume of a person's voice can build up a vivid picture in the patient's mind. The aim should be to ensure that patients think of your staff as confident, competent, and friendly rather than timid or overbearing.
- *Clear, understandable, and unrushed person answering the telephone*: Have you ever experienced the drive-through portion of a fast food establishment when you can only understand 10% of what is being uttered to you over the speaker? If so, you will better empathize with what a patient may feel when a less than understandable dialect answers your telephone. Clear diction in a smiling unrushed tone should be the standard for anyone expected to project the image of the organization on the telephone.

HEALTH CARE FACILITIES/EQUIPMENT

A variety of observable factors and conditions also function as determinants of the overall satisfaction patients perceive when experiencing health care. These include, but are not limited to, the following:

- *Overall outside appearance of the health center:* The general landscaping, maintenance, and condition of the building projects part of the initial impression in the mind of the patient.
- *Appearance of signs on the outside of the building:* Easy readability, sufficient size, and placement in appropriate locations to assist with way-finding are most important to patients. Aside from these functional issues, the overall condition and appearance of signs project either a positive or a negative image.
- *Cleanliness of the reception room:* A lack of cleanliness, even in the reception area, suggests to patients that cleanliness may not be a priority in other (clinical) areas of the health care facility.
- *Cleanliness of the treatment room:* The general concern regarding cleanliness as a priority is replaced by an emphatic panic that *infection* may be a possibility. In a society that is so concerned with the

transmission of acquired immune deficiency syndrome, people are very concerned about clinical treatment area cleanliness.

- *Comfort of the indoor temperature:* It is worthwhile to periodically audit patient perceptions of temperature comfort. Clinicians wearing appropriate clinical jackets over a dress/skirt or shirt and tie may not be aware that the room temperature is particularly cool.
- *Neatness of the reception room:* Neatness and organization have a calming effect on people. Disorganization and clutter can be an unsettling environment to enter for anyone. Patients, who may be anxious to begin with, might find this irritating.
- *Neatness of the treatment area*
- *Noise level (quietness) in the office:* Sudden, unexpected noises can produce anxiety. In an atmosphere that is laden with some level of anxiety already, special attention must be given to keeping noise to a minimum.

In general, these observable health care facility factors and conditions combine to form the surrogate perception component of the patient's mental report card. Although some aspects will vary in relative importance from patient to patient, the optimum approach consists of managing each of these surrogate perceptions positively.

CONCLUSION

In health care, there are six general categories of patient satisfaction elements: *access, convenience, communication, perceived quality of health care received, personal caring,* and the *health care facilities/equipment.* Each element is, in turn, assessed by the patient by observing various associated behaviors, physical appearances, and conditions. The *access* elements include: ease of scheduling appointments—by telephone or in person, waiting time between the preferred day and the visit, waiting time in the reception and treatment rooms, access to emergency medical care, ease of seeing the provider of choice, and ease of using the telephone advice system.

The *convenience* elements include: location and hours of the health care center, parking quality and availability, services available for filling (and refilling) prescriptions, and services for getting the required laboratory and/or radiology work completed.

The *communication* elements include: patient's first impression of the provider, provider's comprehensive and understandable explanation of the medical problem, clear explanation of any needed procedures and/or tests and any prescribed medication, communication between provider and staff, willingness of the provider to listen, explanation of required consent, and education to manage existing health problems and to avoid illness through preventive measures.

The *perceived quality of health care received* elements include: thoroughness of the provider's examination, amount of time the provider spends with the patient, thoroughness of the medical treatment received, and teamwork of the provider with the nursing/supporting staff.

The elements of *personal caring* include: friendliness, courtesy, respect, and personal concern shown by the provider, nursing/ancillary staff, and receptionists, as well as telephone courtesy when calling the office or health care center.

The elements of *health care facilities/equipment* include: overall outside appearance, signage, cleanliness of the reception and treatment rooms, comfort of the indoor temperature, neatness of the reception and treatment rooms, and overall quietness of the office.

ACTION STEPS

1. Review each patient satisfaction element and corresponding behaviors within each of the six listed categories. As you read the description of each behavior, make some notation (i.e., "need to do," "currently doing," "needs improvement," "N/A = not applicable," etc.) to reflect your "gut feeling" assessment of how things are being currently done in your health care organization.
2. Make a list of current patient satisfaction element strengths and weaknesses based on the above assessment.
3. Rank the items in the above list in terms of importance to patients and improvement urgency.

REFERENCES

American Medical Association. (1990). *Risk management principles & commentaries for the medical office.* Chicago: Author.

Bandler, R., Grinder, J., & Andreas, C. (1989) *Reframing: Neuro-linguistic programming and the transformation of meaning.* Milton, WA: Naturesemp.

Baum, N., & Henkel, G. (1992). *Marketing your clinical practice.* Gaithersburg, MD: Aspen.

Covey, S.R. (1989). *The seven habits of highly effective people: Powerful lessons in personal change.* New York: Simon & Schuster.

CRM Films, Inc. (1994). *It's a dog's world.* CRM Films [Videocassette].

Frankel, R. in Shelton, P.J. (1992, May). Communication: A mirror of practice quality. *Podiatry Today, 4*(1), 19–21.

Hayes, J., & Dredge, F. (1998). *Managing customer service.* Hampshire, England: Gower.

Is good communication synonymous with high patient satisfaction? (1996). *The Back Letter, 11*(2), 15.

Katz, J.M., & Green, E. (1997). *Managing quality: A guide to system-wide performance management in healthcare* (2nd ed.). St. Louis, MO: Mosby-Year Book.

Leebov, W., Vergare, M., & Scott, G. (1990). *Patient satisfaction: A guide to practice enhancement.* Oradell, NJ: Medical Economics Books.

Roper Starch Worldwide. (1996, July). *Heads up via business.*

Schauffler, H.H., Rodriguez, T., & Milstein, A. (1996). Health education & patient satisfaction. *Journal of Family Practice, 42.*

Shelton, P.J. (1992, May). Communication: A mirror of practice quality. *Podiatry Today, 4*(1), 19–21, 64.

Strawberry Communications. (1987). *Let's make friends & not lose customers: A workbook on telephone etiquette for better customer relations.* Carrollton, TX: The Zig Ziglar Corp.

SUGGESTED READING

American Health Consultants. (1997). Doctors, not report cards, shape consumer choices. *Patient Satisfaction & Outcomes Management, 3*(2), 18–20.

Bendall, D., & Powers, T.L. (1995). Cultivating loyal patients. *Journal of Health Care Marketing, 15*(4), 50.

Davis, K., & Schoen, C. (1997). *Managed care, choice, and patient satisfaction.* New York: The Commonwealth Fund.

Davis, S.L., & Adams-Greenly, M. (1994). Integrating patient satisfaction with a quality improvement program. *Journal of Nursing Administration, 24*(12), 28–31.

Dube, L., Belanger, M.C., & Trudeau, E. (1996). The role of emotions in health care satisfaction. *Journal of Healthcare Marketing,* Summer 16, no. 2: 45(7).

Genovich-Richards, J. (1995). Member satisfaction surveys: The next frontier. *Managed Care Quarterly, 4*(4), 1–9.

"Hey Doc, let's talk!" (1997). *Peoples Medical Society,* 16, no. 4: 1(2).

James, V. et al. (1997). The telephone advice system. In G.G. Mayer et al. *Making capitation work: Clinical operations in an integrated delivery system.* Gaithersburg, MD: Aspen.

Joiner, G.A. (1996). Caring in action: The key to nursing service excellence. *Journal of Nursing Care Quality,* October 11, no. 1: 38(6).

Katz, J.M., & Green, E. (1997). *Managing quality: A guide to system-wide performance management in health care* (2nd ed.). St. Louis, MO: Mosby-Year Book.

Krueckeberg, H.F., & Hubbert, A. (1995). Attribute correlates of hospital outpatient satisfaction. *Journal of Ambulatory Care Marketing, 6*(1), 11–43.

Los Angeles Times. (1997, December 8). Lessons for HMOs: Time with patients is profitable [editorial], B8.

McKinley, R.K. et al. (1997). Reliability & validity of a new measure of patient satisfaction with out of hours primary medical care in the United Kingdom: Development of a patient questionnaire. *British Medical Journal,* 314, no. 7075: 193(6).

Miles Institute for Health Care Communication. (1992). *Physician-patient communication workshop syllabus.* West Haven, CT: Author.

Mowen, J.C., Licata, J.W., & McPhail, J. (1993). Waiting in the emergency room: How to improve patient satisfaction. *Journal of Health Care Marketing,* 13, no. 2: 26(8).

Naisbitt, J. (1982). *Megatrends: Ten new directions transforming our lives.* New York: Warner Books.

Niles et al. (1996). Using qualitative & quantitative patient satisfaction data to improve the quality of cardiac care. *Journal of Quality Improvement,* May.

Rubenzer, B.E. (1995). The AHRA patient satisfaction survey. *Radiology Management,* Winter, 33–35.

Stewart, M.A. (1995). Effective physician-patient communication and health outcomes: A review. *Canadian Medical Association Journal, 152*(9), 1423–1433.

Thom, D.H., & Campbell, B. (1997). Patient-physician trust: An exploratory study. *The Journal of Family Practice, 44*(2), 176–196.

Waitzkin, H. (1984). Doctor-patient communication: Clinical implications of social scientific research. *Journal of the American Medical Association, 252*(17), 2441–2446.

CHAPTER 4

The Relative Importance Index: Determining the Relative Importance of Each Patient Satisfaction Element

Given the myriad of elements that make up the "service cycle" that drives perceptions of patient satisfaction or dissatisfaction, it is essential that the relative importance of each element be determined. Whether patient satisfaction research is focused on image-related, transaction/process-related, or outcome issues, some components of the overall health care experience will be stronger satisfaction determinants than others. In the context of organizational performance improvement, changes must be targeted toward eliminating dissatisfaction in areas patients consider most important. The challenge, of course, is to identify relative importances for your heterogeneous patient population. In this chapter, several approaches to establishing a *relative importance index* (RII) for the unique patient populations your organization serves will be presented.

THE PURPOSE OF THE RII

RII is a term that was first published by the author in 1997 (Mayer, Barnett, & Brown, 1997). It allows for a relative quantification of the importance of various service indicators within each element (see Chapter 3) of patient satisfaction. Thus, the higher the numerical "rating," the more important the service indicator is in driving patient satisfaction/dissatisfaction. This can be determined separately for various components of the target patient population, based on various clinical or demographic descriptors. For example, patients aged 65+ may place considerably different emphasis on the need for evening appointments than those within the 25–44 age group.

Later in the marketing research process, when the data resulting from a written patient survey are tabulated, attention must be directed to both "satisfaction" and "dissatisfaction" ratings. The percentage of respondents expressing dissatisfaction (a Likert scale rating of "fair" or "poor") on a given item may be referred to as the *dissatisfaction index* (DI) for that item. Why focus on dissatisfaction? Because the more dissatisfied patients are with those items they have indicated are important, the higher the organizational priority to bring about improvement. In fact, in a dynamic continuous improvement environment, there is a constant need for prioritization of improvement projects. Therefore, when you multiply the RII times the DI, the product is what is called the *improvement priority index* (IPI). The following formula summarizes this relationship:

$$IPI = RII \times DI$$

FOCUS GROUP RESEARCH TO DETERMINE THE RII

Service quality expert Karl Albrecht indicated that "the most common method for discovering what is most important to customers is the focus group... you cannot generalize to all your customers on the basis of focus groups, but you will begin to discover the critical factors that are of importance to them" (Albrecht & Bradford, 1990, p. 90). William Fonvielle, a senior vice-president of Forum Corporation, stated that "techniques such as focus groups, customer panels, and individual interviews are most important to answer the question, 'What...service characteristics matter most to your customers?' They're the techniques that let the customer drive what is said" (Whiteley & Hessan, 1996, p. 65).

A focus group consists of a small group of 8–12 volunteers from among your patient population. The group forms its own identity and much of the discussion is among group members. The facilitator functions to focus the discussion on the research topic, directing the group where required, but limiting his or her own involvement as much as possible. Management of the group involves a variety of logistical tasks, including:

- setting the discussion into motion
- keeping track of the progress of the discussion (timekeeping, etc.)

- ensuring that all members of the group are involved in the discussion (some people are shy in groups, yet their knowledge or opinions may be just as valuable as another more outgoing member's)
- bringing the discussion to a close when the topic has been adequately covered
- gathering names and other details related to group members
- recording the discussion using a flipchart or audio- or videotaping

At Friendly Hills HealthCare Network, based in LaHabra California, we conducted focus group research by using computer-based keypad response technology. That is, each participant was provided a keypad with which to enter his or her response to each alternative presented by the moderator. All responses were instantaneously tallied and reported to the group. This afforded the capability of obtaining considerable quantitative information by using focus groups, which traditionally yield primarily qualitative information. Three discrete age-based target patient groups were identified. These included ages 20–44, 45–64, and 65 and older. Within these segments, the additional requirement was that the individual had accessed the Friendly Hills Health Care Network within the past 12 months.

Next, participation incentives in the form of gift certificates were determined and obtained. For the participants in the 65+ age group, these certificates consisted of gift certificates for buffet dinners valued at $10 each. For the remaining two age groups, the incentive needed to be somewhat higher due to the greater inconvenience for these age groups to attend the focus group sessions. Therefore, each participant in the 20–44 and 45–64 age groups was provided with a $25 gift certificate to a local retail clothing store.

Specific participants were randomly selected from the targeted populations who met the selection criteria. This process initially involved obtaining a computer printout from our management information systems (MIS) department, listing the names and telephone numbers of all patients meeting the criteria established. Then, numbers were assigned to each letter of the alphabet, and a table of random numbers was consulted to establish a random sequence of alphabet letters from which to choose participants by their last name. This provided random opportunity for participants with last names beginning with all letters of the alphabet to be selected. At this time, all participants and a list of "backup participants" were randomly selected in the respective age groups. Each participant was then contacted to participate in the focus group research and was provided with a brief background of the research effort and scheduled for the designated times.

Those people who accepted the invitation received a follow-up confirmation letter with specific directions to the location of the research facility.

The objectives for this focus group research consisted of the following:

- Determine the relative importance (weighted contribution to their satisfaction) that representative patients of Friendly Hills HealthCare Network assigned to each of the identified satisfaction elements within the six main categories.
- Determine the relative importance that representative patients assigned to each of the identified service indicators within each satisfaction element.
- Identify any additional service elements or indicators that contribute to patients' overall satisfaction with Friendly Hills HealthCare Network.
- Determine the relative importance that representative patients assigned to each of the newly identified service elements or indicators.

Each focus group was conducted during a 3-hour period. Refreshments were provided to the 65+ age group, whose focus group was conducted during the day. Light dinners were provided to participants in the other focus groups, which were scheduled in the early evening after normal business hours. A *Focus Group Moderator's Guide* was developed to ensure consistency in approach across age groups (see Appendix A). Throughout the process, it was critically important to emphasize and reemphasize that this research was not designed to measure the participants' current level of satisfaction, but rather to better understand what is most important to them in determining their satisfaction with services provided by Friendly Hills HealthCare Network.

During the focus group study for the 65+ age group, it became apparent that patients were having some difficulty with the ranking process. Therefore, a paired choice approach similar to the *conjoint preference analysis* discussed later in this chapter was used to simplify the task. This proved to be very helpful for participants because the challenge of comparing two items is easier than ranking between 6 and 10 items.

The data were reported in the form of bar charts indicating the relative importance of each element within each category of patient satisfaction (Figures 4–1 through 4–6). These charts provided visual evidence of differences in the relative importance of various elements

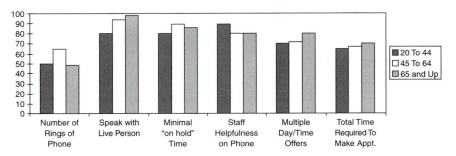

Figure 4–1 Relative Importance of Ease of Scheduling Appointments by Phone. *Source:* Adapted from P.J. Shelton, The Straight-A's Program: A Systematic Approach to Measuring and Enhancing Patient/Member Satisfaction in an Ambulatory Managed Care Setting, in *Making Capitation Work: Clinical Operations in an Integrated Delivery System, Supplement #2,* G.G. Mayer, A.E. Barnett, and N.P. Brown, eds., © 1997, Aspen Publishers, Inc.

between the studied age groups. Additionally, based on a 100-point scale, the relative importance ascribed to each element within each studied age group was tabulated. This tabulation afforded a quantitative representation of the relative importance of each element to each age group studied. These relative numbers made up the RII.

CALCULATING THE RII

The next step was to calculate the RII for each satisfaction element at each of the 41 Friendly Hills health care centers. To accomplish this, the MIS department provided a printout of the quantity (number and

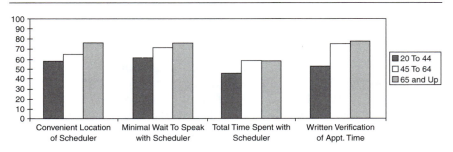

Figure 4–2 Relative Importance of Ease of Scheduling Appointments in Person. *Source:* Adapted from P.J. Shelton, The Straight-A's Program: A Systematic Approach to Measuring and Enhancing Patient/Member Satisfaction in an Ambulatory Managed Care Setting, in *Making Capitation Work: Clinical Operations in an Integrated Delivery System, Supplement #2,* G.G. Mayer, A.E. Barnett, and N.P. Brown, eds., © 1997, Aspen Publishers, Inc.

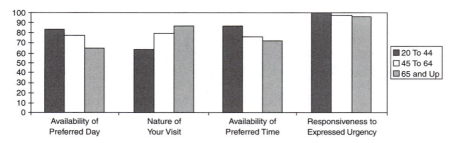

Figure 4–3 Relative Importance of Wait between Preferred Day & Visit. *Source:* Adapted from P.J. Shelton, The Straight-A's Program: A Systematic Approach to Measuring and Enhancing Patient/Member Satisfaction in an Ambulatory Managed Care Setting, in *Making Capitation Work: Clinical Operations in an Integrated Delivery System, Supplement #2,* G.G. Mayer, A.E. Barnett, and N.P. Brown, eds., © 1997, Aspen Publishers, Inc.

percentage) of each of the three age groups represented in the focus group at each of the 41 health care centers. This printout allowed for calculation of the weighted mean RII figure for each element in each category for each health care center. This was accomplished by multiplying the percentage of each age group by the respective RII for the element in consideration. Then, a sum of all the weighted RIIs for each element within each category was created, and finally the sum of the weighted RIIs was divided by three to derive an overall RII for each element within each category for that particular health care center.

The following example, using the service indicator "waiting time in the treatment room," will help illustrate the methodology used for this calculation. Figure 4–1 indicates that the relative importances for the

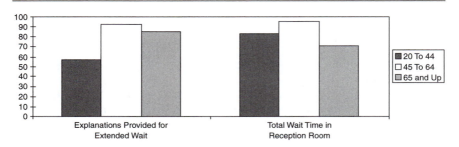

Figure 4–4 Relative Importance of Time Waiting in Reception Room. *Source:* Adapted from P.J. Shelton, The Straight-A's Program: A Systematic Approach to Measuring and Enhancing Patient/Member Satisfaction in an Ambulatory Managed Care Setting, in *Making Capitation Work: Clinical Operations in an Integrated Delivery System, Supplement #2,* G.G. Mayer, A.E. Barnett, and N.P. Brown, eds., © 1997, Aspen Publishers, Inc.

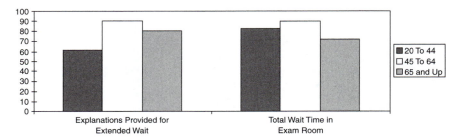

Figure 4–5 The Relative Importance of Waiting Time in Treatment Room. *Source:* Adapted from P.J. Shelton, The Straight-A's Program: A Systematic Approach to Measuring and Enhancing Patient/Member Satisfaction in an Ambulatory Managed Care Setting, in *Making Capitation Work: Clinical Operations in an Integrated Delivery System, Supplement #2,* G.G. Mayer, A.E. Barnett, and N.P. Brown, eds., © 1997, Aspen Publishers, Inc.

three age groups studied were 51.3 for the 20–44 age group, 57.4 for the 45–64 age group, and 26.0 for the 65+ age group. Now, let us assume that the patient population served by the ABC health care center is as follows:

- Eighty-two percent of the patients are in the 65+ age group.
- Nine percent of the patients are in the 45–64 age group.
- Six percent of the patients are in the 20–44 age group.

Thus, the calculation of the overall RII for the element "time waiting in the exam room" within the satisfaction category of "access" at ABC health care center is as follows:

$$51.3 \ (0.06) + 57.4 \ (0.09) + 26.0 \ (0.82) = 3.078 + 5.166 + 21.32 = \textbf{29.564}$$

Therefore, because the vast majority of the patients (82%) is in the 65+ age group, the resultant RII is only 3.56 relative points above the RII of 26.0 identified in the 65+ age focus group.

To further illustrate this point, let us look at the XYZ health care center, serving a very different patient population, as follows:

- Two percent of the patients are in the 65+ age group.
- Seventy-nine percent of the patients are in the 45–64 age group.
- Twelve percent of the patients are in the 25–44 age group.

Thus, the calculation of the overall RII for the element "time waiting in the exam room" within the satisfaction category of "access" at XYZ health care center is as follows:

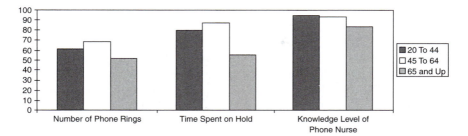

Figure 4–6 Relative Importance of Ease of Using Telephone Advice System. *Source:* Adapted from P.J. Shelton, The Straight-A's Program: A Systematic Approach to Measuring and Enhancing Patient/Member Satisfaction in an Ambulatory Managed Care Setting, in *Making Capitation Work: Clinical Operations in an Integrated Delivery System, Supplement #2,* G.G. Mayer, A.E. Barnett, and N.P. Brown, eds., © 1997, Aspen Publishers, Inc.

$$51.3 \ (0.12) + 57.4 \ (0.79) + 26.0 \ (0.02) = 6.156 + 45.346 + 0.52 = \mathbf{52.022}$$

Therefore, because the vast majority of the patients (79%) are in the 45–64 age group, the resultant RII is only 5.38 relative points below the RII of 57.4 identified in the 45–64 age focus group and 26.02 relative points above the 26.0 identified in the 65+ age focus group. This, of course, seems reasonable because patients in the "retired" 65+ age group typically are less time-constrained and therefore less likely to be seriously inconvenienced by waiting time. If a notable percentage of satisfaction survey respondents from XYZ health care center indicates dissatisfaction with "time waiting in the exam room," this becomes a much higher improvement priority than if the same percentage of ABC health care center patients expressed dissatisfaction with the same element.

When viewing this approach, it is important to recognize that we are deriving the RII using an arbitrary scale of 100. The actual numbers involved are meaningless and provide only relative importances. These numbers cannot be used for any statistical operations whatsoever.

USING CORRELATION ANALYSIS TO DETERMINE WHAT IS MOST IMPORTANT

The American Marketing Association's *AMA Handbook for Customer Satisfaction: A Complete Guide to Research, Planning & Implementation,* authored by research specialist Alan Dutka (1994), states that "correlation analysis is used to determine the performance attributes that have the greatest influence on overall satisfaction" (p. 144). This operation can only be performed after a patient satisfaction survey has been administered and the responses have been tallied. Correlation is the statistical process by which the relationship between different types of data is discovered. The correlation coefficient is a number between –1.0 and +1.0 that indicates the degree of linear association between two variables. Only positive correlations are used for this purpose. In this case, the two variables are

- the percentage of survey respondents who rated the "overall satisfaction" item positively (i.e., "satisfied/very satisfied" or "agree/strongly agree" or "very good/excellent," etc.)
- the percentage of survey respondents who rated another survey item similarly high

It is important to keep in mind that correlation analysis does not prove that a cause-and-effect relationship exists. Leedy (1993) warned that

> finding a coefficient of correlation is not doing research; it is merely discovering a signpost. That signpost points unerringly to a fact that two things are indeed related. It also reveals the nature of the relationship: whether the facts are closely or distantly related. So you come up with a coefficient of correlation. This should spark a barrage of questions in your mind: what is the nature of the relationship; what is the underlying cause of the relationship; if two things are related, how are they related? Answer these questions and you are interpreting what the correlation means. [Now] you are doing research. (p. 274)

For example, it can be very helpful to determine that there is a strong correlation between "overall satisfaction" and "provider's explanation of medical problem—understandable terminology used." This may stimulate further investigation about other aspects of communication between the provider and the patient (back to focus groups again?). In turn, improved communication (and hence, higher patient satisfaction) might be facilitated by developing and presenting special patient communication courses for providers. Or, more basically, using demonstrable communication skills as a provider selection/de-selection criteria.

Generally speaking, improvements in the human-interaction attributes should have the greatest impact on the overall satisfaction rating. Performance attributions with lower correlations with overall satisfaction often may be more related to mechanical or "systems" aspects than to human interactions.

CONJOINT PREFERENCE ANALYSIS

According to Albrecht and Bradford (1990), customers "in a semiconscious way...rank each of the key service attributes according to their importance. The weight is called *valence* and it's a measure of the relative desirability of attributes in relation to each other" (p. 173). The authors recommend using a tool called *conjoint preference analysis* to measure this. In health care, you would simply ask patients to rank a given satisfaction element against all other satisfaction elements within a given category. For example, let us say that within the general satisfaction category of communication, you wish to determine the relative importance of the "provider's explanation of the medical problem." This means that you would need to compare this element to all others within the communication category, one at a time. When preparing to ask patients, you would include a series of comparisons like those listed in Exhibit 4–1 and ask the patients to circle the response that is more important to them when they visit the health care center.

Then, by counting the total number of choices made for each option, you can determine the "valence" or relative importance of "provider's explanation of the medical problem" when compared to the other elements of satisfaction within the category of communication. This procedure can be repeated using each of the other satisfaction elements within the communication category as the "constant" in comparison to the remaining ones. The net result, when this is applied to each element of every category, is a ranking of the relative importance of each element within each category.

The temptation at this point would be to perform a similar operation to compare the relative importance of all of the various satisfaction element categories. This would not provide added value to the research because the satisfaction categories were developed with the understanding that each is important to patients when receiving health care. On the other hand, the tedious task of comparing each element to every other element across categories may be helpful in determining the relative importance of all satisfaction elements.

MOMENT OF TRUTH IMPACT ASSESSMENT (MOTIA)*

An interesting technique for pinpointing the relative importance of various customer interactions was developed by Thomas Connellan

---

Source: This section reprinted from MANAGING KNOCK YOUR SOCKS OFF SERVICE by Ronald E. Zemke, et al. Copyright © 1992 Performance Research Associates. Reprinted by permission of AMACOM, a division of American Management Association International, New York, NY. All rights reserved. http://www.amanet.org.

Exhibit 4–1 Paired Choices To Determine Relative Importances

Provider's explanation of the medical problem *or* Provider's explanation of procedures and tests	Provider's explanation of the medical problem *or* Explanation of prescribed medication
Provider's explanation of the medical problem *or* Willingness of the provider to listen	Provider's explanation of the medical problem *or* Explanation of required consents
Provider's explanation of the medical problem *or* Education to manage health problems	Provider's explanation of the medical problem *or* Education on how to avoid illness
Provider's explanation of the medical problem *or* Communication about health education programs	Provider's explanation of the medical problem *or* Reminders to use preventive services

and Ron Zemke (1993, p. 78). The authors refer to this technique as *Moment of Truth Impact Assessment,* or *MOTIA.* In this context, a moment of truth (MOT) consists of a contact point between the organization and the customer. Essentially, a MOTIA involves focusing attention on those organization–customer transactions that are particularly sensitive to your customers. This process involves three basic steps.

1. Identify those encounters that generate the most praise from and/or problems raised by the customer.
2. Note the key points of customer contact during each of those transactions.
3. Separate the contact points, or MOTs, into high-impact and hardly noticeable events.

In health care as in any other service industry, each service follows a cycle. The cycle begins when a patient recognizes the need for obtaining some form of health care. It ends when the health care is delivered appropriately, safely, and correctly. Each step in the cycle is composed of what patients define as key encounters between themselves and your health care organization. This requires an unusually detailed understanding of what patients expect and an awareness of which steps in the service cycle patients consider to be critical.

In order to create a map of patient-sensitive MOTs, a variety of sources must be used to "listen" to the voice of the patient. Direct sources would include basic marketing research methods, such as patient focus groups, one-on-one interviews, advisory councils, or written surveys. An important, but indirect, source is to review and analyze complaint and/or grievance data. Once each key encounter, or MOT is identified, the component parts of the encounter should be placed into one of three categories.

1. *Patients' standard expectations:* These include the activities that must occur for patients to consider the interaction acceptable.
2. *Experience detractors:* These are patient experiences that have left a less-than-positive assessment of your health care organization, such as examples of events or behaviors that have upset or annoyed patients in the past. (See complaint, grievance, and defection data from your organization.) It is important to focus on both a type of behavior to be avoided and specific behaviors that patients feel detract from their satisfaction with the experience.
3. *Experience enhancers:* These include events and behaviors that patients said exceeded their expectations.

The next step involves the placement of the above information on a MOTIA chart with the experience detractors in the left-hand column, the standard expectations in the middle column, and the experience enhancers in the right-hand column. For example, consider a patient's experience with calling your health care center to make an appointment. Exhibit 4–2 demonstrates how part of such a MOTIA might look.

Using this type of analysis, your health care organization will know what must be done without fail, what should be avoided at all costs, and where it can add value to the MOT "calling to make an appointment." If this approach is taken to analyze each key patient encounter within every service cycle, you will gain valuable insight into patient expectations. In turn, you can "manage" each MOT so as to avoid any experience detractors, provide for all standard expectations, and enhance perceived value by including patient-identified experience enhancers. When translated into employee and system performance, this

Exhibit 4–2 Moment of Truth Impact Analysis

Experience detractors	Standard expectations	Experience enhancers
• The telephone rang nine times before they answered.	• The telephone will be answered within three rings.	• The telephone was answered cheerfully after two rings.
• I couldn't understand what the receptionist was saying.	• The receptionist will speak clearly.	• The receptionist seemed truly concerned about me.
• I was placed on hold before I could say anything.	• I will be asked prior to being placed on hold.	• The receptionist offered a choice of appointment times.
• After holding for 7 minutes, I was cut off!	• I will only be placed on hold for a short time.	• The receptionist seemed friendly and unrushed.

Source: Reprinted from MANAGING KNOCK YOUR SOCKS OFF SERVICE by Ronald E. Zemke, et al. Copyright © 1992 Performance Research Associates. Reprinted by permission of AMACOM, a division of American Management Association International, New York, NY. All rights reserved. http://www.amanet.org.

information can progressively minimize the likelihood of failed patient expectations as well as ensure that you are consistently meeting and frequently exceeding expectations. These are foundational ingredients to preventing dissatisfaction, ensuring satisfaction, and promoting loyalty.

Many years ago, psychologist Frederick Herzberg conducted research concerning motivation in the workplace (Hershey & Blanchard, 1993). This work built on Abraham Maslow's *hierarchy of human needs*, wherein basic physiological needs must be met prior to focusing on higher order needs like belongingness or self-actualization to motivate human behavior. Herzberg discovered that the presence of certain essential workplace provisions, such as "fair pay," did not guarantee employee satisfaction, but absence of them resulted in predictable dissatisfaction. He called these basic requirements *hygiene factors*. In essence, making sure that the hygiene factors are provided serves only to bring employees to "ground zero," that is, neither satisfied nor dissatisfied. According to this theory, only after these factors are in place can employees be motivated by "satisfiers" such as recognition and rewards. Similarly, patients' standard expectations function as hygiene factors that, if absent, result in dissatisfaction.

By conducting a MOTIA, we are determining what patients consider to be their hygiene factors when it comes to the experience of receiving health care. Rust, Zahorek, and Keiningham (1996) support this concept by suggesting that there is a minimum level of service provision that includes elements that, if present, do not cause satisfaction, but, if missing, cause dissatisfaction. In fact, inevitably, there are certain aspects of service encounters that patients take for granted if present and only adversely affect the evaluation if absent. An example of one such hygiene factor may well be the ability to make appointments easily by telephone.

LEARNING FROM EXPERIENCED HEALTH CARE EMPLOYEES

An alternative approach to the systematic identification of the importance of each key encounter for every service cycle is to combine the MOTIA with the five service-quality factors that Zeithaml, Parasuraman, and Berry (1990) identified in their research leading to their SERVQUAL survey instrument (as discussed in Chapter 2). Potentially, every transaction with a patient involves some aspect of those five factors: reliability, responsiveness, assurance, tangibles, and empathy. The combination yields a grid (Figure 4–7) for each MOT within targeted service cycles.

This grid can be used to organize discussions with employees who are experienced with all aspects of interfacing with patients. They should be "customer savvy" so that they can accurately identify enhancing, detracting, and standard expectations for a given MOT. The

	Experience Detractors	Standard Expectations	Experience Enhancers
Tangibles			
Reliability			
Responsiveness			
Assurance			
Empathy			

Figure 4–7 Moment of Truth Grid. *Source:* Reprinted from MANAGING KNOCK YOUR SOCKS OFF SERVICE by Ronald E. Zemke, et al. Copyright © 1992 Performance Research Associates. Reprinted by permission of AMACOM, a division of American Management Association International, New York, NY. All rights reserved. http://www.amanet.org.

employee group should be composed of employees from different departments who share a familiarity with patient complaints, compliments, and preferences. For each MOT, begin with tangibles and brainstorm why each factor is likely to come into play during the MOT being considered. Additionally, this group should be able to provide reasonably accurate insights into which MOTs are most important in making patients happy with the organization.

It is recognized that this approach is a compromise for obtaining first-hand input from patients within your targeted patient population, but it is far better than having senior management assume that they fully understand patient expectations. Perhaps if resources are not available to perform in-depth direct patient research, this approach could be combined with patient input in the form of a single focus group study whereby you check the accuracy of results developed by employee brainstorming.

CONCLUSION

A patient's overall impression of your health care organization is influenced by a wide variety of factors, but his or her attitude of "satisfaction" is ultimately determined by perceptions of those attributes he or she considers to be most important. The RII allows for a relative quantification of the importance of various service indicators within each element of patient satisfaction. This is typically measured in the setting of a focus group (for different targeted groups) where the higher the numerical "rating," the more important the service indicator is in driving satisfaction/dissatisfaction. The RII may vary between focus groups with differing demographic characteristics; this allows for index adjustments to be made for different facilities serving dissimilar patient populations.

Later, when levels of patient satisfaction have been measured (see Chapter 6), the RII can be multiplied by the percentage of patients who are dissatisfied (the so-called DI) to help prioritize improvement needs (yielding the IPI). Mathematically, the formula is: $IPI = RII \times DI$. In essence, this means that you will focus your initial improvement efforts on those areas that the patients consider important and those that they are dissatisfied with. Theoretically, this will yield the greatest increase in patient satisfaction for the improvement resources available.

Other methodologies may be used to determine what is most important to patients. These include correlation analysis, conjoint preference analysis, and MOTIA. *Correlation analysis* emphasizes correlations between positively rated "overall satisfaction" survey items and other survey items. The higher the correlation of the item to overall satisfaction, the more important the patient considers the item to be. *Conjoint preference analysis* is a method of assigning a "valence" to measure the relative desirability of attributes in relation to each other. *MOTIA* involves examining each contact with patients and ascertaining, in a focus group setting, their "standard expectations," "experience detractors," and "experience enhancers."

ACTION STEPS

1. Determine what clinical or demographic factor(s) you would use to group patients when researching the relative importance of various satisfaction elements.
2. Decide how you would gather the data to "adjust" the RII.
3. Determine how you would segment your patient population to compare and contrast the RIIs? (Hint: by facility, department, provider, etc.)
4. Consider the methodology you would use to conduct this research.

REFERENCES

Albrecht, K., & Bradford, L.J. (1990). *The service advantage: How to identify and fulfill customer needs.* Homewood, IL: Dow Jones-Irwin.

Connellan, T.K., & Zemke, R. (1993). *Sustaining knock your socks off service.* New York: AMACOM.

Dutka, A. (1994). *AMA handbook for customer satisfaction: A complete guide to research, planning & implementation.* Lincolnwood, IL: NTC Business Books.

Hershey, P., & Blanchard, K.H. (1993). *Management of organizational behavior.* New York: Prentice Hall.

Leedy, P.D. (1993). *Practical research planning and design* (5th ed.). New York: Macmillan.

Mayer, G.G., Barnett, A., & Brown, N. (1997). *Making capitation work: Clinical operations in an integrated delivery system.* Gaithersburg, MD: Aspen.

Rust, Zahorek, & Keiningham. (1996). *Service quality: New dimensions in theory & practice.*

Whiteley, R., & Hessan, D. (1996). *Customer centered growth.* Reading, MA: Addison Wesley.

Zeithaml, V., Parasuraman, A., & Berry, L.L. (1990). *Delivering quality service: Balancing customer perceptions and expectations.* New York: The Free Press.

SUGGESTED READING

Business Research Lab. (1996–1998). *Measuring what is important to customers* [Web site]. Available: www.corporate@netropolis.net.

Dansky, K., & Brannon, D. (1996). Discriminant analysis: A technique of adding value to patient satisfaction surveys. *Hospital and Health Services Administration, 41*(5), 503.

Delene, L.M., & Lee, H. (1994). The importance of various healthcare quality dimensions from the physician's viewpoint. *Journal of Ambulatory Care Marketing, 5*(2), 47–56.

Glass, A.P. (1995). Identifying issues important to patients on a hospital satisfaction questionnaire. *Psychiatric Services, 46*(1), 83–85.

Hinton, T., & Schaeffer, W. (1994). *Customer-focused quality: What to do on Monday morning.* Englewood Cliffs, NJ: Prentice Hall.

Johnson, B.C. (1996). Achieving patient satisfaction: The relationship between human motivation and outcome optimization. *Journal for Healthcare Quality, 18*(2), 4–10.

Whiteley, R., & Hessan, D. *Customercentered growth: Five proven strategies for building competitive advantage.* Menlo Park, CA: Addison-Wesley.

Woodruff, R.B., & Gardial, S.F. (1996). *Know your customer: New approaches to understanding customer value and satisfaction.* Oxford, England: Blackwell.

Zeithaml, V.A., & Bitner, M.J. (1996). *Services marketing.* London: McGraw-Hill.

The Patient's Mental Report Card: A Model of How Patients Judge Their Health Care Experiences

It is important to think of each patient as carrying around a sort of "mental report card" in his or her head. This is the basis of a grading system that drives patient perceptions of satisfaction/dissatisfaction and behaviors of loyalty/disloyalty. The conceptual model of the patient's mental report card (PMRC) was first developed and published by the author in 1992 (Shelton, 1992a, 1992b, 1993). In this chapter, the two main components of the PMRC—*moments of truth* (MOTs) and *surrogate perceptions* (SPs)—will be presented.

No single MOT or single SP is sufficiently powerful to determine the overall grade on the PMRC; rather, it is the gestalt, or the composite picture, that counts. We will explore a typical PMRC sequence of MOTs and SPs that research has shown to reflect the myriad of patient satisfaction elements presented in Chapter 3. Then, an approach to identifying the MOTs and SPs in your health care organization will be presented. And finally, to ensure that your MOTs and SPs project a positive organizational image, you will learn how to design positive MOT management blueprints and positive SP management plans.

MOTs

In Scandinavia in the early 1980s, a bright service executive formulated a means to bring the "warm and fuzzy" intangible aspects of service into sharp focus so they could be identified and managed to best suit customers' needs and perceived needs. Jan Carlzon, then chief executive officer of Scandinavian Airlines System, created the concept of managing all customer contacts with the organization. He coined the term "moments of truth" to refer to each of these critical contacts. The

imagery suggests that, like the bull and the bullfighter, there are points where the customer comes eye to eye with your organization and something fundamental and memorable takes place (Albrecht, 1989).
    Service quality guru Karl Albrecht indicated that

> Carlzon told his people, "We have 50,000 moments of truth each day in our business." In Carlzon's conception of service, the company exists in the minds of its customers only during those incidents when they come into direct contact with specific aspects of its operation.... In service management terminology, a moment of truth is any episode in which the customer comes in contact with any aspect of the organization and gets an impression of the quality of its service. (Albrecht, 1989, p. 25)

If an airline, with fewer per-person interpersonal contacts than in health care, can substantially improve its overall service quality by engineering each contact to be positive, it would seem that in health care, the opportunity for using a similar approach to improvement is even greater.
    In the context of the PMRC, we shall define a MOT as any interpersonal contact between any representative of the health care organization and a patient. Typically, a MOT is neither positive nor negative in and of itself. It is the outcome of the MOT that counts: Did the patient feel good about the outcome of the interpersonal contact? The MOT functions as the basic "atom" of service, the smallest indivisible unit of value delivered to the patient. In this component of the PMRC, patients are constantly "videotaping" what they observe as they interface with the health care organization, including the process of receiving health care. Each cerebral videotape contains a MOT. The impact of each encounter (MOT) is weighed on the basis of its contribution to an organization's failing, meeting, or exceeding patient expectations.

SPs*

Whereas MOTs are recorded in the PMRC as cerebral "videotapes," SP is the name coined by the author (Shelton, 1992b) to refer to an item that is recorded as a cerebral "snapshot." SPs consist of any conclusion drawn about a health care organization based on the patient's observation of an inanimate object or condition. Each inanimate object may be linked to more than one SP by way of different attributes of

---

Source: This and next two sections reprinted from P.J. Shelton, Surrogate Perceptions, *Podiatry Today*, November 1992, p. 73, © 1992.

that object. For example, if you consider reading materials in the reception room, separate SPs are generated based on the currentness, appropriateness (for your patient population), and accessibility of the book or periodical being viewed.

It is important to keep in mind that SPs may not be fair or accurate, but in the minds of patients (or any consumer, for that matter), perception is reality. Also, an SP can be either positive, neutral, or negative; beyond this designation, there are commonly further descriptors that support why the perception is positive, neutral, or negative. For example, a periodical in the reception room that is 2 years old projects a definite "negative" SP. Furthermore, the surrogate (hidden) interpretation may be "not up-to-date," which is quite significant in a field where state-of-the-art current technology is of utmost concern to patients.

Recall that, when it comes to health care service, patients expect certain minimums to be provided for consistency. However, if these minimums are present, there is no guarantee of satisfaction, but the moment one of them is not present, you can bet that dissatisfaction will occur! For example, competent medical care is expected; when it is present, patients feel that they sort of "got what they paid for." If, on the other hand, this minimum expectation is not provided, dissatisfaction is inevitable.

Appendix 5–A provides a detailed overview of the most common MOTs and SPs that make up the PMRC. This overview serves to cross-reference the patient satisfaction element with each MOT or SP, along with the corresponding specific attributes that patients observe.

A TYPICAL PMRC

Let us examine a typical PMRC to give you a better feeling for how the overall conceptual model applies in practice.

Print Media Promotion

The first SP of your health care practice or organization may well be some form of print media promotion. This promotion could be in the form of a *Yellow Pages* listing/ad, direct mail, and so forth. The first attribute is the design and layout of the promotion. If the piece was produced in-house by someone who was not specially trained in marketing or graphic design and layout, the SP will likely be negative, registering an "unprofessional" caption beneath the snapshot in the patient's mind. On the other hand, if a marketing professional working in conjunction with a graphic artist created the design and layout, the SP is likely to be "professional." In other words, you and your health care organization could be very professional in every sense of the word, but this important first impression remains negative because you were not perceived as professional! Not fair, is it? Probably not accurate, right? Sorry, but perception is reality in the minds of your patients.

The next attribute of your print media promotion consists of claims of "competence, convenience, and caring" (which are high on patients' lists of desirable characteristics in a health care provider). When you make these claims and fail to substantiate them with tangible evidence of your sincerity, the SP is "huckster" or "typical marketing hype." Why? Because the consumer is accustomed to reading marketing claims that contain empty promises. On the other hand, if you claim to be "convenient" and you substantiate the claim with, for example, early morning, evening, and Saturday hours; user-friendly no-cost parking; and a handy location (near major freeways/motorways and public transportation), the SP will be positive, or "credible."

The third SP-linked attribute of your print media promotion is the orientation of the text that makes up the message you send. When it is feature-oriented, such as a litany of conditions you treat, offering a limited service mix, the SP is neutral, with a descriptor like "average" attached. When it is focused on benefits that are important to patients and offers a wide service mix with many types of services, the SP is now positive. Indeed, it is in alignment with the number one objective of marketing—differentiation; simply, in the mind of the patient, you or your health care organization are viewed as "different and better" than your competitors.

Telephoning the Health Care Facility*

The next contribution to your PMRC (and perhaps the first, if print media marketing is not a part of your repertoire) is in the form of a critical MOT—the telephone during normal business hours. This occurs while the patient is external to the health care center, it is typically health-related, and it involves the staff—not the provider. This information was originally published by the author (Shelton, 1993). "ABC Health Care Center... hold please...CLICK" followed by a long black-hole silence may have been an appropriate response to consumer demands during the early 1960s. However, this hurried, abrupt, and impersonal approach has no place in the new millennium. What about the telephone MOT during nonbusiness hours? Whether you

*Source: Reprinted from P.J. Shelton, The Patient's Mental Report Card - Part 3, Podiatry Today, January 1993, p. 19, © 1993.

like it or not, the image of your practice/organization is projected here as well—regardless of how the telephones are managed (by your staff or an outside answering service). Keeping tabs with how your competitors meet the telephone challenge can be valuable and enlightening. After all, how can you do better than them if you don't even know what they are doing?

When it comes to the telephone, rest assured that patients have experienced first-class organizations managing the process with elegance. Try calling any service business that has impressed you within the last 90 days. See how they manage the telephone. Then call an organization that has turned you off with inefficiency, poor service, or even rudeness. Chances are that you will experience a striking contrast between the two responses. What difference does this make? In a word, a lot, because patients' expectations are largely shaped by their experiences. In Bob Cialdini's (1988) classic perception experiments, an individual faces three pails of water: one cold, one at room temperature, and one hot. After holding one hand in the cold water and the other hand in the hot water for a period of time, both hands are simultaneously placed in the room temperature water. As you might expect, the hand from the cold water perceives a change to hot water, whereas the hand moving from the hot water now feels cold. What's the point? The same experience can be made to seem very different depending on the nature of the event that precedes it. Thus, particularly on the telephone, patients' service quality expectations are, in large part, influenced by the service quality they have experienced elsewhere.

A variety of attributes related to how the telephone is managed contribute to the overall grade a patient gives to this "MOT package." First, the telephone should be answered within two to three rings. If this is consistently not happening in your health care organization, it may well be that you are understaffed. Next, the manner in which patients are consistently spoken to makes a real difference. A courtesy-based standard sequential response, such as "Good morning/afternoon/ evening, ABC Health Care Center, this is (staff member's name) speaking, how may I help you" sounds far better than a more abbreviated and abrupt format. Remember that, for all intents and purposes, the callers are "blind." They don't care how busy your office is or what kind of day you are having. They just want to accomplish their communication mission, which assumes that your employees are service/ convenience-oriented.

Next, consider the tone with which telephones are answered at your facility. In fact, consider the facial expressions of employees when they answer the telephone. Because emotions are easily detectable by auditory perception alone, a smile is the ideal. If you have any doubt about this, just tune in to your favorite radio talk show personalities and see how easy it is to detect their emotional feelings about various issues. The fact is, you can "see" a smile (and the associated friendly attitude) over the telephone lines. Some health care practices/organizations even go so far as to place small mirrors near each telephone with a clearly visible sign reading "Smile, the patient signs your paycheck."

Continuing the telephone "experience" from the patient's perspective, the manner with which the dreaded "hold" button is used (or misused) can make a big difference. Placing a patient on hold without permission or, worse yet, asking "Would you hold, please?" and giving the patient no chance to decline (just pressing the hold button) can be quite aggravating. This MOT is managed much more positively by waiting for the caller's permission to put him or her on hold and then checking back with the caller every 20–30 seconds to give the option to continue holding or to leave a message. In the event that the patient opts for leaving a message, this leads to another MOT to be managed. Providing a realistic time frame within which the return call can be expected, promptly posting the message to the intended call recipient, and returning the call as promised all create the framework for this MOT to be deemed acceptable by patients. Also, if the caller is provided with pleasant, soothing music interspersed with periodic brief educational health information, the perceived holding time can be somewhat minimized.

Scheduling an Appointment by Telephone*

The next MOT on the PMRC occurs when the patient schedules an appointment by telephone. In the case of a large health care network in the United States, or the National Health Service in Great Britain, the first patient concern is the classic access factor: "How long will I have to wait to get an appointment?" Of course, this applies to smaller group practices as well, especially if they are traditionally handling high patient volumes. If the overall delay is inversely proportionate to the patient's sense of urgency, then it is deemed "acceptable." Once the basic urgency-delay concern is resolved, the next observation is whether or not the patient is given multiple day and time options to choose from. When there are no alternative time slots available, the impression is one of a negatively managed "take it or leave it" MOT.

---

*Source: This and next two sections reprinted from P.J. Shelton, Surrogate Perceptions, *Podiatry Today*, November 1992, p. 73, © 1992.

Conversely, when patients are given options to choose from, there is a clear sense that the patient's convenience truly matters.

Finding, Parking Near, and Observing the Health Care Facility

Now that the patient has scheduled an appointment, the next series of MOTs and SPs continues to impact the grades established thus far on the PMRC. First of all, were the directions provided clear and accurate? Is there ample convenient parking available? If the appointment is in the evening, is the parking lot well lit and safe? Then, a series of attributes related to the physical facility itself begins to be scrutinized. The first attribute is one that will stay with us throughout the patient's sequential tour—cleanliness. A dirty facility creates the negative SP of "infection-prone," whereas a spotlessly clean facility suggests "infection-free." Then there is maintenance to be observed. An unkempt building that is in disrepair projects the powerful negative SP of "inattention to detail." Would you want to be operated on by a surgeon who doesn't give attention to detail? A neat, well-kept building with neatly groomed grounds registers as "meticulous" in the patient's mind.

The Reception Room

At this point, the patient is ready to enter the office/health care center reception room (bus stations have "waiting rooms"). This is the first internal SP/MOT-fertile territory encountered during a patient's visit. The first object patients are likely to observe is the receptionist's window. The significant attribute is that of openness. If the window is small, closed, or frosted, the SP is negative, with the interpretation that "patients are an intrusion"; a large, wide-open receptionist's counter implies the positive message, "Welcome to our office."

The first MOT occurs with the receptionist's greeting of the patient. Initially, is the patient's presence acknowledged with some form of verbal greeting? I'll never forget the small sign located outside the frosted receptionist window of the first office I remodeled; it read, "Ring bell and be seated." Sounds more like a Pavlovian training session than a proper welcome into the practice. Needless to say, that sign ended up in the same trash barrel as the bell and the frosted window. Dale Carnegie (1989, p. 45) stated many years ago that the sweetest sound to anyone's ears is the sound of his or her own name. Therefore, the optimum greeting includes the patient's name. A first name basis should remain at the discretion of the patient; the best policy is for patients to be respectfully greeted as Mr. or Mrs. (last name), unless sufficient rapport has been previously established (or the patient has requested).

The next SP is the room decor. If the interior design is "mix and match," the SP is "economy class." Conversely, a nicely decorated and color-coordinated room says "first class." The neatness attribute can either say "disorganized" or "meticulous." In many reception rooms, this depends on where the mental "snapshot" was exposed. The message here is clear: The reception room must be checked for neatness throughout the day, not just in the morning at the start of clinical hours. Also, be mindful of the temperature: Is it set to keep clinical personnel with their clinic jackets and uniforms comfortable, whereas patients consider it too cold?

The Receptionist's Work Area*

As patients stand at the receptionist's counter, desk, or window, their gaze naturally turns toward the receptionist's behind-the-counter work area. Organization is the first appearance SP attribute. A cluttered, disorganized area projects the negative SP of "inefficient business management." In today's complex health care systems, patients are increasingly concerned with how well you handle their paperwork, including referral letters, medical records, and finance-related forms. As you might expect, a well-organized work area projects the SP of "efficient business management." The next appearance SP attribute is cleanliness. In today's infectious disease-conscious society, a dusty, dirty appearance sends an unwanted SP: "infection-prone." A spotlessly clean receptionist area suggests "infection-free."

What more could the patient be observing at this point? How about the technology of the business equipment within patient view? This is no time to reflect the good old days. If your health care organization is fully equipped with a manual typewriter, rotary dial telephone, and manual adding machine, don't expect patients to perceive your facility as "state of the art." What does this have to do with the patient's clinical treatment? Absolutely nothing, but the SP of obsolete business equipment is: "This provider/health care organization uses old technology (business and medical)." Conversely, when patients see a front office with a computer terminal, modern telephones, fax machine,

---

*Source: This and next three sections reprinted from P.J. Shelton, The Patient's Mental Report Card - Part 2, *Podiatry Today*, December 1992, p. 19, © 1992.

and so forth, reflecting modern times, they assume that your medical equipment is equally high-tech.

Patient Information Forms

After making the above SP-laden observations, a new patient is likely to be asked to fill in one or more forms. Patient information forms are carefully observed, with several attributes projecting various SPs. The first attribute is print quality, which has both functional and aesthetic implications. Character size smaller than 12 points is impossible for many people (especially senior citizens) to read; in fact, if you have a significant patient population in the 65+ age group, it may be much better to opt for 14-point type. If you are not sure of the value of this effort, simply witness the success of large-print *Reader's Digest* for seniors and others with impaired vision.

Next, turn your attention to the aesthetic component of forms. Are your patients handed a fifth-generation photocopy of a patient information or medical history form to complete in the reception room? Not only is it difficult to read, but the SP is "cheapskate...quality is unimportant here." With instant print shops (or in-house printing capabilities) readily available and affordable, there is simply no excuse for not having all information forms projecting a positive image. Next, patients view the clarity and organization of your information forms. If they contain medical jargon and confusing language, or reflect illogical organization, patients may form the SP: "Look for hazy communication in this office." If you need further justification for making this effort, look at printed materials from some excellent and some not-so-good businesses; you will surely want to imitate the excellent ones.

Reception Room Seating

Typically, the forms to be completed are somewhat lengthy, so patients prefer to be seated during the process. This is the next "challenge" to be faced. Because the population is graying, with the anticipated growth of the senior citizen segment to exceed 20% by the year 2000, seating should reflect the needs of the elderly (whenever appropriate). This means no couches, a minimum chair height of 17 inches, firm but comfortable cushions, and sturdy armrests to enable these patients to get in and out of the seat. Ignore these factors and patients may believe that the provider/health care organization has no concern for patient comfort. Couple this with patients' inherent fear of discomfort, and this seemingly innocuous impression can pave the way for expectations regarding your concern for their comfort during treatment.

Reading Materials

Once patients have quickly glanced at the overall decor of the reception room, been appropriately or inappropriately greeted by the receptionist, taken a seat, and completed the necessary information forms, their attention turns to whatever can help them pass the time. If there is to be any wait at all, reading material becomes their next focus of attention. Is it current? Is it appropriate? Is it health-related? Is it accessible? Currentness projects the SP that the health care facility/organization is up-to-date. A rule of thumb: Monthly periodicals should be the current month; weekly materials should be no older than 2 weeks. Appropriateness refers to how well the reading materials match your patients' demographics. Providing *Field & Stream, Sports Illustrated,* and *Macho Monthly* in the reception room of a gynecologist projects the negative SP: "provider first, patient second." Next, the provision of specialty-specific reading materials projects the SP that "the doctor/provider values patient education," and general health reading materials suggest that "the doctor/provider is part of the health care team, concerned with my overall well-being." Finally, the attribute of accessibility (and variety) can project a positive SP—"convenience/options"—or a negative SP—"inconvenience/limited choices."

Waiting Time

Recall that the number one patient complaint is "waiting time." Although delays longer than 15–20 minutes are bound to occur from time to time, this should be the exception rather than the rule. Why is this so very important? A number of studies reported in the literature demonstrate a correlation between waiting time and overall customer/patient satisfaction. In a study conducted by Mowen, Licata, and McPhail (1993), one of the central concepts they embraced is that waiting time is an important indicator of the responsiveness of a service provider. "The time spent waiting can be psychologically painful because it causes the consumer to give up more productive, rewarding activities and increase the investment required to obtain a product or service.... Researchers found that the longer a customer waited, the less satisfied he or she became with the service" (p. 26(8) Of course, other variables appear to influence this relationship as well, such as the consumer's prior experience, expected waiting time, situational context, time of day or day of week, and importance of time to the consumer.

Mowen et al. cited the works of Maister (1985), who discussed several effects of waiting, including the following:

- Anxiety increased the perception of the length of waiting time.
- Unoccupied waiting time seems longer than occupied time.
- Uncertainty increases the perception of waiting time.
- Unexplained waiting time is perceived as being longer than explained waiting time.
- Unfair or unjust waits seem longer than justified waits.
- Waiting alone seems longer than waiting with a group.

Indeed, waiting for health care is situationally stressful. The wait is usually unoccupied time, waiting mostly for preprocess services, the personnel too busy or unconcerned to inform the patient of the reason for the wait. This failure to provide information causes uncertainty.

The true MOT contribution of this matter to the PMRC consists of the manner in which delays are managed by staff. This begins when the patient arrives at the reception desk to check in for an appointment. If there is an anticipated delay (greater than 20–30 minutes), you should inform the patient of the delay and apologize for any inconvenience. Ignoring this delay is blatantly discourteous and leaves the patient wondering, "What other surprises will I not be told about?" The key to appropriately managing this MOT is to provide patients constantly with updated, honest information in a timely manner. If a new delay develops after the patient has checked in, you should announce the delay along with an accurate estimation of how much longer the wait will be. Again, an apology for the delay coupled with an offer to reschedule the appointment shows respect for the patient's time. Research clearly demonstrates that patients' perceptions of waiting time are influenced (positively or negatively) by the manner in which they are treated by staff during the delay. The power of clearly communicating expectations to patients can be manifested by observing a "satisfied"/informed patient waiting 30 minutes versus a "dissatisfied and disgruntled"/uninformed patient waiting 20 minutes.

The Patient Is Escorted to the Treatment Room

Once the reception room waiting time is over, the next combined MOT/SP contribution to the PMRC occurs when the nurse or medical assistant calls the patient and escorts him or her to the treatment room. Is the patient's name enunciated clearly or mumbled inaudibly? Is the name pronounced correctly or mutilated? Is the patient greeted in a friendly and enthusiastic manner or by using a lifeless, boring monotone? Each of these considerations contributes to the patient's grade of this MOT. The first set of SPs generated during this trip concerns the appearance of the back office staff. When they are provided with color-coordinated (and preferably style-coordinated) uniforms, the SP is "team of professionals." Uncoordinated and inappropriate attire appears unprofessional and may even be in violation of the Occupational Safety and Health Association's bloodborne pathogen standards. The next staff appearance attributes are grooming and jewelry. Neat and clean grooming combined with a minimum of jewelry creates a professional SP, whereas wrinkled (or worse yet, dirty) uniforms and excess jewelry synergize to project unprofessionalism.

Once the staff appearance has been observed, patient attention turns back toward the interior facility details, such as the hallway carpeting/flooring. Excessively worn carpeting/flooring leads patients to ask, "What else isn't being maintained in this facility?" If the carpet is not spotlessly clean, patients may believe the facility is infection-prone. If it is immaculately cared for, patients register an "infection-free" check on their mental report cards.

The patient's next observation may be photographs, decorative items, and paintings hanging on the walls along the way to the treatment room. These are evaluated in terms of their orientation, as we noted with reading materials.

The Treatment Room

Alas!...the patient arrives to the treatment room. The first and most powerful SP observation is cleanliness. Here, fastidious attention to detail is essential to earn an SP of "infection-free." This attention applies to everything in the room, from instruments to the treatment chair and waste container. Next, the treatment chair or table is evaluated from the standpoint of mechanical operation; deficient function leads to the familiar SP question: "What other equipment (especially treatment-related) is not properly maintained?" Now, take a look at the instruments that are visible to the patient while he or she is waiting for treatment. Remember that all instruments suggest an SP of "pain/shots." Finally, patients pay particular attention to all dressings applied to them by the physician/provider. Neat and methodical application says "neat/methodical physician/provider." Neat and methodical application by the nurse or medical assistant says "competent/well-trained staff."

Waiting in the Treatment Room

While the patient is in the treatment room, waiting time once again becomes an issue. This occurs in several segments: waiting for the nurse or medical assistant to obtain and chart basic information about the patient's symptoms, condition, or progress; waiting for the health care provider to enter the room; waiting for staff to "set up" for any special diagnostic or therapeutic procedures ordered by the provider; waiting for the provider to reenter the room, and so forth. As in the reception room, the grade received from the patient on the PMRC is, in large part, related to how the waiting time is managed.

The best overall approach to handling wait time in the treatment room is to schedule in such a fashion as to minimize waiting time in the first place. Unfortunately, health care practices/organizations seldom have an accurate understanding of the total waiting time patients experience once they are placed in the treatment room. This can be understood best by conducting a treatment room (and reception room, for that matter) waiting time audit. While visiting the Eye Hospital in Birmingham, England (yes, as a patient), I was impressed to note that just such an audit was a part of their ongoing efforts to improve the quality of service. A sequence of checkpoints was listed on a small sheet of paper; each component process step was followed by a blank line for the current time to be entered. These included:

- appointment time
- time checking in with receptionist
- vision check completed
- time in to see the ophthalmologist
- time clinical visit completed
- time patient checkout process (and reappointment) completed

Only with this type of approach can process bottlenecks be identified accurately and corrected. When observed waiting times in a particular area are either consistently long or highly variable, further investigation is needed. By flowcharting the processes involved with patients moving to and through each sequential "checkpoint," a more objective understanding of delay-causing step(s) is possible. Once these delay-causing steps have been identified, you should enlist the assistance of all employees involved in implementing the procedures and performing the process tasks to brainstorm possible root causes of delay. If any obvious inefficiencies are occurring, the same group can use its collective creativity to streamline the process. Once the change is implemented, continuous time audits will document whether or not the desired effect has been achieved.

The Noise Level

The next significant SP is a "condition" that is observed, rather than an inanimate object, that contributes to the mental report card of patients throughout the course of their health care center visit—noise. Our lives are full of distracting, unwanted sounds: horns blowing, children yelling at play, sirens blaring, auto and home burglar alarms discharging, doors slamming, and so forth. However, people expect a medical office to be relatively quiet. I can recall repeatedly admonishing surgical residents to avoid making unnecessary noises in the presence of patients during procedures performed under local anesthesia. It went something like this: "Sudden, unexpected noises are anxiety-producing. Patients have enough stress as it is. We needn't add to it!"

When patients are asked about their tolerance for noises in a medical office, they are typically willing to accept those sounds that are "necessary" for normal office functions. This would include such things as computer printing, deliveries, patient conversations (loud or soft), staff speaking softly, and telephones ringing (few rings before being answered). On the other hand, patients resent those noises that they perceive as "unnecessary." This category includes such things as loud staff talking, yelling down the hall, outbursts, heavy footsteps, doors banging, and boisterous laughter. Leebov and colleagues (1990) found that noise in medical settings causes a number of adverse effects on patients, including the following:

- an increase in patient's perception of pain
- an interference with relaxation and rest, which, in turn, interferes with recovery
- an increase in irritability and anxiety
- a stimulus to blood pressure elevation
- an insult to patients—they find it intrusive and inconsiderate (p. 85)

Just as we recommended a waiting time audit, it may be a good idea to perform a noise audit. This may be accomplished best by having a nonstaff, objective "outsider" positioned in an unobtrusive office location (reception room or within easy earshot of a treatment room) listen intensely to each and every sound that surrounds him or her. These sounds would include such noises as telephone rings, staff conversations, staff removing or replacing items from cabinets, banging and slamming, and so forth. Once problem areas are identified, noise reduction strategies can be developed by those employees involved in the high noise area(s).

Medical Equipment

The next SP is based on observations of the equipment that is present in the treatment room. This isn't to suggest that patients can accurately judge the true technical/medical value of that equipment. Rather, they form an impression of whether or not these items appear to be modern and "state of the art." Remember, SPs don't have to be accurate or fair, but they are *perceptions* in the minds of patients and, well, that is their reality. These perceptions are, in part, driven by expectations that are built by medical external marketing, wherein advertisements may make claims of various scientific and not-so-scientific equipment representing the elusive concept of "state of the art."

Provider Appearance

As we continue our journey through a typical patient's health care experiences, a critical series of high-impact SPs and MOTs begins when the physician/provider first enters the treatment room. First, there is the appearance of the doctor/provider. Seem ridiculous? An unfair and inaccurate judgment factor, you say? Patients repeatedly indicate that this has a significant bearing on their overall impression of the physician/provider. I will never forget the comments my then 75-year-old mother made when an on-call surgeon visited her in the hospital on a Saturday afternoon to do a consultation: "He was wearing Levi's and a sweatshirt.... If he doesn't take his job any more serious than that, there's no way I'd let him operate on me!" Granted, little actual correlation exists between a provider's appearance and his or her clinical (or surgical) competence, but nevertheless, this adverse SP led her to request consultation from a different surgeon.

Provider Friendliness

The next general, but important, physician/provider characteristic observed by patients is friendliness. Merriam-Webster's Collegiate Dictionary (1993) defines friendly as "showing kindly interest and goodwill;...a favored companion;...serving a beneficial or helpful purpose" (p. 246). Recall that friendliness is one of the behaviors that contributes to satisfaction/dissatisfaction within the category of "personal caring." During any two-way verbal communication between two people, there are two dimensions: content and relationship. In the context of health care, the *content* dimension focuses on a conversational exchange of information pertaining to the patient's health problem. The *relationship* dimension defines the relationship being developed between the patient and the physician/provider. Every time something is said during the conversation, there is the potential for either positively or negatively influencing the evolving relationship.

Provider Communication with the Patient

In Chapter 3, the fundamental importance of and elements of the communication process were presented. Both physicians/providers and patients rate communication-related characteristics as extremely important, but they differ on what constitutes good communication. According to Wendy Levinson, professor of medicine at the Oregon Health Sciences University in Portland, "Patients tend to look at communication from a broader perspective than their doctors, rating interactive discussions about their current condition and overall health as most important...on the other hand, physicians tend to concentrate on the specific reason for the patient visit, as well as their own ability to explain and discuss treatment options and outcomes with the patient." Tom Campbell, associate professor of family medicine and psychiatry at the University of Rochester (New York) School of Medicine, expressed it this way: "Different expectations about what constitutes good communication tell us that as we move forward to find ways to measure quality of care, we must recognize that open, back-and-forth communication about the patient's general health and emotional well-being ranks as high as the doctor's technical skills and other criteria to the patient."

A recent study conducted by Johns Hopkins University (1997) examined different communication styles of practitioners and polled both physicians and patients about their communication preferences. The researchers listened in on office visits between 127 physicians and 527 patients, then analyzed the conversations. They discovered that in 32% of the visits, physicians asked simple yes-or-no questions and primarily used medical jargon to communicate. In 33% of the visits, this communication style was combined with slightly more personal communication. Twenty percent of the visits involved equal amounts of medical talk and personal conversation. Eight percent of the conversations were dominated by personal exchanges—small talk, encouraging phrases, and open-ended questions for the patient regarding lifestyle and general well-being. Though in this pattern, the physicians did most of the talking, the study found that patients whose physicians communicated in this way were the most satisfied.

Marshall Zaslove (1998) described this as psychosocial talk.

> Research shows the one type of physician communication that patients find most satisfying is "psychosocial" talk about function and feelings.... It's vastly more popular with patients than the strictly "biomedical" style of most physicians: lots of diagnostic questions and instructions on regimen, but little interest in how they're actually functioning and feeling.... It's unfortunate that when physicians have to speed up their visits, psychosocial communication is the first thing to be eliminated. Very few docs [providers] now use it, but patients definitely prefer it, and research indicates that the psychosocial style visit actually does not take any longer than the biomedical type. (p. 226)

If the only conversation between physician/provider and patient relates to the health problem that brought the patient in, minimal relationship or rapport develops. On the other hand, if the content dimension is consistently preceded by a brief discussion of other matters affecting the patient's life—vacations, children, hobbies, and so forth, this provides the relationship dimension and projects an image of friendliness. A strategy that I have found to facilitate this process in a busy clinical practice is the use of a *personal reference notes* page. This page should be placed in the very back of each patient's medical chart and should be a different color than other papers in the chart. Then, either the provider or the supporting staff can jot down a brief nonclinical, personal note each visit that pertains to something the patient mentioned in conversation. For example, "Going to grandson's wedding on October 6th" or "Vacationing for 2 weeks in France," and so forth. Then, prior to the visit, a 2-second glance at the note allows you to focus immediately on the relationship dimension of your visit communication. Patients sincerely appreciate your personal interest; it contributes significantly to continually building rapport. This is clearly a win-win situation that costs little in terms of time or money.

Before moving on to other MOTs related to the patient's encounter with the provider, a brief word about the focus of attention is in order. We have all met people (all too often) who routinely enter a room delivering the nonverbal message, "Here I am. Pay attention to me." Others more graciously emanate the message, "There you are" and make you the center of attention. An excessive dose of physician/provider self-disclosure overemphasizes his or her own importance and precludes patients from getting the attention they deserve. This is an example of improperly using the relationship dimension of communication because it backfires, causing patients to feel intimidated rather than building rapport. It is best for physicians/providers to make it clearly understood that the patient is the most important thing during the visit, keeping the focus of the conversation on him or her. What may seem like a small matter to the provider may be of monumental proportion to the patient; in short, if the patient thinks something is important, it is important. The entire subject of provider communication has been studied intensively by the Miles Institute for Health Care Communication. They offer a highly interactive workshop entitled "The Miles Physician-Patient Communication Workshop." The highlights of this workshop are discussed in Chapter 9.

The Medical Examination

Following the initial conversation between provider and patient, the next MOT occurs during the actual examination process. The degree of practical sensitivity to the comfort/discomfort inherent to the examination provides a patient with the first behavioral indicator of the provider's humanistic concern. The shock of a cold stethoscope or, worse yet, speculum sets the stage (and rightfully so) for the provider to be labeled "inconsiderate." The impression can be much more favorable if the provider takes the time to warn the patient in advance: "This is going to feel a little cold" or, better yet, "This is quite cold. I'm going to warm it a bit before it touches you."

The same holds true when it comes to examining a patient with a problem that, by it's very nature, is painful—the complaint that brought the patient to the facility in the first place. Granted, some palpation may be necessary in order to pinpoint the anatomical basis of the pain, but this too requires some degree of sensitivity. It never ceases to amaze me when I observe a provider repeatedly pressing on an obviously painful problem like an abscess, contusion, or infected ingrown toenail! I have found it very helpful in such circumstances, where patients are anxious to start with, to take a few seconds to reassure the patient by saying something like, "I want to take a close look at this, but we already know it hurts, so I'll be as gentle as possible." More often than not, this simple phrase is followed by a sigh of relief from the patient. Or, in those cases where pressing and probing are essential to making a diagnosis, simply warning the patient in advance, as in "I need to examine this carefully to determine (what tissues are involved). If I cause you any discomfort, I apologize in advance," clearly demonstrates your sensitivity.

Thoroughness of Examination

The next attribute of the clinical examination MOT series relates to the process (vs. outcome) component of perceived quality of care. Although there are a variety of processes involved in the patient's health care experience, the initial evaluation/examination process is typically judged on the basis of thoroughness. This begins with the medical and clinical history interview—discussing previous health problems, medications, allergies, and previous treatment(s) (and response to each) for the presenting complaint. Next should come a focused and detailed discussion of the history of the chief complaint, including factors that have either relieved or exacerbated the symptoms in the past. This is the primary indication to the patient that his or her health problem is being taken seriously.

Cursory evaluations give the impression of low concern and that time efficiency is more important than clinical accuracy. This, in turn, spells "poor quality" in the mind of the patient when "grading" the provider's role of the process component of health care. Even though many routine diagnoses can be made "at a glance" by an experienced provider, patients ought not be made to feel that their chief complaint is not worthy of the clinician's full attention. If this occurs, patients feel shortchanged, having received less than expected value for their health care dollar.

The next aspect of the clinical evaluation/examination that is observed by patients consists of inquiries related to the underlying cause of the presenting symptoms. These may take the form of any current or future recommended clinical or laboratory tests, radiography, bone scans, magnetic resonance imaging, and so forth. The impact this has on the PMRC is dependent on the nature of the complaint; the more serious the diagnosis is, the more careful diagnostic testing is expected by the patient.

Provider's Explanation of the Patient's Condition

Once the provider has completed the evaluation/examination, the next important MOT on the PMRC occurs during the explanation of the patient's condition. The most important overall consideration in this process is to have the provider adjust the "level" of the explanation to the patient's apparent capacity to understand. In other words, if two very different patients enter at different times with the same basic problem, each should receive an explanation in terms he or she can easily comprehend. For example, the explanation of an orthopaedic problem such as achilles tendonitis should be tailored differently for a mechanical engineer than for the average patient. For the former, a discussion of the origin of the gastrocnemius and soleus muscles along with their mutual contribution to the achilles tendon and the lever function of the ankle joint would be reasonable. In the case of the latter, simply explaining that there is an excessive amount of strain on the achilles tendon that leads to inflammation of the tissues adjacent to the tendon that, in turn, causes pain, would be sufficient.

Once the proper level of explanation is established, a number of items should be included to facilitate the patient's understanding. These include, but are not limited to, the following:

- Provide a functional (basic anatomical and physiological) background related to the presenting symptoms.
- Relate the patient's presenting symptoms to some deviation from normal function.
- Describe what the body is doing in response to the trauma or deviation from normal function.
- Present the rationale for considering treatment, including the "downside" of no treatment at all.
- Discuss any lifestyle factors that may have contributed to the problem.

In health care today, there are a variety of modalities that can be used to aid patient understanding. Professionally produced anatomical charts assist with explanations that show the relationship between adjacent tissues and structures. Similarly, Krames Communications produces excellent condition-specific booklets that contain both text explanations in laymen's terminology and anatomical drawings. These serve well to supplement explanations provided during the visit, and to clarify any misunderstandings. Anatomical models are especially valuable for clarification because they offer three-dimensional viewing.

When the condition is somewhat complex, requiring a rather elaborate explanation, professionally produced videotapes can be very helpful. Using this approach, every patient receives the same thorough explanation of the particular condition. It is not dependent on how rushed the provider is on a given day. It must, however, be kept in mind that patients do not want this sort of presentation to be a substitute for the provider's explanation. I have found that placing a blank white drawing board in each treatment room adjacent to the exam chair/table is extremely helpful. Patients expect the provider to "custom-make" some aspect of the explanation of the problem spontaneously. This allows for a convenient, focused, and simplistic diagram to be drawn that demonstrates how/why the symptoms are occurring. Ideally, all of the above-mentioned modalities should be combined to make the process of explaining the patient's condition truly educational. This leaves the patient with the correct impression that the provider really cares about the patient's understanding of his or her health problem.

Discussion of Treatment Options

Now that the diagnosis has been made and the condition has been explained to the patient by the provider, the next MOT occurs during the discussion of treatment options. Naisbitt said, in 1982, that people want to play an active role in making decisions about their well-being. Therefore, they expect to be given sufficient information to allow them to make an informed decision in conjunction with the provider. This should include an appropriate range of options from most to least conservative. The potential complications associated with failure to treat the problem and/or failure of the patient to comply with treatment instructions should be discussed as well. When done in a pleasant way, this discussion serves to underscore the provider's concern for resolving the patient's health problem. Recall from Chapter 3 that the provider's explanation should have the following characteristics:

- use of understandable terminology
- use of visual aids to aid in the explanation
- adequate amount of time spent on the explanation
- answering of patient questions

Patient Health Education

The overall management of many health problems commonly includes certain lifestyle changes. In order to motivate patients to comply rationally with recommendations for change, some form of health education and behavior modification is often needed. Therefore, the next MOT/SP combination may consist of the availability, distribution, and quality of health education resources that are available for patient use. The diagnosis of a complicated disease process or condition, coupled with the provider's relatively brief explanation, is insufficient to give patients the extent of information they truly need to understand their condition thoroughly. For example, a diabetic patient who is suffering from a painless sensory neuropathy may consider the lack of pain to be a beneficial feature of the condition. In reality, this can be very dangerous—pain provides us with a valuable warning system because minor cuts or injuries can go unnoticed and go on to develop infections and other complications. Generally speaking, if a patient emerges from the visit confused about his or her condition or overwhelmed with the information that was given verbally, the health education MOT will surely register a negative on the PMRC.

Traditionally, health education has been associated with any change in behavior, conducive to health, that takes place as a result of learning. The World Health Organization believes that health education and health promotion are inextricably linked; health promotion programs promote health and health education is an integral part of that activity. Most health educators agree that health education shares the following characteristics:

- Health education focuses primarily on the individual and his or her lifestyle.
- Health education literature and programs are concerned with the transmission of health-related information.
- Any change in behavior occurring as a result of health education is voluntary.

Furthermore, one of the major shifts in American health care has been from illness response to health promotion. In a managed care environment, there is considerable financial incentive to reduce costly medical care through health awareness and education. How people live has an important impact on their health. Whether people smoke, whether they are physically active, what and how much they eat and drink, their sexual behavior, and whether they take illicit drugs—all these factors can have a dramatic and cumulative influence on how healthy people are and how long they will live.

Patient education truly functions as a vital component of the broader concept of health promotion. The prevention of disease and the promotion of good health are largely dependent on the informed and willing contribution of individuals to their own health. In the field of patient health education, there are two general types of approach—compliance-based and patient-centered.

1. *Compliance-based* patient education aims to provide information for people in the hope that they will change their behavior in the light of knowledge about potential health problems. The most common assumption associated with this approach is that people can be treated as empty buckets into which the appropriate information regarding their health can be poured.

   The failure of traditional compliance-based educational programs is widely recognized. Verbal patient education is of limited value where individuals find they are unable to remember much of what has been said. Furthermore, lack of understanding of information imparted by providers helps explain poor levels of compliance. Thus, it would appear that a purely didactic approach to patient education can have only a limited potential to influence patient behavior.

2. *Patient-centered* health education aims to empower people by helping them understand their own illness and where they are in their "readiness" for change and action. This enables patients to identify the benefits and develop the skills of contributing to effective self-care wherever possible. The basic principles of a patient-centered approach to health education include the following:
   - Promote patients' sense of ownership over the behavioral changes needed. This can be accomplished either by motivating patients to want to know more about the needed changes or by providing them with a greater understanding of their condition or illness.
   - Identify where patients are in their readiness for change and provide appropriate information and support to bring about the desired behaviors.
   - Assist patients with the process of developing their own objectives, setting goals to take a particular course of action (which includes overcoming any recognized weaknesses), and evaluating the consequences of taking the action.
   - Encourage patients to contribute to the learning process.
   - Incorporate behavior modification techniques into the office visit.

- Take a needs-based approach to providing new information, building on patients' existing knowledge and only adding new information when the learner identifies a reason for needing it.
- Support and praise change and the achievement of goals.

Funnel (1991) summarized the value of a patient-centered education as follows:

> The patient-centered approach is widely adopted in the management of many chronic illnesses, e.g., Diabetes, rheumatoid arthritis and asthma. This approach is becoming increasingly popular with regard to the management of patients with diabetes, where the patient's contribution to their own care…is vital to their overall well-being. (p. 82)

Explanation of Recommended/Prescribed Medications

Following the majority of visits to a provider, patients leave with a prescription in hand. According to Nelson, Wood, Brown, and Bronkesh (1997), up to one-half of all prescription medications are taken incorrectly. Patients get confused or overwhelmed, or they just plain forget. Of course, patients are interested in deriving the potential benefits of taking the medication. Therefore, the process of carefully explaining the important details pertaining to the medication constitutes another MOT on the PMRC. A brief rapid-fire recitation of the dos and don'ts of taking a medication may be somewhat informative at the time of the visit, but it may not be sufficient to ensure that the well-intentioned patient will take the medication correctly. When the outcome of this mismanaged MOT is uncertainty, confusion or, worse yet, a preventable side effect, patients may rightfully become upset. This, then, reflects on their PMRC in a negative light.

New Orleans urologist Neal Baum uses a medication form that he gives to patients during their visit. This form lists the following information:

- patient name, date, and diagnosis
- medication name
- dosage
- route of administration
- possible side effects—emphasizing those warranting a phone call to the doctor (Baum & Henkel, 1992)

The American Medical Association (1990) recommends that instructions and explanations pertaining to medication should contain the following information:

- proper use of the medication
- potential adverse effects of the drug
- potential adverse effects of not using the prescribed drug
- potential adverse effects of not using the drug as prescribed

Explanation of Recommended Radiographs or Laboratory Tests

Very often, laboratory tests and/or radiographs are needed as part of the diagnostic workup or to assess the progress of a treatment regimen. "Go to the radiology department and give them this note" hardly informs the patient about the purpose for which the radiograph is being ordered. Rest assured that this approach will get a negative grade on the PMRC. On the other hand, taking a few moments to explain the rationale for and importance of obtaining additional information is what patients expect. "In order to make sure that the fractured bone is healing as it should be, I need to have another x-ray taken. Please take this form to our radiology department; it tells them exactly how I want the x-ray taken. We'll notify them that you are on your way. Then, I should be able to review the radiographs this Wednesday. I'll give you a brief call to let you know my findings. Then, during your next visit, we'll review them together so you can see the healing progress."

It really doesn't take that much additional time to exceed patient expectations by taking a more caring approach. This becomes even more critical when the diagnosis of a potentially serious disorder is contingent on receiving the results of a laboratory or radiographic evaluation. When providers go out of their way to ease a patient's anxiety, a high PMRC grade for that MOT can usually be anticipated. To ensure that the patient's experience at the laboratory or radiology went smoothly, ask the patient during a follow-up visit, "How did they treat you in [the laboratory/radiology department]? Did everything go all right?" Keep in mind that patients hold the referring provider partially accountable for everything that occurs during that experience. By getting feedback, you will know if your positive efforts are being supplemented or undermined by the referral process.

Explanation of Recommended Surgery

A recommendation for surgery may or may not come as a surprise to the patient. The manner in which the provider explains the proposed surgery will drive the PMRC grade of this important MOT and often determine whether the recommendation is followed. More importantly, this establishes the foundation for patients to give both an informed and an educated consent. An informed consent functions as a legal document containing certain minimum information.

- the risks and benefits of a proposed treatment or procedure
- alternatives to a proposed treatment or procedure
- the risks and benefits of the alternative treatments or procedures
- the risks and benefits of doing nothing ("watchful waiting")

An educated consent relates to the ability of the patient to arrive at a reasoned decision about whether to proceed with the recommended surgery. This is of even greater importance when the surgery is of an elective nature. In order for an educated consent to be given, the patient needs to know (in addition to informed consent information mentioned in Chapter 3) additional things in laymen's terminology:

- the anatomical context in which the surgery is to take place
- specifically how the patient's anatomy differs from the "normal" or optimum
- what the surgery will attempt to accomplish to restore near-normal or optimum status
- how the operative site structure(s) are likely to appear if the surgery goes as planned
- approximately where the incision(s) will be made
- the likelihood of recurrence of the preoperative state
- evidence suggesting that this surgical approach is the optimum one for his or her disorder
- whether this is to be performed under local, general, or other anesthetic
- where the surgery will be performed
- what the anticipated surgery and related fees are; what, if anything, needs to be paid "out-of-pocket"; and what is covered by a third-party payer, if applicable
- directions to the surgery facility (hospital, surgicenter, etc.)
- what should be brought or not brought with the patient to the surgery facility

- what other people they are likely to encounter (admitting clerk, surgical nurse, anesthetist, etc.) prior to seeing the surgeon on the day of surgery
- how much discomfort can be anticipated postoperatively and for about how long
- what provisions will be made to control the postoperative pain
- what type of dressings or cast will be applied when the surgery is completed
- when the first postoperative visit will be and how often the patient will be seen by the surgeon thereafter
- what can be anticipated during the postoperative visits (dressings removed, wound cleansed with antiseptic solution, sutures removed, topical antibiotic applied, fresh dressings applied, altered mobility restrictions, etc.)
- what mobility limitations can be expected immediately following surgery, and throughout the postoperative course
- if mobility assistance (crutches, walker, wheelchair, etc.) will be required, what information about their proper usage will be provided
- whether the patient will be able to drive immediately following the surgery; if not, within what time period during the postoperative course
- whether and how much time the patient will need to arrange to be off work
- about how long the postoperative disability will last; how long before normal basic activities of living (bathing, eating, grocery shopping, dressing yourself, etc.) and desired exercise (running, cycling, swimming, skiing, etc.) can be resumed (These should be presented in conservative and realistic time frames!)
- what measures will be taken to prevent the occurrence of possible complications
- specifically what the patient is expected to do or refrain from doing in order to facilitate the postoperative healing process (i.e., detailed postoperative instructions)
- in general terms, how possible complications would be managed if they did occur
- the circumstances under which the patient should contact the surgeon, and what signs, symptoms, or problems should prompt this
- specifically how the patient can contact the surgeon, if needed, between visits

- whether the patient is psychologically prepared for coping with the overall experience of undergoing surgery. Patients in a seriously depressed state or grieving should defer elective surgery until such time as this status changes.

Given this extent of information, the patient is in an ideal position to make an intelligent and informed decision about whether to proceed with the surgery. As is the case with other aspects of provider-patient interaction, the best approach is to establish realistic expectations in the mind of the patient. The objective should be to never have a patient be able to rationally think or say, "If I had known all this, I never would have had the surgery done."

Such statements elevate the stress level of providers and patients alike. A much more proactive approach consists of setting the stage for exceeding the patient's expectations—providing more provider caring, less discomfort than expected, faster healing than estimated, and so forth.

The above sections have provided the reader with a typical series of MOTs and SPs that combine to form the patient's grading on his or her mental report card. The cerebral videotapes of each MOT and the cerebral snapshots of each SP play over and over to influence perceived satisfaction continually. Granted, not all MOTs and SPs carry the same relative weight (as we saw in Chapter 4), but they each have some influence in driving your organization's grade on the PMRC.

IDENTIFYING THE MOTs AND SPs IN YOUR HEALTH CARE ORGANIZATION

Many aspects of a patient's overall health care experience are somewhat "generic" and universal from organization to organization. For example, patients will always be involved in calling the health care center for an appointment, spending time in the reception room, communicating with the staff and provider, and so forth. Of course, each of these activities must be examined in the context within which they occur in your organization. Other aspects may be much more specific or unique to your organization, such as a telephone advice system that is staffed by specially trained registered nurses from early morning until late at night.

All MOTs and/or SPs involved with each generic and each unique service offering need to be carefully identified. Appendix 5–A may be used as a guide while attempting to identify all component attributes of your PMRC. Using this as your foundation, it is best to involve all staff members, each contributing to the identification of MOTs and SPs that are within their normal work area. This can be efficiently accomplished by using a group brainstorming format, keeping in mind standard procedures:

- Clearly define MOTs and SPs so staff know exactly what they are supposed to be brainstorming about (with emphasis on all aspects of your organization).
- Allow think time prior to beginning group discussion.
- Get everyone involved via random contributions or "round robin."
- Post all ideas on a flipchart to validate each contribution.
- Refrain from judging the value/importance of each contribution.
- Place emphasis on the quantity of ideas.

When summarizing contributions from all staff members in the various departments, you may use the table in Figure 5–1 to organize the information.

DESIGNING POSITIVE MOT MANAGEMENT BLUEPRINTS

In order to design a comprehensive service strategy that accounts for all important-impact MOTs, both patients and employees must be in-

Moments of Truth	Surrogate Perceptions

Figure 5–1 Format for Patient's Mental Report Card Brainstorming Exercise.

volved. Albrecht recommends the development of a "moment of truth chart" for each important MOT in your organization (1992, p. 220). This should contain three columns (Figure 5–2). The central column should contain the customer's standard expectations for that MOT, the left column should list the negative factors that could happen or not happen to make the MOT fail expectations, and the right column should list the positive factors that would add value to the MOT in the eyes of the patient.

Wexler, Adams, and Bohn (1996) modified Carlzon's original concept of a MOT into three distinct kinds of "moments" reflecting the customer's perception of the interaction. When the experience is positive, they refer to a "moment of magic"; when it is negative, it is a "moment of misery." On the other hand, when the interaction is aligned with the customer's expectation, the result is a neutral "moment of truth." Although this semantic twist is creatively descriptive, the underlying meaning remains consistent with Carlzon's original concept.

An interaction between any representative of the organization and the customer is a MOT, which can be grossly mismanaged, adequately managed, or managed exceptionally well. The key is to identify each organization-to-patient personal interaction (a slight modification of

Negative Factors	Standard Expectations	Positive Factors

Figure 5–2 Moment of Truth Analysis Chart.

Carlzon's idea that we shall persist in terming a "moment of truth") and determine how expectations could be (and have been) failed, met, or exceeded. This requires input from those most intimately involved in the process—patients and employees.

Not only are patients highly qualified to provide input, but they are generally willing to do so to provide value to the health care organization. This input can be used to help you figure out what patients want and don't want, how they do and don't want health care delivered, and what elements of the health care experience could be changed, improved, or removed to serve them better. Employees are armed with an incredible amount of valuable information about patients and the characteristics of service that leave a lasting positive impression on them. They know, from firsthand experience, where the weak points are in the most carefully designed service delivery system. A variety of formats for getting input from both patients and employees will be explored in Chapter 6.

The next step is to create a process flowchart of each MOT as it is routinely experienced by patients currently. (See Chapter 10 for detailed guidelines for the creation of process flowcharts.) As you examine each MOT flowchart, identify where in the process your organization has failed patient expectations (based on patient complaint and grievance data, employee input, and informal patient input). Then look for the underlying causes of service breakdowns, with the objective of error-proofing the process by redesigning it. Next, reference your MOT chart to include feasible positive MOT management factors as part of the process redesign. Pilot test the new MOT management process for a period of time and monitor patient reaction (less complaints, improved satisfaction scores, etc.). If the improvement is reflected positively, then develop behavioral standards that incorporate the new process into all employee training, reward, and recognition programs.

DESIGNING POSITIVE SP MANAGEMENT PLANS

Recall that an SP is a patient's impression of your health care organization based on his or her observation of an inanimate object or condition either before, during, or after visiting your facility. The best way to appreciate the wide variety of SPs that contribute to your PMRC is by photographing each one. Begin with your print media promotion, external health care center signage, and facility; then follow the typical service cycle (see Appendix 5–A) through until the patient makes an appointment for the next visit. Each photograph should be taken as a representation through the eyes of the patient. For instance, seated in the reception room, take snapshots of various items within the gaze of a patient sitting in the same place. This is to be done strictly on a candid basis because advanced preparations would not accurately reflect what the patient typically observes.

Next, develop a list of conditions within your organization that create SPs on the mental report cards of your patients. This would include such items as temperature, odors, sounds, overall noise level, and so forth in various locations throughout a typical patient's sequential experience. Then, using the tables in Figures 5–3 and 5–4, combine the photographed SPs with the list of SP conditions to form an SP chart, including the positive and negative factors that influence the patients' perceptions.

Once again, it is important to get feedback from both employees and patients in order to accurately identify which factors would contribute negatively and positively to each SP. This process can also be used to gain an understanding of the relative importance of those factors that can be changed. Then, using a format similar to the table in Figure 5–5, develop a gap analysis that identifies the gaps between SPs as they currently exist and how they should ideally be (at least, the ones most important to patients).

Based on the identified gaps between what is and what should be, management can embark on a prioritized plan of action to allocate needed resources to continuously improve the SP component of the PMRC. This process will be discussed in greater detail in Chapter 11.

Negative Surrogate Perception Factors	Neutral Surrogate Perception Description	Positive Surrogate Perception Factors

Figure 5–3 Surrogate Perception Analysis Chart—Inanimate Objects.

Negative Surrogate Perception Factors	Condition Description	Positive Surrogate Perception Factors

Figure 5–4 Surrogate Perception Analysis Chart—Conditions.

Surrogate Perception Object or Condition	Current Surrogate Perception Projected	Current-to-Ideal Gap	Ideal Surrogate Perception Projected

Figure 5–5 Surrogate Perception Gap Analysis.

Similarly, a careful analysis of the overall impact of each MOT, based on feedback from patients using a variety of mechanisms (see Chapter 6), forms the basis for bringing about both behavior-based (see Chapter 9) and systems- and process-based (see Chapter 10) organizational improvements.

CONCLUSION

The PMRC is a model of how patients judge their health care experiences on an ongoing basis. The PMRC is made up of MOTs and SPs. A MOT, for our purposes, is an impression of the organization based on any interpersonal contact between any representative of the health care organization and the patient. In essence, patients retain a sort of "cerebral videotape" of each MOT they experience, weighing it on the basis of its contribution to your organization's failing, meeting, or exceeding their expectations. An SP is an impression of your health care organization based on the patient's observation of an inanimate object or condition. SPs are "recorded" in the PMRC as cerebral "snapshots." Each inanimate object may be linked to more than one SP by way of different attributes of that object. In this chapter, we took a detailed sequential look at a typical PMRC.

By combining all of a patient's impressions (MOTs + SPs) of your health care organization in sequential order, it becomes evident that the elements of satisfaction described in Chapter 3 and the service quality descriptors discussed in Chapter 2 are actually only component parts of the PMRC. By carefully itemizing and assessing (via gap analysis) the current quality of each MOT and SP in your health care organization, you can begin the process of positively managing each of them—with special emphasis on those your research demonstrates to be of high priority. Everyone throughout your organization, whatever its size, should "internalize" this model so they can fully appreciate how patients arrive at the PMRC "grades" that surface as satisfaction/dissatisfaction ratings and loyalty/disloyalty behaviors.

ACTION STEPS

1. Design a means of introducing and simply explaining the PMRC (i.e., MOTs and SPs need to be clearly distinguished) to everyone in your organization so they "internalize" and remember it.
2. Using Appendix 5–A as a guide, organize one or more groups to brainstorm a list (using the format in Figure 5–1) of the specific MOTs and SPs that patients experience when interacting with your health care organization.
3. Representatives of all who have regular direct patient contact should work in groups from various "patient experience areas" (i.e., different departments, facilities, reception, back office, etc.) to brainstorm the specific MOTs and SPs that patients are likely to be using in their area to form your organization's "grade" on their mental report cards.
4. Develop a PMRC that uniquely represents the way patients experience your health care organization.

REFERENCES

Albrecht, K. (1989). *At America's service*. Homewood, IL: Dow Jones-Irwin.

Albrecht, K. (1992). *The only thing that matters*. New York: Harper Business.

American Medical Association. (1990). *Risk management principles & commentaries for the medical office*. Chicago: Author.

Baum, N., & Henkel, G. (1992). *Marketing your clinical practice*. Gaithersburg, MD: Aspen.

Carnegie, D. (1989). *How to win friends and influence people*. New York: Simon & Schuster.

Cialdini, R.B. (1988). *Influence: Science and practice*. New York: Harper Collins.

Funnel. (1991). Empowerment: An idea whose time has come in diabetes education. *Diabetes Education*.

Johns Hopkins University. (1997, January). How doctors and patients view communication styles. *Journal of the American Medical Association*.

Leebov, W., Vergare, M., & Scott, G. (1990). *Patient satisfaction: A guide to practice enhancement*. Oradell, NJ: Medical Economics Books.

Merriam-Webster's Collegiate Dictionary (10th ed.). (1993). Springfield, MA: Merriam-Webster.

Mowen, J.C., Licata, J.W., & McPhail, J. (1993). Waiting in the emergency room: How to improve patient satisfaction. *Journal of Health Care Marketing, 13*(2), 26(8).

Naisbitt, J. (1982). *Megatrends: Ten new directions transforming our lives*. New York: Warner Books.

Nelson, A.M., Wood, S.D., Brown, S.W., & Bronkesh, S.Z. (1997). *Improving patient satisfaction now: How to earn patient and payer loyalty*. Gaithersburg, MD: Aspen.

Shelton, P.J. (1992a, December). The patient's mental report card—Part 2. *Podiatry Today, V*(7), 19–22.

Shelton, P.J. (1992b, November). Surrogate perceptions. *Podiatry Today, V*(6), 73–75.

Shelton, P.J. (1993, January). The patient's mental report card—Part 3. *Podiatry Today, V*(8), 19–20, 72.

Wexler, P.S., Adams, W.A., & Bohn, E. (1996). *The quest for quality: Prescriptions for achieving service excellence*. New York: St. Martin's Griffin.

Zaslove, M.O. (1998). *The successful physician: A productivity handbook for practitioners*. Gaithersburg, MD: Aspen.

SUGGESTED READING

Albrecht, K., & Bradford, L.J. (1990). *The service advantage: How to identify and fulfill customer needs*. Homewood, IL: Dow Jones-Irwin.

Albrecht, K., & Zemke, R. (1985). *Service America! Doing business in the new economy*. Homewood, IL: Dow Jones-Irwin.

American Health Consultants. (1997, February). Doctors, not report cards, shape consumer choices. *Patient Satisfaction & Outcomes Management, 3*(2), 13–20.

American Health Consultants. (1998, January). Can you give your patients the ideal visit? *Patient Satisfaction & Outcomes Management, 4*(1), 1–9.

Anderson, K., & Zemke, R. (1991). *Delivering knock your socks off service.* New York: AMACOM.

Baggott, R. (1998). *Health and health care in Britain* (2nd ed.). London: MacMillan.

Conomikes, G.S. (Ed.). (1998). *Successful practice management techniques: 329 ideas from Conomikes Reports.* Los Angeles: Conomikes Reports.

Disend, J.E. (1991). *How to provide excellent service in any organization: A blueprint for making all the theories work.* Radnor, PA: Chilton Book.

LeBoeuf, M. (1987). *How to win customers and keep them for life.* New York: Berkley Books.

Mayer, G.G., Barnett, A., & Brown, N. (1997). *Making capitation work: Clinical operations in an integrated delivery system.* Gaithersburg, MD: Aspen.

Murphy, K.J. (1992). *Effective listening: How to profit by tuning into the ideas and suggestions of others.* Salem, NH: ELI Press.

Schaaf, D. (1995). *Keeping the edge: Giving customers the service they demand.* New York: Penguin Books USA.

Shelton, P.J. (1993). *Managed care participation guide: A workbook designed to help podiatric physicians successfully navigate the managed care environment.* Anaheim Hills, CA: Innovative Management Systems.

Strawberry Communications. (1987). *Let's make friends & not lose customers: A workbook on telephone etiquette for better customer relations.* Carrollton, TX: The Zig Ziglar Corp.

Whiteley, R., & Hessan, D. (1996). *Customercentered growth: Five proven strategies for building competitive advantage.* Menlo Park, CA: Addison-Wesley.

Zeithaml, V.A., & Bitner, M.J. (1996). *Services marketing.* London: McGraw-Hill.

Zeithaml, V.A., Parasuraman, A., & Berry, L.L. (1990). *Delivering quality service: Balancing customer perceptions and expectations.* New York: The Free Press.

Zemke, R., & Schaaf, D. (1989). *The service edge: 101 companies that profit from customer care.* New York: NAL Books.

The Patient's Mental Report Card

PMRC	Category	Description	Specific Attribute
SPs	Communication	Print media promotion	Professional design/layout
			Claims substantiated
			Benefit-oriented
MOTs	Communication	Patient calls HCC on telephone	Answered promptly
		(normal business hours;	Answered appropriately
		general impression)	Speak w/ "live" person
			Clear & understandable
			Pleasant voice tone
			Staff seem unrushed
			Ask before place on "hold"
			Minimum "on-hold" time
			Music/info. while "on-hold"
			Efficient call transfer
MOTs	Access	Patient calls HCC on telephone	Staff helpfulness
		(purpose: to make an appointment)	Resp. to expressed urgency
			Multiple day/time offers
			How soon appt. available
			Preferred date available
			Preferred time available
			Preferred provider available
			Minimum time required
		Patient informed of HCC location	Convenient to home
			Convenient to work
	Convenience	Patient informed of HCC hours	Convenient provider hours
			Convenient staff hours
			Early morning hours offered

PMRC	Category	Description	Specific Attribute
			Evening hours available
			Weekend hours available
MOTs	Access	Patient calls HCC on telephone	Speak w/ "live" person
		(nonbusiness hours;	Able to contact provider
		non-emergency)	Getting telephone advice
MOTs	Access	Patient calls HCC on telephone	Responsive to caller needs
		(nonbusiness hours; emergency)	Arranges for getting care
			Arranges for transporting
MOTs	Convenience	Patient travels to HCC	Clear directions provided
			Main thoroughfare access
			Public transportation access
SPs	Communication	Patient views HCC exterior signage	Easily visible from street
			Appearance of signage
MOTs	Convenience	Patient parks vehicle for HCC visit	Parking provided at N/C
			Ease of finding space
			Closeness to HCC entrance
MOTs	Personal caring		"Disabled" spaces available
			Lighted during evening hours
			Security personnel on site
SPs	HCC facility	Patient views HCC facility	Appearance—decor
		from exterior	Appearance—cleanliness
			Appearance—maintenance
SP	HCC facility	Patient views receptionist's	Openness (vs. small/
		"window"	frosted)
MOTs	Personal caring	Greeting of patient by receptionist	Patient soon acknowledged
			Patient greeted by name
			Receptionist's tone cheerful
SPs	HCC facility	Patient views receptionist's	Well-organized
		work area	Cleanliness of area
			Modern equipment
SPs	HCC facility	Patient views reception room	Decor—nicely decorated
			Color-coordinated
			Neatness of room
			Cleanliness of room
SPs	HCC facility	Patient sits down	Enough seating available
			Comfort of seating
			Cleanliness of seating
			Condition of seating

PMRC	Category	Description	Specific Attribute
SP	General	Patient notices temperature in reception room	Comfortable level maintained
MOT	Communication	Patient asked to complete information forms	Requested courteously
SPs	Communication	Patient views information forms provided	Print quality
			Print size (12–14 point)
			Neatly organized
			Logically arranged
			Easy to read
			Easy to understand
SPs	Personal caring	Patient looks over reading materials in reception room	Accessible
			Up-to-date
			Appropriate
			Sufficient variety
			Health-related
MOTs	Access	Patient waiting time in reception room	Apology made
			Patient informed of wait
			Explanation(s) provided
			Delay changes updated
			Total waiting time minimal
MOT	Personal caring	Patient's name is called by nurse/ medical assistant	Staff smiles, greeting patient
			Name pronounced correctly
			Name enunciated clearly
	Personal caring	Nurse/medical assistant speaks with patient	Friendly
			Treated as welcome visitor
			Staff—pleasant tone of voice
			Staff—listens attentively
			Respectful to patient
			Personal concern evident
SPs	General	Patient views b/o staff appearance	Professional/uniformed
			Clothing clean & neat
			Grooming clean & neat
			Minimal jewelry worn by staff
	HCC facility	Patient views carpeting	Spotlessly clean
			In good condition

PMRC	Category	Description	Specific Attribute
		Patient views photographs, paintings, etc. on wall	Appropriateness
			Oriented to patient population
SPs	General	Patient hears noise level throughout office	Quiet (acceptable noises only)
SPs	HCC facility	Patient views treatment room	Cleanliness of everything
			No signs of previous pt.
	Quality	Patient views equipment	Modern, "state-of-the-art"
			Cleanliness of equipment
			Mechanical operation
MOTs	Access	Patient waits to be seen in treatment room	Patient informed of wait
			Explanation(s) provided
			Waiting for nurse to enter
			Waiting for tx "set-up"
			Total waiting time minimal
MOT	Communication	Patient speaks with staff nurse/assistant	Friendly staff
			Knowledgable staff
			Staff prepares pt for visit
SP	General	Patient notices air quality in treatment room	Fresh, no "clinical odors"
SP	General	Patient observes appearance of provider	Professional appearance
			Clothing clean & neat
			Grooming clean & neat
MOTs	Personal caring	Patient greeted by provider	Greets patient by name
			Smiles when greeting patient
			Makes patient feel welcome
	Communication	Patient observes provider working w/staff	Communication
			Teamwork
MOTs	Communication	Patient observes provider willingness to listen	Eye contact maintained
			Provider clarifies understanding
			Provider appears unrushed
		Patient experiences rapport-building	Relationship dimension emphasized
			Conversation focused on patient
			Cultural sensitivity
			Provider professional attitude

PMRC	Category	Description	Specific Attribute
			Pleasant tone of voice
			Timely return of calls
MOTs	Quality	Provider obtains history of	Detailed history taken
		main complaint	Considers overall health
MOTs	Personal caring	Patient views provider's	Empathy demonstrated to
		personal concern	patient
			Caring attitude displayed
			Exhibits interest in problem
	Communication	Nursing staff communicates	No need to "repeat story"
		with provider	
MOTs	Personal caring	Patient observes provider's	Minimize patient discomfort
		humanistic side	Sensitive to patient pain
			Patient confidentiality respected
MOTs	Quality	Patient notes thoroughness of	Sufficient time spent with
		examination	patient
			Provider focuses on problem
MOTs	Quality	Provider recommends diagnostic	Rationale explained to
		testing/x-rays	patient
			Results impact on treatment
	Personal caring		What to expect during test
	Communication		Logistics of getting test done
	Quality		Prompt results available
	Convenience		Convenient lab location
			Convenient lab hours
	Access		Minimum waiting in lab
		Provider explains diagnosed	Understandable
		problem to patient	terminology
			Visual aids used
			Patient's questions answered
			Adequate time spent
			Written information given
			References for education
MOTs	Quality	Provider explains treatment options	Consequences—no treatment
			Conservative option offered

PMRC	Category	Description	Specific Attribute
	Communication		Understandable terminology
			Treatment success likelihood
			Supp. treatment measures
			Adequate time to explain
			Patient's questions answered
	Personal caring		Empathy re: treatment concern
MOTs	Quality	Process of patient receiving treatment	Immediate treatment
			Provider's hands washed
			Explained during process
			Sensitive to patient pain
			Dressings carefully placed
SPs	Quality	Process of patient receiving treatment	Dressings neatly applied
			Referral given if needed
MOTs	Quality	Provider gives patient prescription for drug(s)	Rationale explained to patient
	Communication		Understandable terminology
	Quality		Proper use of medication
			Possible side effects
			Possible adverse reactions
			Problem of not taking drug
			Problem—incorrect drug use
	Communication		Cost to patient, if applicable
			Patient questions answered
			Written instructions provided
	Convenience	Patient getting prescribed medication	Conven. pharmacy location
			Conven. pharmacy hours
			Rx filled quickly
MOTs	Communication	Patient gives educated consent for surgery	Anatomical context explained
			Likely outcome of surgery
			Explained risks of surgery
			Likely outcome if no surgery

PMRC	Category	Description	Specific Attribute
			Alternative procedures
			Anesthesia (L/G/R) to be used
			Where surgery to be done
			Possible out-of-pocket costs
			What to bring to surgery
			Directions to surgery location
			What people they'll encounter
			Accurate discomfort estimate
			Accurate disability estimate
MOT	Quality	Outcome or result following treatment	Obtained desired result
			Printed post-tx instructions
			Any complication(s) explained
			Complication managed well
MOTs	Access	Patient schedules follow-up appt. w/ receptionist	Conven. scheduler location
			Min. wait to see scheduler
			Multiple day/time offers
			How soon appt. available
			Preferred date available
			Preferred time available
			Preferred provider available
			Written appt. received
			Minimum time required
			Informed what will be done
	Personal caring	Patient sees receptionist's friendliness	Greets patient by name
			Smiles when greeting patient
			Treats patient as guest
		Patient sees receptionist's courtesy	Pleasant tone of voice
			Professional attitude
			Listens attentively
		Patient feels respected by receptionist	Privacy & confidentiality respected
			Tactful handling of financial issues
			Cultural sensitivity

PMRC	Category	Description	Specific Attribute
		Receptionist personally concerned	Empathy demonstrated to patient
			Caring attitude displayed
			Exhibit true interest in patient
		Patient informed of laboratory results	Prompt results available
			Patient privacy respected
			Compassionate communication
	Convenience	Reminders for upcoming scheduled visit	Telephone reminder
			Written reminder
		Preventive care acquisition	Telephone reminder
			Written reminder
			Printed educational materials
			Available education references

CHAPTER 6

Measuring Patient Satisfaction: Determining an Organization's Grades on the Patient's Mental Report Card

Now that you are equipped with an understanding of the moments of truth (MOTs) and surrogate perceptions (SPs) that drive the grades your organization receives on the patient's mental report card (PMRC), the next logical step is to find out what those grades currently are. Seeking and responding to patient feedback regarding their perceptions of service quality are two of the most essential nonclinical endeavors a health care organization can undertake in the new millennium and beyond. Osborne and Gaebler (1994) identified three important principles that underscore the importance of measuring organizational performance.

1. If you can't see success, you can't reward it.
2. If you can't reward success, you are probably rewarding failure.
3. If you can't recognize failure, you can't correct it. (p. 15)

By measuring patients' degree of satisfaction with the way all MOTs and SPs are currently being managed, you can determine your organization's current grades on those (PMRC). This, then, forms the foundation for you to identify specific action(s) needed to increase patient satisfaction and loyalty. In this chapter, an overview of various mechanisms for obtaining patient satisfaction feedback will be presented. Then, practical survey and focus group research methodologies will be discussed in detail, with "mini case studies" of how these have been applied in both small and large health care settings.

OVERVIEW OF MECHANISMS FOR MEASURING PATIENT SATISFACTION

There are a variety of methods that can be used to directly or indirectly measure patient perceptions of satisfaction with your organization. By combining more than one source, you will develop a better overall understanding of how patients are thinking and feeling about their experiences in your facility. The following is a brief list of methods commonly used:

- *Postappointment telephone survey:* This survey should be conducted within 2–3 days of the patient's most recent visit to your health care center. Although anonymity is sacrificed, the response rate is high (which eliminates nonresponse bias), information is gathered rapidly, and an opportunity to solicit open-ended responses is provided. It is best to open the telephone conversation with a scripted introductory dialogue that should include an introduction of the calling staff member as well as identification of your organization. This prevents a premature "solicitation phone call response" hang-up. Then, make sure this is not a "bad time to call" and generically inquire about the patient's progress. Capture whatever comments are made and move on. Once a cooperative spirit is detected with the patient, explain the "other reason for calling"—to ask them about their most recent visit: (1) "What did you like about your most recent visit to our health care center?"; (2) "Did anything concern or bother you about your most recent visit?" and (3) "What can we do to provide better service to you?"

  Upon completion of the telephone call, thank the patient profusely for his or her cooperation and document the responses on a prepared telephone survey response form. Telephone survey response rates can exceed 85%, whereas typical response rates for mail questionnaires are in the 20% to 30% range.

- *Open-ended questionnaire:* This type of questionnaire is a valuable source of qualitative information. It may be distributed to current patients who have visited your facility two or more times in the recent (6 months) past. This ensures that their responses are based on multiple experiences rather than a single visit. The questions asked may be the same as those listed above for the postappointment telephone survey. The most candid answers will be obtained when the respondent's anonymity is preserved. This can be accomplished by giving the patient a postage-paid envelope in which to mail back the completed survey. Again, it is best if this envelope is addressed to an "outside party" rather than to the address of your health care facility.

- *Objective survey questionnaire:* This type of questionnaire is considered by many to be the best instrument for obtaining quantifiable response data. The most meaningful and valid data will be collected when respondent anonymity is preserved and responses are sent to an outside market research or consulting firm. Patients may fear some form of retribution if they believe the provider will know how they responded, especially if low ratings or critical responses are given. This process will be explored in depth later in this chapter.
- *Lay advisory panel:* This method is better suited for smaller organizations. It consists of four or five patients who are relatively articulate and representative of the demographics of your organization's patient population. You may wish to schedule regular (quarterly) meetings for their advice regarding current service quality and needed improvements. Hold the meetings in a location away from your facility, perhaps in a small private area of a restaurant. Each panel member should be compensated for his or her time with dinner and an appropriate gift. Also, panel members should be rotated periodically so as to gain new perspectives.
- *Patient focus group:* This consists of a group of patients who are representative of your organization's patient population being led through a focused discussion that is structured to evoke suggestions and perceptions from them. This is a well-respected and proven qualitative market research technique. With certain modifications (see later this chapter), a quantitative component can be introduced that, when aligned with your research objective, can enhance the value of the focus group process outcome.

  Another useful application of focus groups is to solicit patient reactions to new plans and ideas your organization has for change. This affords the opportunity to refine the plan on a proactive basis before it is implemented, obviating the need for later "knee-jerk" reacting to patient complaints. When several people interact in a focused discussion, there is a synergy that develops whereby the participants piggyback on one another's views and creative ideas.
- *Computer-based patient input:* It is becoming more and more common for health care and other organizations to have internet web sites available for patients/customers to voice their concerns re-

lated to satisfaction issues; alternatively, the use of dedicated computer kiosks/terminals within the organization is another potential method of obtaining patient information.

- *Complaint analysis:* One of the oldest forms of consumer satisfaction measurement involves various efforts to record, categorize, analyze/track, act on, and solicit customer complaints. When a trend of complaints is recorded and related to an area that patients consider to be of high relative importance, elimination of the underlying cause of dissatisfaction becomes an improvement priority. Because most unhappy customers don't complain, but just leave, an assertive program of patient complaint management is in order. As a patient satisfaction measurement tool, complaint analysis has severe limitations regarding the representativeness of the problems reported and the patients who complain. Nevertheless, it provides a supplemental source of dissatisfaction tracking.

THE SATISFACTION SURVEY RESEARCH PROCESS

The term *survey* is derived from the Latin *super,* meaning "above," "over," or "beyond"; the element *-vey* comes from the Latin verb *videre,* meaning, "to look" or "to see." Thus, the word means "to look or to see over or beyond" the casual glance or superficial observation. This observation, although not restricted to perception through the physical eye, is always accompanied by some record, or preservation of fact. The physician "looks" at the patient's heart using a stethoscope and records findings in the medical record; this "observation" can then be enhanced (and recorded) by means of an electrocardiogram.

A survey is the most commonly used method of gathering quantitative patient satisfaction data. These data are considered descriptive because they come to the researcher through observation, as compared with historical data, which come to the researcher through written records. Because of the complexity of a survey research project and the importance of gathering quality data, considerable attention will be devoted to this process. It is essential to approach the design and administration of surveys in a structured way so as to avoid errors, wasted time, and poor quality responses.

Your organization may not have the time or internal resources to "build your own" survey instrument. Rather, you may prefer to purchase an "off-the-shelf" version or have a consultant develop one. This is clearly the better choice for solo or group practices, as well as for many smaller health care organizations. In either case, the more you know about the overall development, sampling, administration, and data collection processes, the better equipped you will be to make educated choices along the way. After all, what you really want "at the end of the day" is reliable, valid, and credible data on which to base your improvement efforts.

A systematic approach to patient satisfaction survey research should generally occur in the following sequential fashion:

- Establish your survey project objectives—what you want to learn.
- Determine your sample—who you will ask to get the information you want.
- Select your specific survey methodology—how you will ask for the information.
- Design your survey questionnaire—what you will ask to get the information you want.
- Pilot test or pretest the survey questionnaire.
- Translate the questionnaire into one or more foreign languages.
- Develop response incentives or inducements.
- Administer the survey—ask the questions.
- Enter and tabulate the data.
- Analyze the data.
- Communicate the data throughout the organization (see Chapter 7).

Establishing Survey Project Objectives

Before any form of research can be undertaken, the scope and objectives must be clearly defined. All too often, research surveys are conducted with insufficient clarification of their objectives, resulting in findings that are too vague, too narrow, or entirely inappropriate. The investigator must have a clear understanding as to what information is needed and how each item will be analyzed. The analysis must be determined in the planning stage, not after the data have been gathered. Will responses merely be described by listing the percentages of subjects who responded in certain ways, or will the responses of one group be compared with those of another?

Two questions should be answered to help arrive at your specific research objectives.

1. What is the problem? This question is best asked as specifically as possible. For example: "We currently have no standardized mechanism for measuring perceived service quality for patients" or "We don't really know what our patients consider to be our

service strengths and weaknesses" or "Our patient disenrollment numbers are up (or new/reenrollment numbers are down); we don't know whether patient dissatisfaction or other market forces are behind this decline."

2. What data are needed to find a solution? The first step would be to review any existing information. For example, is any segment (age group, gender, clinical diagnostic category) of your patient population more represented in the recent decline? Next, generate a list of necessary information. This could include such items as the following:

   - area(s) of their health care experiences (with us) that patients are most satisfied or dissatisfied with
   - a comparison of patient satisfaction levels between various departments or facilities
   - any relationship between age or gender and the current level of satisfaction with our services
   - whether some employees or providers are contributing more to patient satisfaction/dissatisfaction than others
   - whether recent organizational changes have increased or decreased patient satisfaction (assuming previous satisfaction data are available for comparison)
   - what important elements of patient satisfaction we should target our improvement efforts toward

The outcome of this procedure should be a clear and concise written statement of the objective(s) of the proposed research survey and its scope. For example, at Friendly Hills HealthCare Network, our 1996 patient satisfaction survey research objectives included the following:

- to develop and administer a means of measuring current patient satisfaction that is network-wide, regional-, health care center-, department- and provider-specific
- to include the elements of patient satisfaction identified in our initial research [see Chapter 3] in the survey instrument and...
- to obtain a minimum response rate of 25 percent at each of the 41 health care centers participating in the survey

In addition to this, it is important to spell out any constraints at this early stage because they are likely to materially affect the nature of the research that can be undertaken. Of course, the two most important constraints are typically time and money. Is your organization prepared to commit the needed resources to support the many tasks involved in conducting comprehensive patient satisfaction survey research? Or more importantly, does senior management consider the findings of this research a high enough priority to respond to identified weaknesses with whatever it takes to bring about measurable improvement? It should be kept in mind that it is worse to ask patients their opinions and attitudes with no intention of changing anything than it is to never ask them in the first place.

Determining Your Sample—Who You Will Ask

Most researchers who use questionnaires have in mind a specific population to be sampled. Of course, the subjects selected must be the ones who have the answers to the questions. This is referred to as the *target population*. Proper selection is important because a poorly defined target population will result in unrepresentative results. The results of a survey are no more trustworthy than the quality of the population or the representativeness of the sample. Your sampling procedure could be likened to looking through the wrong end of a telescope, wherein you see the world in miniature. This is what should be achieved with a well-planned survey sample. According to Leedy (1993), "The sample should be so carefully chosen that through it the researcher is able to see all the characteristics of the total population in the same relationship that they would be seen were the researcher in fact to inspect the total population" (p. 199).

It may seem intuitively obvious that a patient satisfaction survey will be targeted toward patients being served by your organization. A closer look, however, asks "Which patients will actually be called on to participate in the survey research?" To determine this, we need to consider the two basic types of sampling: probability and nonprobability. The subject of sampling is described in detail by Phipps and Simmons (1998). The following discussion is derived from excerpts of that work (pp. 92–93):

- *probability (or random) samples:* where individual patients are drawn in some random fashion from among the population of all of your organization's patients
- *nonprobability (or nonrandom) samples:* where patients are selected on the basis of one or more criteria determined by the researcher

There are four probability sampling methods that may be employed in patient satisfaction research.

1. *Simple random sampling:* In this type of sampling, individuals are drawn randomly from the population at large. In order to accomplish this, it is necessary to construct a sampling frame, which consists of a list of all the known patients within the population from which the selection is to take place. Then, each patient is assigned a unique number (often this is already done by the database containing enrollment information—each patient is automatically assigned a number). Finally, specific patients are selected using a random number table or the computer equivalent, a random number generator.

2. *Systematic sampling:* In this type of sampling, patients are sampled at intervals based on a random start point. For instance, it might be decided to survey every twentieth patient on the total patient list starting at number 8. Thus, the patients that would be sampled are numbers 8, 28, 48, 68, and so forth.

3. *Stratified random sampling:* In this type of sampling, the patient population is first divided into groups based on one or more criteria (e.g., age, gender, primary health care facility or provider) and, from within these groups, individual patients are randomly selected. In order for this method to be used, the data available on each patient must contain information about the criteria to be used to stratify the groups.

4. *Multistage sampling:* In this type of sampling, the patient population is divided into quite large groups, usually based on geography. Then, a random selection of patients from each of these large groups is made and the resulting list is subdivided again. A random selection of groups is again made from the resulting subdivisions and the process is repeated as many times as required by the survey. Eventually, patients are sampled randomly from the small groups arising as a result of the final subdivision.

As a result of either the inability to establish a sampling frame or simply time and/or financial constraints, it may be necessary to consider using a nonprobability sampling method. There are four basic nonprobability approaches.

1. *Judgment sampling:* In this type of sampling, the researcher selects the patients that he or she feels are representative of the population or have a particular expertise or knowledge that makes them suitable. This type of sampling is commonly used with small sample sizes.

2. *Convenience sampling:* In this type of sampling, the most convenient group of patients is selected. This group may be the patients

who happen to be scheduled for clinical visits during specified convenient calendar dates. This approach is often used to save time and financial resources.

3. *Cluster sampling:* In this type of sampling, the patient population is divided repeatedly into groups rather like the process for multistage random sampling. However, cluster sampling differs in that all patients from the remaining small groups are surveyed, rather than just a random sample of those remaining.

4. *Quota sampling:* In this type of sampling, the researcher selects a predetermined number of patients from different groups (i.e., based on age, gender, clinical condition, etc.). This is the most popular nonprobability sampling method used. For example, if you know that your current patient population demographics include 38% male patients and 62% female patients, a gender quota reflecting this could be chosen. Additionally, you may wish to impose other quota criteria, such as that 90% of the patients you survey have been treated by your organization within the past 6 months.

Table 6–1 provides a comparison of the various sampling methods on the basis of sampling frame requirement, cost, representativeness, and likelihood of bias.

Determining Sample Size—How Many You Will Ask

The next important consideration in determining your patient population sample is *sample size*. The number of completed survey questionnaires required to produce a statistically valid sample is based on three main factors.

1. *Variability in the population:* This factor refers to the proportionate distribution of the characteristics one is interested in. When the proportion is either small or very large, the size of the sample required in order to measure this accurately is smaller than when the population is more or less equally split between having and not having the attributes under consideration. In other words, the more respondents are likely to differ on the key items of the survey, the larger the sample must be in order to reach a given level of confidence.

2. *Required level of confidence:* This factor refers to the level of confidence one can have that the results achieved by the sample are likely to provide a true indication of results in the underlying population. Common sense, and a statistical formula, indicate

Table 6–1 Comparison of Sampling Methods

Sampling Method	Sampling Frame	Cost	Representativeness	Likelihood of Bias
Simple random	required	high	may not be representative	low
Systematic random	required	moderate	may not be representative	low
Stratified sampling	required	moderate	representative	low
Multistage sampling	required	moderate	may not be representative	low
Judgment sampling	not required	low	may not be representative	high
Convenience sampling	not required	low	may not be representative	high
Cluster sampling	not required	moderate	may not be representative	moderate
Quota sampling	not required	moderate	representative	moderate

Source: Adapted with permission from R. Phipps and C. Simmons, *Understanding Customers 1998–99*, p. 92–94, 99, and 109, © 1998, Butterworth-Heinemann.

that the higher the level of confidence required in the results, the larger the size of sample necessary. A more careful look from a statistical standpoint shows that to increase the level of confidence from the 68% level (a one-in-three risk of the sample not being representative of the population) to the 95% level more commonly used (only one-in-20 risk that the sample is not a good one), it is necessary to multiply the sample size by a factor of four. If a survey of 100 patients indicated that 28% of the patient population rated "overall satisfaction" as "excellent" at a 68% level of confidence, to increase the level of confidence in the results to the 95% level, a survey of 400 respondents would be required.

3. *Required limits of accuracy:* Intuitively, the larger the sample size, the more accurate the results are likely to be as a predictor of population values. The statistical formula of sampling theory makes it possible to quantify this relationship. The relationship is inverse and square. In other words, to double the accuracy in the

results (i.e., to halve the allowable range in the limits of accuracy), it would be necessary to multiply the size of the sample by four. Continuing the example above, if the sample of 400 patients indicated that at the 95% confidence, 28% of the patient population rated "overall satisfaction" as "excellent" within limits of accuracy of 10%, this would indicate that between 25.2% and 30.8% of the patient population would rate overall satisfaction as excellent. For greater precision, the limits of accuracy must be reduced. To halve this to ±5% (i.e., between 26.6% and 29.4%), a sample size of 1,600 patients would be required.

As illustrated above, a number of factors are relevant to determining sample size. However, from a very practical standpoint, several "rule-of-thumb" guidelines may be helpful.

- In general, for acceptable statistical validity of results generated from quantitative surveys, any subgroup containing less than 100 respondents should be treated with extreme caution in statistical analysis.
- Respondent numbers less than 50 should not be subjected to statistical analysis at all.
- Minimum sample sizes for quantitative consumer surveys are of the order of 300–500 respondents.
- The maximum practical size of a sample is approximately 1,000 respondents; contrary to popular belief, this has nothing to do with the size of the population, provided that it is many times greater than the sample.

These guidelines have been derived from sampling theory, which forms the basis for random sampling. In the case of quota sampling or other nonprobability sampling methods, it is usual to increase the size of the sample in order to compensate for any inaccuracies that may have been introduced by the sampling procedure. Finally, it should be mentioned that the only time the size of the underlying population needs be taken into account in considering the size of the sample required is when the size of the sample required (i.e., for the desired accuracy and confidence levels) is likely to account for 10% or more of the population.

Avoiding Bias in Your Research

The next sampling concern relates to the avoidance of bias. In this context, a *bias* occurs when a sample of the overall patient population is not truly representative of that wider population. More specifically, bias is any condition or influence that distorts the data from what may have been obtained under conditions of pure chance. In addition to this, bias could be in the form of anything disturbing the randomness by which the choice of a sample population has been selected. There are three main sources of bias.

1. *Incomplete coverage:* This may occur if the sampling frame is incomplete (i.e., not every member of a population is included in a sample), certain outlying areas are excluded, or the survey method used limits those that can be sampled (i.e., a telephone survey requires that the respondent own a telephone).
2. *Nonresponse bias:* Low response rate is a challenge for any survey research project.
3. *Overrepresentation:* Deliberate overrepresentation of certain groups is inherent to the nonprobability sampling methods. For example, if the sample consists of existing long-term patients, their loyalty to your organization may bias the data in that more favorable responses may be given; former patients, who have defected from your organization due to dislike of your service, may bias the data in the direction of less favorable results.

Additionally, there are two potential sources of response error.

1. *Respondent errors* arise when respondents give inaccurate information because of misunderstandings or loss of interest when participating in lengthy surveys.
2. *Questionnaire errors* occur when the wording and order of questions affect the accuracy of the results.

The following checklist for avoiding sample selection bias was adapted from *The Survey Research Handbook,* written by Alreck and Settle (1985, p. 77).

- Are some patients in the population more visible than others? If so, be sure the more visible patients are selected in the same proportion as the more obscure ones.
- Are the patients in the sample frame presented in systematic order? If so, the sequence must not alter the probability of selection of some patients over others.
- Are some respondents more accessible than others? When they are, controls and incentives must be used to obtain equal proportions of those with high and low accessibility.

- Are sample patients clustered, either deliberately or accidentally? When clusters exist, there must be no more interaction or similarity within clusters than between clusters.
- Will your survey administrators have more affinity for some respondent patients than others? If so, incentives and controls must be used to avoid overselecting those with greater affinity.
- Is there an opportunity for respondents to select themselves or decline? If so, the opportunity should be reduced or concealed from potential respondents.
- Will there be a high proportion of nonrespondents? If so, there should be as little interaction as possible between nonresponse and the issue being surveyed.
- Are some types of respondents both more or less likely to respond and likely to respond in a certain way? If so, the nonresponse bias must be reduced or controlled.

Totally excluding all sources of bias is extremely difficult but worth trying for whenever feasible. By being aware of potential bias, you can make an effort to avoid the more obvious sources and interpret your results cautiously. Furthermore, the researcher should always acknowledge the possibility of biased data and recognize the likelihood of bias in the survey project. Forming conclusions about the data without acknowledging the effect that bias may have had in distorting them is naive.

In a patient satisfaction survey research project undertaken at Friendly Hills HealthCare Network in 1996, we used a convenience form of nonprobability sampling. The patients visiting each of the 41 health care centers on specified, randomly selected days within a 6-week time frame were asked by trained survey administrators to complete a satisfaction survey questionnaire (Appendix B). Fortunately, 3,123 patients completed surveys, so that the sample size somewhat compensated for the inherent statistical concerns associated with nonprobability sampling.

Selecting Your Specific Survey Methodology—How You Will Ask

Earlier in this chapter, we discussed a variety of methods available for soliciting and obtaining satisfaction feedback from patients. Once you have decided that an objective survey questionnaire will be used, the next decision is whether to use the mail or some form of interview to obtain responses. The mail survey is self-administered so that the preparation and mailing of the survey must receive very careful attention. Interview surveys, on the other hand, are ordinarily administered entirely by the field or telephone worker. Therefore, with an interview survey, the questionnaire plays an important role, but it is not the key element. Because there are significant differences in the two methods, several key points pertaining to each approach will be examined.

When using a mailing piece for data collection, the cosmetic aspects are critical because this is the only contact that respondents will have with you as the researcher and your research project. The appearance and quality of the mailing piece and its contents have a very important effect on mail survey response rates. It is best to plan and create a mailing piece (and all associated printed materials—envelope, cover letter, return envelope) of the highest possible quality permitted by your budget. If some components are done very well and others are done cheaply, the overall image of the project will diminish considerably—effectively offsetting any advantages of the higher quality components.

The survey questionnaire should be mailed in a standard business envelope. The back of the envelope should be blank, with the front containing only the return address, potential respondent address, and postage. The return address should be printed on the envelope versus affixing a return address label. Also, in most cases, the return address printed on the mailing envelope should be the same as that appearing on the return envelope. The exception to this would be in the circumstance in which your health care organization's stationery is being used to mail the surveys out, but they will be returned to an independent outside researcher for analysis; this preserves anonymity for the respondents.

The next consideration with a mailed survey questionnaire is the postage. Of course, the postage must be prepaid by the researcher (or sponsor)—the important factors relate to response rate influence and cost. The highest response rate can be anticipated with the use of regular first class stamps. The second highest response rate can be achieved by acquiring a bulk mailing permit and purchasing so-called "precanceled" stamps. Metered postage, even if first class, provides a lower response rate than the use of stamps. This response is associated with the patient's perception that an actual stamp enhances the value of the item (survey questionnaire) contained in the mailing. With a bulk mailing permit (which is printed on the envelope), the researcher can anticipate the lowest response rate. Bulk mail is also slower than first class mail, but it costs just more than half as much per piece.

Finally, the letter of transmittal (commonly referred to as the "cover letter") introduces a mail survey to respondents. Because there is no personal contact involved, this letter must explain the rationale behind the project and obtain the cooperation of the potential respondent. Therefore, it should answer the following questions:

- What are this mail and survey all about?
- Who wants to know the information?
- Why is the information needed?
- How did I get selected to receive this survey?
- How important is this survey?
- How much of my time will this take?
- Is the survey going to be difficult to complete?
- Will it cost me anything?
- Will they be able to identify me?
- How will my responses be used?
- What do I get out of taking the time to complete and return this survey?
- When does this have to be returned by?

General conventions for a cordial business letter should apply to the cover letter. That is, it should not be too formal or demanding, nor should it beg the recipient to complete the survey. Also, the letter should not be written using vocabulary or sentence style that is "over the head" of the least sophisticated respondents. It is equally important that the letter not appear condescending or patronizing to the most sophisticated respondent. Show respect for the reader's time and effort. Remember that, within the first few seconds, the reader will decide whether or not to cooperate. Finally, thank the recipient profusely for his or her anticipated cooperation.

An alternative to the mail survey is the personal or telephone interview. Although every respondent to a mail survey receives exactly the same information in the same way, interviewers introduce the element of variation. Interviewers are likely to vary from one interviewer to another and from one interview to the next. The more variation present, the greater the incidence of random error and systematic bias—and the lower the validity and reliability of the data.

Random error reduces the reliability of the results, whereas systematic bias diminishes the validity of the results. Some of the more common sources of interviewer error include the following:

- *Instruction error:* It is common for interviewers to "ad lib" the instructions rather than present them in the precise way they appear on the questionnaire. Moreover, this ad-libbing typically is done in an inconsistent way, so that the interviewer inaccurately "memorizes" instructions that may be quite different from the written form intended.

- *Interrogation error:* Even subtle differences in the wording of questions can have an impact on how patients will respond. If the same question is asked differently from one patient to the next, then error is introduced into the process. This holds true for simple factual information like "How old are you?" (vs. "What is your age?"), as well as more complicated questions. Thus, interviewers must be admonished about the error potential of modifying any aspect of the questions.
- *Response option error:* It must be specified whether interviewers are to read or not read the response options; if they fail to follow these instructions explicitly, error is introduced into the results.
- *Scale interpretation error:* Whenever there is a numerical equivalent to each verbal response, such as a "5" associated with "strongly agree" and a "1" with "strongly disagree," there is likely to be error, particularly if the number and corresponding response are not listed together on the questionnaire. That is, the "strongly agree" may be reported as a "1" and vice versa.
- *Recording error:* This type of error is much more likely when verbatim responses are to be recorded. The more the interviewer is required to write, the greater the likelihood of error. This potential exists to a much lesser degree with structured response options.
- *Interpretation error:* Whenever an interviewer is asked to interpret the responses, then "translate" the response into one present on the questionnaire, errors are likely. Very seldom will responding patients use the same words as those that appear in the response options. In effect, the interviewer is asked to make judgments about the responses and then record them.

Survey results are affected randomly by interviewer error. In other words, these errors are just as likely to distort the results in one direction as another. This distortion reduces the reliability of the data (and therefore, indirectly, the validity as well). Systematic bias, on the other hand, directly reduces the validity of data by consistently distorting the data in one particular direction. As a result, bias is a much more serious and damaging problem. Two important potential areas of interviewer bias to prevent are *amplification of response bias* and *creation of response bias.*

Although the same potential biases for mail surveys also apply to interview surveys, the very presence of interviewers is likely to amplify (i.e., increase the tendency toward) or create additional response bias. New response bias can be created based on the verbal or nonverbal actions of the interviewer. For instance, an intimidating interviewer may create a threat to the responding patient, whereas a rude or pushy interviewer would introduce a hostility bias.

In a written survey, the major contributor to *nonsampling* error and specifically to *response errors* is faulty questionnaire design. Response errors occur because responding patients do not give accurate answers to questions that have been asked. Furthermore, many factors that lead a respondent to give inaccurate responses can be traced directly to improper questionnaire design and construction. The format of a question, the content of a question, or the organization of the questions can induce a responding patient to give an inaccurate response. The resulting response errors are of particular significance because evidence indicates that nonsampling errors are a much larger part of total survey error than sampling errors.

The Purposes of a Survey Questionnaire

Crouch and Housden (1998, p. 137) identified four main purposes of the questionnaire data collection process.*

1. *To collect relevant data:* The data quality depends entirely on the design of the questionnaire and the questions it contains. Once you as the researcher (or your team) have decided on the questionnaire objectives, they form the framework for all decisions about the questionnaire structure and question content. Data relevance, then, is determined both by your questionnaire objectives and by the analysis and interpretation to which it will be subjected. There is no point in asking about a patient's age (or age range) if you don't intend to distinguish patient satisfaction strengths and weaknesses by age group, or at least provide an age distribution of all respondents.
2. *To make data comparable:* The questionnaire must be constructed in such a way that the words have the same meaning to all respondents. Thus, among hundreds or even thousands of respondents, the main variable is the variation in response to each question.

---

*Source: S. Crouch and M. Housden, *Marketing Research for Managers,* 2nd ed., pp. 137 and 140, © 1996. Reprinted by permission of Butterworth Heinemann Publishers, a division of Reed Educational & Professional Publishing Ltd.

3. *To minimize bias:* Any tendency for some extraneous factor to affect the survey question answers is considered bias. By using wording that respondents clearly understand, each response will reflect the true opinion of the respondent completing the survey.

4. *To motivate the respondent:* The format and type of questions used should be varied and interesting for the respondent. If you ask a patient to take his or her time, attention, and thought to complete the questionnaire, you need to make the questions as easy to understand and answer as possible.

Validity and Reliability

A survey can be considered *valid* to the degree that it measures only what it is supposed to measure. For example, if you purport to be determining provider-specific patient satisfaction, yet no means of identifying the provider appear on the questionnaire (i.e., only the provider type… if there is more than one), the validity of the research is lessened. Furthermore, the survey must not be influenced by any extraneous factors that distort the results in one direction or another.

Reliability refers to "repeatability"—the ability to get the same results/data from several measurements made in a similar manner. This can occur with the same respondent on repeated occasions or among respondents. Reliability *over time* means that if the same respondent were asked the same question several times throughout a month, the same response would be given. Reliability *among respondents* means that all respondents who have the same opinion about a particular issue (e.g., "the doctor explained my health problem clearly") would respond the same to any question pertaining to that issue.

Figure 6–1 demonstrates the concepts of validity and reliability using a star as the target. The star located at the center of each quadrant represents the actual average of some value of a given population. The small circles represent the bullet holes made from shooting a pistol at the target. These "bullet holes" are analogous to the averages that might be obtained from several measurements from sets of people in the same population.

Both targets on the top row of Figure 6–1 contain bullet holes that are centered on the star/target. Even though the bullet holes in the upper right-hand quadrant are spread over a wider area, there is a random pattern centered around the center of the star/target. Nothing is "pushing" or "pulling" all of the bullets toward one direction. The lower row of the same diagram represents the results of survey data that are typical of low validity. In the lower left-hand quadrant, the shooter constantly shot below and to the right of the star/target. The

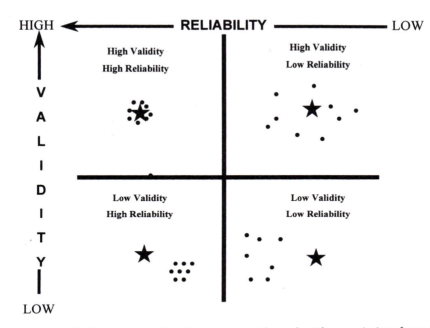

Figure 6–1 Validity and Reliability. *Source:* Adapted with permission from P. Alreck and R.B. Settle, *The Survey Research Handbook,* p. 64, 77, 98, 104, 159, 193, 194, 207, 214, 237, and 255, © 1985, The McGraw-Hill Companies.

shooter aiming at the lower right-hand quadrant's target persistently shot too high and to the left of the target. Thus, the effect of systematic bias is to "push" or "pull" the results in one or another direction.

In the upper left-hand quadrant, the bullet holes are closely clustered about the target. In other words, the person shooting consistently hit on or very near the target. If the bullet holes represent averages obtained from different measurements from the same population, the reliability is quite high because the results are very similar. There is little "random error" in the data. On the other hand, the upper right-hand quadrant shows the bullet holes to be randomly scattered on the target; they are spread over a wider area rather than being clustered near the target. The shooter is not doing the same thing with each shot. If the bullet holes were different patient satisfaction survey measurements, they are not very good representations of one another. Reliability is said to be low, whereas the random error is quite high.

It is important to keep in mind that, technically, no data can be more valid than they are reliable because validity means hitting the target consistently. Surveys on sample populations are said to be invalid if their findings are not to be generalized to the whole population. Good questionnaires are both valid and reliable; they measure what they purport to measure and do so reliably.

TYPES OF DATA OBTAINED USING QUESTIONNAIRES*

According to Crouch and Housden (1998), there are basically three types of data gathered using questionnaires—fact, opinion, and motive. Factual information is typically easy to ask and to answer, provided the respondent knows and can remember. This includes the so-called "demographic" information like age, sex, insurance company, and so forth. Facts may include information that is relevant to the survey, such as an answer to the question, "Have you ever visited our clinical laboratory for testing?" Fact may also refer to specific behavior: "Do you test your blood sugar at least once each week?" All factual information can be described as "hard data" because they are data that can be relied on. This allows for reasonable quantitative estimates for the patient under study, providing some basis for cross-tabulation of research results.

The second type of information gathered by patient satisfaction surveys relates to patient *opinion.* This includes the beliefs, attitudes, feelings, and knowledge of the respondent. Because patient perceptions are dealt with in the PMRC model, using a survey questionnaire to determine your organization's grades on the PMRC, this type of information is of critical importance. Feelings and attitudes are generally rather complex, having a number of dimensions. Therefore, it is best to use multidimensional scaling techniques in patient satisfaction survey research. The results of opinion questions are often described as "soft data" because they are less valuable in decision making than factual information. Nevertheless, opinion data can be extremely helpful in identifying service quality strengths and weaknesses.

The third type of information gathered by questionnaires relates to *motive.* Health care organizations wish to influence patient behavior; therefore, it is important to know why people believe or do something. The challenge with this lies in the fact that it is often hard to explain fully why one does or thinks a particular thing. The answers are likely to be so diverse that they are difficult to compare and analyze; the analysis is inevitably subjective. Therefore, for patient satisfaction sur-

---

Source: S. Crouch and M. Housden, *Marketing Research for Managers,* 2nd ed., pp. 137 and 140, © 1996. Reprinted by permission of Butterworth Heinemann Publishers, a division of Reed Educational & Professional Publishing Ltd.

vey research, it is advisable for motive information to be gathered in a more qualitative research setting, such as a focus group or in-depth interview. From this, categories of reason that are most relevant to the objectives of the survey can be determined. Then, specific survey questions designed to measure how many people share these motives can be included in a representative sample survey that will produce quantifiable data.

ORGANIZATION AND CONTENT OF PATIENT SATISFACTION SURVEY QUESTIONNAIRES

The questionnaire itself consists of three main parts: the initiation, the body, and the conclusion. The first part initiates the task for the respondent and sets the stage for the kind of questions to follow. It indicates the type of information that is sought and provides some insight into the response task. This segment typically contains the most general questions that will be asked. At all costs, poor initial impressions must be avoided. The opening questions should be easy (close-ended) and nonthreatening and, if possible, significant to the respondent. It is important to include only questions that are applicable to all respondents. This is not the place to seek "sensitive" information or ask "delicate" questions.

Typically, the *funnel sequence* is followed when the respondent is assumed to have some ideas about a topic. This is the procedure of asking the most general question about the topic under study first, followed by successively more restricted questions. This approach prevents early questions from conditioning or biasing responses to questions that come later.

The body of the questionnaire is the larger, middle portion that contains items dealing with the substance of the research—patient satisfaction. The rule of thumb for this section is that the questions should be in a sequence that appears to be logical and meaningful to respondents. There should be a clearly identified and smooth transition from one section to the next. By grouping questionnaire items, the task becomes simpler and easier for respondents. Additionally, the entire survey becomes more efficient.

Survey questions may be grouped by topic, content, or scaling technique. Topic grouping is one of the most common criteria for organizing items. For example, patient satisfaction survey items may be logically grouped into: access (arranging for and getting health care), convenience, communication, perceived quality of health care received, personal caring, health care center facilities, and demographic sections.

Questionnaire items can also be grouped logically by the content of the questions. Once a respondent's mind is focused on one particular area of inquiry, his or her mind will have turned to that issue. Patients can easily respond to additional items about the same issue, but may find it difficult to keep "shifting" their attention from issue to issue. Therefore, it would not be appropriate to jump around from one content category to another, with no logical sequencing.

Survey questionnaire items can also be grouped by scaling technique. Often, the majority of a given survey can be answered using a single scale. Not only is this logical, but it is also an efficient use of the respondent's time and attention. For example, if all items are written as statements with which respondents can express the degree to which they agree or disagree with the statement, a Likert scale is used. The response range typically would include: "strongly agree...agree... neutral...disagree...and strongly disagree." Or, if you wish to have patients rate your health care organization in terms of the various MOTs and SPs that make up their mental report card, you may wish to use a different Likert scale: "poor...fair...good...very good...excellent... and...does not apply." This approach saves time and space and makes the response task easier as well. The respondents only need to read the instructions and learn the use of the scale one time, and they can proceed through the list of all such items rapidly.

The final or concluding portion of the survey is best reserved for two item types: (1) those that deal with sensitive or delicate issues or topics and (2) demographic or biographic questions that measure the attributes or characteristics of respondents. This information helps the researcher more accurately portray the nature of the sample population. It also allows for comparison of the demographic profile of the sample to that of the population as a whole. Finally, these items can be used to divide the sample into subsamples by age, sex, and so forth.

Demographic items should be clustered together in a single section and included at the end of the questionnaire. This facilitates response, and respondents are less likely to refuse or terminate the process if they have been cooperating for some time. If you wish to include income, which is considered the most sensitive and threatening demographic item (possibly driven by pride or fear of some Internal Revenue Service "connection"), place this last on the survey. Racial or ethnic identity, if needed, or religious preference information, would best be placed second to last—just before income information.

Typical patient satisfaction questionnaire "general information" items would include the following:

- Was this your first visit to ABC Health Care Center?...Y/N
- How often have you seen a health care provider in the past year?...x1, x2, x3+
- Are you...M/F?
- What is your age?...under 6, 6–15, 16–25, 26–35, 36–45, 46–55, 56–65, 66–75, 75+
- How long have you been using ABC Health Care Organization?...less than 1 year, 1–2 years, 3–5 years, 6–10 years, 11+ years
- Do you intend to remain a patient of ABC Health Care Organization?...Y/N
- All things considered, how satisfied are you with ABC Health Care Organization?...completely satisfied, couldn't be better, very satisfied, somewhat satisfied, somewhat dissatisfied, very dissatisfied, completely dissatisfied, couldn't be worse, neither satisfied or dissatisfied
- Would you recommend ABC Health Care Organization to your family and/or friends?

Types and Composition of Survey Questions

Open-ended questions are questions that ask the respondent to answer in his or her own words. *Close-ended questions,* by contrast, are questions that ask the respondent to choose from specific, predetermined answers, giving the one that is closest to his or her own opinion, attitude, or viewpoint. Open-ended questions, such as "Please provide comments or suggestions about your physician based on your most recent visit," can enhance a survey's usefulness and value. The responses to these types of questions may clarify the reasons for "very poor" or "very good" ratings. Also, this type of question could function as a warning signal that one of your close-ended questions has been misunderstood by the respondent. Even if the intent of a question is clear, sometimes respondents reverse the rating scale, indicating a "1" for a rating of "excellent," when it should have been a "5."

If you choose to include open-ended questions in your patient satisfaction survey research, several guidelines should be kept in mind.

- Do not suggest alternatives in the question. Bias will be introduced if the patient is led or prompted into a response.
- Record responses verbatim. Summarizing comments can introduce bias because various recorders may have variable editing skills.

- Do not begin open-ended questions with "Why?" because defensive barriers are often created when the word is used. "Why" implies that a rational explanation for the patients' opinions or attitudes should be provided. Such perceptions are not always formed in a completely rational manner.

There are several significant drawbacks to using open-ended questions in your survey. First, they are not very well suited for self-administered surveys, simply because most respondents will not write elaborate answers. Second, answers to open-ended questions may be a more direct result of the respondent's ability to articulate than a measure of the respondent's knowledge, attitude, or interest in the issue being researched. Finally, open-ended questions must be coded or categorized for analysis purposes, which can be a tedious task.

Itemized or close-ended questions come in a variety of forms including ranking, scaled items, and categorical responses. A ranking forces the patient to place responses in a rank order according to some criterion. For example, when determining the relative importance of certain elements of patient satisfaction, the respondent may be asked to rank order the relative importance of several items. As a result, value judgments can be made and the rankings can be summed and analyzed quantitatively.

Scaled close-question items are the most commonly used types of questions. With this type of question, subjects are asked to indicate the strength of their agreement or disagreement with a statement or to indicate the frequency of some behavior, like visiting the health care center. The Likert scale is a 5-point scale in which there is an assumption of equal intervals between responses (strongly disagree... disagree...neutral...agree...strongly agree). The difference between "agree" and "strongly agree" is considered to be equivalent to the difference between "disagree" and "strongly disagree."

Categorical responses, also known as "dichotomous questions," offer the subject only two choices: "yes" or "no"; "true" or "false." The limitation of this approach is the lack of other options available to the respondent, such as "sometimes" or "it depends." For completeness in recording responses, a "don't know" category should be included on the questionnaire. Although categorical responses take less of the respondent's time, thought, and attention, they do not provide as much information as the patient's degree of agreement or frequency of behavior, as determined with scaled items.

Multiple-choice questions offer the respondent a range of answers. In order to design such an item, the researcher needs to know what to ask, as well as the range of all possible answers, which must be comprehensive, so that no respondent should want to give an answer that is not offered, and mutually exclusive, so that no respondent should believe that his or her answer could be in more than one category.

The danger with multiple-choice questions is that people are classified into neat and tidy "boxes" that may not reflect the true response of the patient accurately. This can be somewhat overcome by including a category labeled "other... please specify." Tabulating and analyzing well-designed multiple-choice questions is easy, thereby making them a challenging but worthwhile addition to the questionnaire.

The most effective survey questions, according to Alreck and Settle (1985), have a variety of attributes in common—focus, brevity, and simplicity.

Each question should focus on a single, specific issue or topic. The best way to make sure that a question is focused directly on the issue at hand is to ask as precisely as possible exactly what you, the researcher (in alignment with your research objectives), need to know.

The next important question attribute is brevity. Not only are long questions more likely to lack focus and clarity, but they are more cumbersome to answer because respondents are likely to forget the first part of the question by the time they read the last part. In general, the longer the question, the more difficult the response task becomes. Short questions are less subject to error on the part of the researcher or respondent.

Next, the meaning of the question must be clear to all respondents. That is, virtually all respondents must interpret the question in exactly the same way. It is advisable to have multiple people read over the proposed questions to make sure all opportunities for improvement are identified. If different readers report dissimilar interpretations of what exactly is being asked, reword the question to enhance clarity. This is important, because the researcher knows exactly what he or she is attempting to ask, but an independent reader must rely solely on the content and wording presented on the proposed question.

The building blocks of clarity in communication are made of vocabulary and grammar. In order to obtain meaningful responses, questions must be expressed with the appropriate words, with the words combined to clearly communicate with respondents. It should be kept in mind that all individuals have essentially three levels of vocabulary.

1. *Core vocabulary:* These are words with which individuals are very familiar; they are used in everyday speech.
2. *Recognizable vocabulary:* These are words that individuals recognize when they are read or spoken, but they are seldom spoken by

the individuals themselves; there is a fairly good understanding of the meaning (perhaps by contextual interpretation alone).
3. *Unfamiliar vocabulary:* These are words that the individual does not recognize or understand.

The researcher should restrict question composition to the usage of core vocabulary of virtually all respondents. If common words from the core vocabulary of the least sophisticated or educated respondents are used in the questions, everyone will understand them. If bigger words or words that are seldom used in speech are used in the questions, many people will not know what they mean or what is being asked. It should be recognized that there may be a temptation on the part of researchers to use "sophisticated" vocabulary in order to appear well educated, so they use fancy words or complex sentences. However, speaking the common language means finding synonyms for the polysyllabic and Latinate constructions that come easily to the tongue of the college educated. One need not use "principal" because "main" will do as well. "Intelligible" is rarely as good as "clear" or "understandable." The real measure of educated survey research is that the researcher generate data that are reliable and valid, data that are free from error and bias. This can be accomplished best by using simple, core vocabulary.

Once we accept the limitation of core vocabulary use, the next important consideration is grammar—how the words are arranged within each question. Recall that there are four basic sentence types: simple, compound, complex, and compound-complex. *Simple* sentences have a subject and a predicate, and sometimes an object or complement. *Compound* sentences are just two simple sentences connected together by a conjunction. *Complex* sentences are simple sentences with a dependent clause taking the place of a word, and *compound-complex* sentences are a combination of the two. The most effective survey questions are simple sentences.

The next important consideration in survey question development is to make sure the questions are composed in such a fashion as to avoid instrumentation bias. Alreck and Settle (1985, p. 104) specifically mentioned several types of instrumentation bias and how to avoid them.

1. Un-stated criteria—If the criteria by which respondents must judge some issue or respond to some question are not completely obvious, the criteria must be stated in the question. If an item might be judged by multiple standards and the criteria are not explicitly stated, some re-

spondents will use one set of criteria and others will use another.... Thus, some people may respond based on their own needs and others may consider what the [health care organization] needs to do to win [patients] in general.

2. Inapplicable questions—The questions must be applicable to all respondents in the sense that they can reply, based on their own experience or condition.

3. Example containment—When the question contains an example that consists of a response alternative or identifies a class or type of response alternative, it is likely to interject a bias. Because the example brings that particular response or type of response to mind, many may choose or include it but fail to include others.... It is important to identify the entire class of alternatives and avoid examples that are among the possible choices for the respondents.

4. Over-demanding recall—The researcher must not assume that respondents will recall their behavior or feelings over an extended period of time. Often the topics or issues of the survey are very important to those conducting the project, and so the researcher assumes that they are equally as important and memorable to respondents. This is seldom ever the case.

5. Over-generalizations—There are times when it may be appropriate and acceptable to ask respondents for generalizations. When a survey question seeks a generalization, it should represent a policy, strategy, or habitual pattern of the respondents, rather than specific behavior.

6. Over-specificity—A survey question is overly specific when it asks for an actual or precise response that the respondent is unlikely to know or unable to express.

7. Over-emphasis—If the wording of a question is over-emphatic, it is likely to introduce bias by calling for a particular type of response. When it is necessary to describe some condition in the question, it is advisable to use words that lean toward understanding, rather than overstating the condition. Respondents are then free to reach their own conclusions about the degree of severity. If the condition is described in overemphatic terms, a judgment or conclusion is imposed on the respondents.... Each question must be examined carefully to avoid wording

that over-emphasizes or over-states the condition. Words that are overly dramatic or constitute a conclusion must be avoided.

8. Ambiguity of wording—There are many words and phrases that designate different things for different people. Often those who write questions are totally unaware of the fact that others may have a completely different understanding of the term. To avoid such ambiguity, virtually every questionable word or phrase must be checked carefully to be sure that it has a common meaning for everyone in the survey sample.

9. Double-barreled questions—When two questions are both contained within one item, the item is known as a double-barreled question.... Probably the most common form of the double-barreled question includes both the action and the reason or motive in the same item. This is certainly not the only form of double-barreled question, however.... The key to detecting double-barreled questions is to determine if part of the item might be true and part false.

10. Leading questions—When questions lead the respondents to a particular answer, they create a very strong bias and often result in data that are completely invalid.

11. Loaded questions—While leading questions direct the respondents' attention to a specific type of response or suggest an answer, loaded questions are less obvious. The loaded question includes some wording or phrase that constitutes a more subtle form of influence. Often loaded questions take the form where a "reason" for doing something is included in the item.

Cosmetic Aspects of the Patient Satisfaction Survey

The appearance and quality of the patient satisfaction survey questionnaire (and any associated envelopes, cover letter, etc.) must be viewed through the eyes of your patients as the basis of another SP. Not only will this project a segment of the image of your organization, but response rates (particularly if you are mailing your survey) will be affected as well. Therefore, attention to the details of quality (printing and paper stock) and overall appearance are well worth the effort.

The first cosmetic attribute is the quality of the paper stock used. More specifically, the paper's weight, cotton content, and texture drive quality perceptions. The paper should be of 20-pound stock or heavier because lighter paper has a tendency to allow the printing to "bleed through" to the other side. Also, the same stock should be used for the outer mailing envelope, the postage-paid return envelope, the cover letter, and the survey questionnaire itself. It doesn't make sense to economize on one component while having all other aspects of high quality because this will diminish the positive image projected. The texture should be smooth or subtly textured, but not slick.

The next considerations are paper and ink color. Intuitively, it may be tempting to place the survey on a brightly colored paper stock in order to attract more attention. This should be avoided because the overall perception is likely to be negative and "unprofessional." Although white paper is always acceptable, alternative considerations such as off-white, pale gray, or beige are also appropriate. With regard to print color, economic constraints typically preclude the use of two or more colors. The use of screening to highlight instructions or a section change can be just as effective as using different colored ink. The only exception to this is the signature on the cover letter; if the letter is printed in black, the signature portion should appear in blue, to emphasize the hand signature.

The next cosmetic consideration is the print size, pitch, and quality. Although a business letter may be well accepted when printed with a normal 10-point font, for ease of reading, particularly if your sample population contains a significant number of patients age 65 and greater, a 12-point font is recommended. The tradeoff, of course, is that less information can be gathered per unit of space; however, readability is of paramount importance. Thus, this recommendation is not universally followed by patient satisfaction researchers. In fact, Atlantic Information Services presented the patient satisfaction surveys of a wide variety of health care organizations (1996). Many of them appear to have fonts in the size range of "8 or 9"; expecting anyone with even the mildest degree of uncorrected visual impairment to read this is simply unreasonable in the author's opinion. The pitch (letters per inch) also contributes to the readability of survey documents; a 10 pitch is easier for seniors to read, but a 12 pitch is acceptable. The use of 15 pitch is to be avoided on any printing intended for reading by patients.

The quality of the printing is determined by the mechanism used to print the document. The use of a dot-matrix printer, or electric typewriter (yes, there are a few still around!), projects the image that quality is not very important in this survey. With the affordability, availability, ease-of-use, and high quality of printing with an ink-jet or laser printer, coupled with computer-based word-processing software, there is simply no excuse for projecting a second-rate image with the printing. Professional typesetting is always a high-quality option, but the use of left- and right-justification along with proportionate spacing typically found with popular word-processing software creates a very similar appearance. Bold or italicized type can be used to highlight certain words or phrases where needed.

Next, consider the size of the paper for the survey instrument as well as for any envelope(s) needed for mailing and/or return. Standard 8½" x 11" letter size (A4 210 x 297mm in the United Kingdom) is ordinarily best because people are accustomed to reading from this size correspondence. When multiple pages are required for your survey questionnaire, they should be printed on both sides and attached. Ideally, you should use a folded 11" x 17" piece of paper that produces two 8½" x 11" sheets that can be printed on four sides (booklet style). This projects a much better image than stapling pages together. Envelopes for sending the survey should be either a standard #10 business size envelope or a large envelope allowing for flat document placement if budget permits and the mailing piece is relatively thick. The postage-paid return envelopes should be slightly smaller, say size "9," so as to easily fit within the original mailing envelope.

Finally, the layout of all patient satisfaction research documents should be simple, clean, and conventional. Avoid a dense, cluttered appearance by using ample white space. It is much better to use more pages than to attempt to condense too much information into less space. Use one-and-one-half-spaced or double-spaced type, with sections separated by double or triple spacing. This approach makes the response task appear simpler for the respondent, which can increase the response rate, validity, and reliability of the data. The mailing envelope should display the potential respondent's address centered on the front, with the return address on the upper left-hand corner. Nothing should appear on the back of the envelope, not even to reemphasize the importance and value of the contained survey questionnaire.

When the patient opens a mailed survey questionnaire, the first thing encountered should be the cover letter, which sets the tone for the patient's perception of your survey research project. This letter should be followed by the survey questionnaire itself. This is not the time to enclose other items, such as vouchers or health care newsletters.

Survey Completion Instructions

It is extremely important that the respondent be spared from confusion while undertaking the response task. Therefore, wherever there is a task initiation or change, specific instructions must be provided. Generally speaking, these instructions should be written at a level that meets the comprehension requirements of the least sophisticated respondents. The more complex the scaling technique and the less sophisticated the responding population, the more in-depth the instructions should be. When rating scales are used, respondents need to be told what items or elements are to be rated, what criterion or standard should be used for judgment, how the scale is to be used, and exactly how and where the responses are to be reported.

Exhibit 6–1 contains portions of introductions and instructions from a variety of patient satisfaction survey studies conducted by or for various health care organizations.

The Stages of Responding to a Survey Question

As we review the various steps involved in developing a valid and reliable patient satisfaction survey questionnaire, it is important to

---

Exhibit 6–1 Sample Patient Satisfaction Survey Introduction and Instructions

Sponsoring Organization	Sample of Survey Introductions/ Instructions
Colorado Department of Health Care Policy and Financing; "The Colorado Medicaid Primary Care Physician Program Patient Survey"	• Please fill out this survey for the person to whom the survey is addressed. If it is addressed to a child, please fill it out for the child regarding the care he or she receives. • On average, please rate your health care based on the following statements. • Please circle the number that corresponds with your answer.
The George Washington University Health Plan Member Satisfaction Survey	• Please complete the following survey to help us assess your satisfaction with your health care. The survey is anonymous so please respond openly. Your responses are important to our efforts at improving the quality of services at the Health Plan. Please feel free to write additional comments below. • How would you rate the following? (Please circle one number on each line.)

continues

Exhibit 6–1 continued

Sponsoring Organization	Sample of Survey Introductions/ Instructions
Harvard Community Health Plan Member Survey	• The opinions of all of our members are important to us as we work to provide members with high quality medical care and service. You can help us determine how well we are serving your health care needs and how to improve our services by taking just a few minutes to complete this questionnaire. If the envelope is addressed to your child, please complete the questionnaire with your child's health care in mind. Otherwise, please complete the questionnaire based on your experiences. We would like your opinions about your care to be based on the primary medical site/doctor's office that you (or your child) had the most experience with during the past year. Be assured that your answers and comments will remain confidential and reported in summary form only. Please return this questionnaire in the enclosed, postage-paid envelope. Thank you for letting us know how well we are doing in meeting your health care needs.
National Research Corporation: "The NRC Listening System" for MeritCare Hospital	• MeritCare Hospital is committed to improving the care and services our patients receive. As part of the improvement process, we are asking for your help to identify areas that need improvement. Recently, you were a surgery patient of our hospital from May 1 through May 5. Please take a few minutes to answer a few questions about your stay. We are able to sample only a small number of patients, so your response is very important. • After you have completed this brief questionnaire, simply return it in the enclosed postage-paid envelope. • Your responses are confidential. Results are reviewed in summary form with answers from

continues

Exhibit 6–1 continued

Sponsoring Organization	Sample of Survey Introductions/Instructions
	many other patients. Thank you for your help. • Marking instructions: INCORRECT MARKS [demonstrated] CORRECT MARK [demonstrated] –Please use a pen or pencil. –Fill the circle completely. –Erase cleanly any marks you wish to change. –Do not make any stray marks on this form. • Mr. XYZ, how would you rate MeritCare Hospital on the:
Parkside Associates, Inc. "Physician Office/Clinic Quality of Care Monitor"	• Directions: Below are a number of questions about your recent physician office visit. Please answer each question by checking the box that best indicates your opinion about the service you received. If a question does not apply to your situation, check "Does Not Apply." If the patient is a minor/child or cannot complete the survey, a family member is encouraged to do so for him or her. • Please check here if someone other than the patient is completing the survey.
Friendly Hills HealthCare Network Patient/Member Satisfaction Survey	• Dear Patient: As part of our continuing effort to improve quality and services, we ask that you assist us by participating in this survey about your recent visit to one of our health care providers. • Below are a number of questions about your most recent visit. Please answer each question by checking the box that best describes your opinion. If the patient is a minor child or cannot complete the survey, please make sure that it is completed by a family member. If you have visited a Friendly Hills HealthCare Center in the past, please answer only about your most recent visit to a health care provider.

continues

Exhibit 6–1 continued

Sponsoring Organization	Sample of Survey Introductions/ Instructions
	• Please express your opinions openly and honestly. Your responses will be kept completely confidential, so you are assured that your identity and responses will not be shared with your health care providers at Friendly Hills HealthCare Center. • When making your selection, please fill in the box representing your rating: [demonstration diagrams]. • Thank you for participating in this survey. Your input is very important in helping us improve our services.

Source: Adapted with permission from *A Guide to Patient Satisfaction Survey Instruments*, pp. 15, 31, 35, 55, and 83, © 1996, Atlantic Information Services, Inc.

keep in mind how a typical respondent approaches each question. Research in cognitive psychology applied to questionnaire deficiency has identified four distinct stages that combine to provide the selected response. Jobe and Mingay (1998, pp. 1053–1055) summarized these stages as follows:

1. comprehension—in which the respondent interprets the meaning of the question
2. retrieval—in which the respondent searches long-term memory for relevant information
3. estimation/judgment—in which the respondent evaluates the information retrieved from memory and its relevance to the question; the respondent may then combine the separate items of information to form a response or, alternatively, the respondent may decide that the recalled information is inadequate and use that information as a starting point in forming an estimated response
4. response stage—respondent weighs factors such as sensitivity of the question, social desirability of the answer, probable accuracy of the answer, and so forth, and then decides what answer to provide.

During each of these stages, there is the potential for erroneous reporting. By carefully designing questions following the principles discussed in this chapter, the likelihood for response bias can be decreased. Exhibit 6–2 offers a variety of general guidelines for questionnaire design. These are based on recommendations of The Chartered Institute of Marketing (Phipps & Simmons, 1998).

Pilot Testing Your Patient Satisfaction Survey Questionnaire

A pretest or pilot study is of particular importance when contemplating the distribution (by any means) of a patient satisfaction survey questionnaire. This testing may be accomplished best in two stages. First, obtain input from several colleagues and front-line employees.

Exhibit 6–2 Guidelines for Questionnaire Design

- Keep the survey short, because an excessively long survey is often indicative of poorly defined survey goals. As a rule of thumb, keep the number of questions less than 40. Go through each question. If you do not know or care what you will do with the result, then leave the question out.
- Design the questionnaire to match the survey method being used.
- Keep the questionnaire simple. Do not mix topics, because this may serve to confuse the respondent.
- Do not combine two questions into one.
- Avoid unnecessary terminology, abbreviations, technical words, and jargon—these should only be used where questions are intended for a specialist group that would be expected to understand (unlike patients).
- Do not present biased questions. For example, "How satisfied are you with the way you were treated by the receptionist?" assumes that people already have a positive perception of the receptionist and thus biases their response. A more correct way to phrase this would be to ask, "How satisfied or dissatisfied are you with the way you were treated by the receptionist?" A suitable response scale would then be provided.
- Make sure your questions are grammatically correct—poor grammar can lead to confusion. It also annoys certain people and creates a poor impression.

continues

Exhibit 6–2 continued

- Each question should have a "Don't Know" or "Not Applicable" response unless you are absolutely certain that you have covered all possibilities.
- Provide example questions at the beginning of the questionnaire to demonstrate the method of completion. If a number of different question formats are used, provide examples of each and instructions for completion within the body of the questionnaire to avoid confusion.
- Be specific in your questioning. Vague, nonspecific questions lead to vague, nonspecific results.
- Always allow for respondents to make their own comments at the end of the questionnaire—this will often provide useful leads for follow-up studies or allow you to interpret more accurately the data you collect.
- Take care when laying out your questionnaire—a neat and tidy layout creates a good impression and reduces error.
- Take care with the ordering of your questions—make sure that the response on a question is not affected by a previous answer or pre-empts a response to a later question.
- Always start your questionnaire by explaining who you are and what you intend to do with the data you collect. This is polite as well as being ethically correct.

Source: Adapted with permission from R. Phipps and C. Simmons, *Understanding Customers 1998–99*, p. 109, © 1998, Butterworth-Heinemann.

These people can provide valuable critiques about the questionnaire. Then, after revising the questionnaire in accordance with the criticisms received in the first "trial run," a representative sample of respondents can be selected who are a part of the intended population for the second pilot study.

Dillon, Madden, and Firtle (1990, p. 399), discussed five types of decisions involved in pretesting.

1. *What items should be pretested?* All aspects, including layout, question sequence, word meaning, question difficulty, branching instructions, and so on should be part of the pretest.
2. *How should the pretest be conducted?* To whatever extent possible, the pretest should involve administering the questionnaire in an environment and context that is identical to the one that will be used in the final survey. An essential feature of conducting the pretest involves debriefing and/or protocol analysis. *Debriefing* takes place after a respondent has completed the questionnaire; it

involves asking respondents to explain their answers, to state the meaning of each question, and to describe any problems they had with answering or completing the questionnaire. In *protocol analysis*, the respondent is asked to "think aloud" while completing the questionnaire.

3. *Who should conduct the pretest?* The survey project team director and several members of the research team should participate in the pretest so that they can combine their observations in a debriefing following the pretest meeting(s).

4. *Who should be the respondents in the pretest?* The respondents included in the pretest should be as similar as possible to the target population in terms of familiarity with the topic, attitude, and behaviors associated with the topic; general background characteristics; and so forth. This is absolutely critical to performing a pretest.

5. *How large a sample is required for the pretest?* Unfortunately, there is no one answer to this question. To a large degree, it depends on the variation of the target population. With a heterogeneous target population, a larger pretest sample will be required. Also, the more complex the questionnaire, the larger the sample needed.

Translating the Questionnaire into a Foreign Language

It may seem obvious to suggest that you produce your patient satisfaction survey questionnaire in more than one language, particularly if you have a culturally diverse patient population. However, this process deserves more than a casual approach because mistakes can be (and have been) made in a variety of settings when literal equivalence is used as the sole approach to translation. For example, the Portuguese translation for a U.S. airline's Boeing 747 "rendezvous lounge" was "prostitution chamber." At Friendly Hills HealthCare Network, a literal translation of the Likert scale designation of "poor" (on the scale: "does not apply...excellent...very... good... fair...poor") was "pobre," which refers to economic depravity versus a low quality rating. Fortunately, this was detected and corrected (to read "mal," depicting a low rating) by a Spanish-speaking staff member after the "professional" translation vendor returned the literal translation, but before printing.

A combination of several translation methods should be considered in order to prevent potentially embarrassing errors.

- *Direct translation:* With this method, the instrument undergoes a single translation from one language into another by a bilingual translator. Using this method alone, however, exposes the instrument to all of the problems discussed above.
- *Back translation:* This is a variation of direct translation in which the translated survey instrument is translated back into the original language by another bilingual translator. This allows the researcher to identify and correct any discrepancies that arise in the meaning between the original and the retranslated instruments. Note that back translation requires that equivalent terms for words or phrases exist in the other language, which may not be possible.
- *Decentering:* This method is a hybrid of back translation that involves a successive iteration process of translation and retranslation of an instrument each time by a different translator. The back-translated versions in the original language are compared sequentially. If discrepancies occur, the original is modified and the process is repeated until both show the same or similar wordings. Generally, each iteration should move the instrument closer and closer to the intended meanings.

The quality of the translation can be evaluated by first having a monolinguist review the clarity and comprehensiveness of the translated questionnaire and then having bilingual evaluators determine the extent of change in the meaning between the two versions. You should also assess an appropriate respondent's ability to answer the translated questions correctly. And finally, you should pretest both the original and the translated questionnaire with a bilingual individual. This helps avoid the problems associated with literal translation of idiomatic or colloquial expressions.

Developing Response Incentives or Inducements

Generally speaking, response rates for mail surveys are rather low. Therefore, the researcher needs to mail several times as many questionnaires as the required number of respondents. In turn, this increases the overall research costs. Furthermore, low response rates increase the likelihood of response bias, which reduces the validity of the research data.

In an attempt to improve response rates, your organization may wish to provide some sort of incentive to complete the survey questionnaire. This functions to get the potential respondent's attention, set a positive tone for undertaking the response task, and establish a sense of obligation to cooperate. The latter is especially the case when the "reward" is included in the original mailing. If receipt of the "token of appreciation" is contingent on the questionnaire being completed, and there is a perceived possibility that the respondent may be identified, an element of bias is introduced. The sense of obligation may not influence only the decision to respond, but also the manner in which the survey is completed. This could be based on the respondent's erroneous assumption that the researcher/organization seeks, and is rewarding, favorable ratings/responses.

If you decide to use an incentive to boost your response rates, several factors need to be taken into consideration when selecting the incentive.

- *Cost:* Besides the normal budgetary limitations, there is another reason to keep the reward inexpensive. You are only providing a *token* of your appreciation; anything greater suggests that you are attempting to pay the respondent (albeit meagerly) for his or her time and effort. Therefore, it is best to avoid the use of cash. The risk here is that respondents could feel that their time has been grossly undervalued.
- *Perceived value:* Make sure your incentive item has sufficient value to the potential respondent so that it doesn't diminish rather than enhance goodwill for your organization.
- *Nonbiasing factor:* The incentive item should not be directly associated with any of the topics or issues found within the survey questionnaire because such inducements could influence one or more responses.
- *Uniqueness:* An item can be much more attractive if it is not readily available through normal retail stores.
- *Self-indulging:* The item should be some form of luxury or treat the respondent would enjoy but is not likely to purchase for him- or herself.
- *Personalized:* The item should be something that either has the respondent's name on it (risky because the benefits of anonymity are erased) or relates to a special interest the respondent is known to have.

At Friendly Hills HealthCare Network, we developed a response incentive that met several important criteria.

- It would be perceived as valuable to the respondents.
- It was considered highly likely to increase patient participation in the survey research, thus enhancing overall response rate.
- Total incentive costs were less than $2,500.
- It preserved the responding patients' anonymity.

The incentive consisted of a raffle scheme wherein responding patients were given a chance to win 1 of 20 $50 gift certificates. Upon placing a completed survey into a slotted box labeled "completed surveys," one of our survey administrators gave the patient a "raffle ticket" (green-colored index card). Respondents were instructed to write their name and any contact mechanism they felt comfortable with (address, telephone number, etc.) on the index card and place it in the slotted box labeled "raffle entries." It was made very clear to patients that the information on the raffle entry could not be linked to their survey responses in any way.

For those patients who simply could not take the time to complete the survey while at the respective health care center, a survey questionnaire, postage-paid return envelope, and yellow "raffle ticket" were provided to them. And, they were informed that they could still be eligible (even though they had a lesser chance than those completing the survey on-site) to win one of the prizes if they returned the completed survey within 2 weeks. The return envelopes were addressed to the outside data collection agency used for optically scanning the completed questionnaires. Their staff were instructed to send all completed yellow "raffle tickets" to us; this allowed for respondent anonymity to be preserved because there was no correlation between the yellow cards and each participant's survey responses.

This approach effectively met our response incentive objectives. Patient anonymity was virtually preserved, although one could argue that we knew the collective name list of those responding. This could be countered with the observation that a small percentage of the respondents simply completed the survey without entering the raffle— with no possible link to their identity as participants in the research. At a total cost of $2,000 for prizes and an additional $100 worth of supplies, we remained under budget. And finally, the chance to win a $50 gift certificate must have been perceived as reasonably valuable because the overall response rate for the project was 49%. We considered this quite respectable in view of the fact that the survey questionnaire contained 60 items.

Preparing the Survey Instrument for Data Scanning

If your health care organization serves a large patient population (and therefore the survey sample size is likely to be large), it is advisable to consider the services of an outside market research agency to scan and tabulate the data. At Friendly Hills HealthCare Network, we contracted with Pine Company, a well-respected firm based in Santa Monica, California. Their research staff reviewed the survey instrument to ensure that the layout and design were appropriate for intelligent character recognition, the recommended high-accuracy, high-speed scanning technology. As a result, position markers were added to the survey to ensure accurate alignment during the scanning process.

Administering the Survey—Asking the Questions

The 1996 Friendly Hills HealthCare Network patient satisfaction survey was distributed on-site at each of the involved 41 health care centers. In order to facilitate survey administration, we contracted with a private temporary employment agency to screen and provide us with 10 individuals who met the following requirements:

- personable, friendly, and outgoing
- professional in appearance and demeanor
- bilingual (English and Spanish)
- prepared to travel (via their own transportation) within all areas of southern California, covering all 41 health care centers to be studied

These individuals were brought into the Friendly Hills HealthCare Network Education and Research Building to receive 4 hours of training in the process of survey administration. During this workshop, all materials including surveys, survey collection boxes, survey mailing boxes, raffle insertion boxes, card tables, signage (see Exhibit 6–3), and additional supplies were provided. To facilitate participants' recollection of the information presented, a *Survey Administrator's Training Guide* was provided for each attendee. The information presented in this guide, reflecting the overall contents of the workshop, is presented in Exhibit 6–4.

The survey administrators were assigned a series of health care centers in rotation. Prior to each patient's visit on the designated survey day, patients were asked to do the following:

Exhibit 6–3 Survey Administration Desk Sign

> # Help us serve you better.
> ## You can win $50.00 for
> ## sharing your opinion today.
>
> – Complete our *Patient Satisfaction Survey* (immediately following today's visit).
> – Fill out a raffle card to enter the drawing.

- Help us improve services by participating in our survey study.
- Pay particular attention to the name of the provider they were seeing today.
- Stop by the patient satisfaction survey desk (well-identified and standardized from health care center to health care center) following their visit.
- Complete a patient satisfaction survey.
- Place their completed survey in the box labeled "completed surveys."
- Take a survey questionnaire with them (along with a self-addressed stamped envelope provided) in the event that they were in a rush, with the request to return it within 2 weeks. The survey completion instructions were contained on the survey instrument (see Appendix B), eliminating potential instruction error on the part of the survey administrators. Prior to the onset of the survey project, the organizational standard for all providers to wear name badges at all times when treating patients was reinforced. At this point, it was necessary to assign numbers to an alphabetical listing of the cities representing each health care center. Additionally, a numbering scheme had to be developed to represent each provider at each health care center. This allowed for the generation of a master health care center list as well as a list containing the names and codes of all providers.

Prior to the onset of survey administration at each health care center, the appropriate health care center number code was penciled onto the appropriate space on all survey questionnaires to be used that day. Of course, the initial amount was simply an estimate, and additional

Exhibit 6–4 Survey Administrator Workshop Outline

Topic Sections	Specific Topics Discussed

Introduction	• Welcome and introduction to staff members
	• Thank you for your willingness to participate in our patient satisfaction survey research
	• The purpose of this workshop
	• The role of a survey administrator
	• A word about your appearance and professionalism
	• The Health Care Centers (HCCs) you will be working in
	  – Locating the HCC (see directions and maps provided)
	  – Allowing sufficient driving time
	  – Parking at the HCC

Organizing your time	• Arrival to and departure from the HCC
	  – Arrive a minimum of 15 minutes prior to starting time
	  – Depart after end of business day for that HCC
	• Breaks
	  – Lunch - 30 minutes - 2+ survey administrators - separately
	  – Coffee breaks - 15 minutes in AM + 15 minutes in PM

Setting up and getting ready for the day	• Introducing yourself to the HCC supervisor, manager, and front office staff
	• Setting up your area
	  – Selecting your location - near reception room
	  – Signage placement
	  – Table placement
	  – Table-top arrangement
	  – Separating Completed Surveys box from Raffle Entry box
	  – Clipboard placement
	  – HCC code number (see list) penciled onto all surveys

Steps for doing the job the "right" way	• Initiating previsit contact with the member/patient – Introducing yourself and stating why you are there

continues

Exhibit 6–4 continued

Topic Sections	Specific Topics Discussed
	– Dialogue for talking with member/patient, instructing him or her to pay attention to the name of the provider he or she is to see during their clinical visit today
	– Ensuring patient of confidentiality (and anonymity)
	• Postvisit contact
	– Ask patient name of provider he or she saw
	– Check the provider code list to determine code number
	– Place provider code in appropriate space at top of survey
	• Explaining to the member/patient what is needed
	– Tone of voice and professionalism
	– Getting the member/patient's cooperation
	– Making sure the member/patient understands what is needed and reference instructions for survey completion
	– Answering any member/patient's questions related to the survey research project
	– Meeting resistance and responding appropriately
	• Administering the survey questionnaire
	– Being properly prepared (plenty of sharpened pencils, surveys available in both English and Spanish)
	– Dealing with patient who does not have time to complete the survey on-site, but would like to provide feedback (give survey, SASE, yellow "raffle ticket")
	– Working with member/patient with visual impairment
	– Working with member/patient with hearing impairment
	– Working with illiterate member/patient
	– Be prepared to answer "How long will this take?"
	– Answer questions re: eligibility for $50 prize
	• Ensure confidentiality while completing survey

continues

Exhibit 6–4 continued

Topic Sections	Specific Topics Discussed

	• Ensure confidentiality during placement of survey into Completed Surveys box
	• Provide member/patient with appropriate "raffle ticket"
	  – Instructions to place name and any preferred method of contacting him or her in the event his or her ticket is selected to win
	  – Instructions to place completed raffle ticket in Raffle Entries box
	• Thank the member/patient for his or her time and input during the survey process

What you should do at the end of the day	• Clean up your area, making sure it is left in the same condition in which you found it upon arrival in morning • Remove all completed surveys from Completed Surveys box (count them) and place them in the Survey Mailing Box provided, and seal it • Give the Survey Mailing Box to the HCC supervisor • Call total number of completed surveys in to Friendly Hills HealthCare Network, using the assigned telephone number

surveys had to be prepared throughout the day based on demand. Then, in keeping with the research objective of producing provider-specific data, the predetermined provider number was encoded on each survey by the survey administrator prior to giving it to the patient.

Completed surveys were placed in a large "completed surveys" container, rather than given to the survey administrators, thereby preserving respondent anonymity, which is very important in the health care setting. Patients often welcomed the opportunity to "be heard" regarding their satisfaction perceptions. Furthermore, long-term patients welcomed the opportunity to contribute to our overall improvement efforts.

At the end of the survey day, all completed surveys were placed in a survey mailing box and given to the health care center supervisor to be delivered to the Friendly Hills HealthCare Network Education and Research Building. Patients who preferred to take the survey with them for completion at home were instructed to use the provided self-addressed stamped envelope (addressed to Pine Company Market Research) to return their completed survey and yellow "raffle ticket." Pine Company was instructed to place all received yellow raffle tickets in a separate mailer (with no connection whatsoever with the returned completed survey questionnaire) and send them to the aforementioned location.

After the administration of surveys at three pilot test locations (one small-sized health care center—with fewer than 100 scheduled patients, one medium-sized health care center—with 100–200 scheduled patients, and one large-sized health care center—with more than 200 patient visits scheduled), all survey administrators were brought in for a debriefing of their respective survey administration experiences. At this time, all logistical challenges were discussed and appropriate solutions were developed using structured brainstorming. The remainder of the health care centers were then surveyed according to schedule.

The next steps of any patient satisfaction survey research are to scan or otherwise tabulate the data, to analyze the data, and to communicate the data throughout the organization. Each of these steps will be discussed in detail in Chapter 7.

USING FOCUS GROUP RESEARCH TO DETERMINE PATIENT SATISFACTION

Focus groups are "focused" discussions that are structured and led so as to evoke the perceptions and suggestions of patients. They can also be used to solicit reactions to plans and ideas your organization has, enabling you to make any needed modifications prior to implementation. Researchers often prefer the focus group format to individual interviews because participants actually trigger memories and suggestions in one another. According to Smith, Scammon, and Beck, "Focus groups are 'safe' for patients because they allow talking with other patients whose experiences are likely to be similar to theirs... patients seem to find group discussions particularly cathartic because of the 'support group' feeling created when discussing their hospital stays" (1995, p. 23).

Typically, focus groups are composed of 6–12 persons who share common characteristics such as "current patients of your health care organization." Focus group sessions generate information that is not easily obtainable using other methods. Interactions among the group members often stimulate thinking in a manner that is not possible with other interviewing techniques. Most people who conduct qualitative market research would classify focus groups into three different types:

1. *Full group* consists of a discussion of approximately 90–120 minutes, led by a trained moderator, involving 8–10 persons who are recruited for the session based on their common demographics, experiences, or attitudes.
2. *Mini-group* is essentially the same as a full group, except that it generally contains 4–6 individuals.
3. *Telephone group* involves individuals participating in a telephone conference call, wherein they are led by a trained moderator for 30 minutes to 2 hours. These individuals are recruited according to the same parameters as full and mini-focus groups.

Some researchers prefer to use mini-groups to full groups because they feel they can gain more in-depth information from a smaller group. The reason is that a group session lasts approximately 100 minutes; if 10 people are involved, the average individual (assuming he or she is not attempting to dominate the discussion) gets only 10 minutes to participate. With a mini-group, the time per person is doubled, thus (theoretically) enabling the moderator to get more information from each individual. Other researchers prefer to use mini-groups because they find that it is not feasible to recruit more than six persons for a particular group.

Patients are invited by letter (usually followed with a confirmation phone call) to participate in a focus group designed to gather their input regarding experiences with your health care organization. Typically, if meetings take place during the working day, breakfast or lunch is served. If sessions are to be held in the evening, light refreshments (or dinner) should be served. Three components are important to the success of a focus group: (1) recruitment of the correct participants, (2) quality of the questions, and (3) skills of the moderator.

In selecting your focus group participants, you should first identify the selection criteria—for example, "ages 65+ who have visited your health care facility within the past 6 months." Then, make sure that once you have developed a list of individuals meeting the criteria, the actual participants are chosen randomly from that list. Then, there is the female:male ratio of your patient population; if it is 60:40, then 60% of your participants should be randomly selected from the list of females who meet the participation criteria.

The questions being used to orchestrate the focus group discussion should be derived from or directly related to your overall research objectives. Additionally, they should be designed in such a fashion as to identify new ideas or concerns. This can usually be accomplished best using open-ended questions coupled with the interactive discussion.

The success of any focus group depends largely on the moderator's skill. The moderator can be an external consultant or someone from inside your health care organization. Armed with several predesigned questions, the moderator's main role is to

- Ensure that everyone around the table has an opportunity to speak.
- Keep the group on track.
- Probe for the most in-depth information possible.
- Take detailed notes (along with audio- or videotaping) that can be transcribed after the meeting.

A good rule of thumb is to invite approximately 50% more patients than you want to attend. This allows for the typical one-third "no-show" rate.

Focus groups can be conducted in a variety of locations. The most common locations include a designated market research facility, a hotel meeting room, or an on-site meeting room in your health care organization. Market research facilities are designed specifically for collecting feedback from small groups of people. Typically, there is a large meeting table, microphones for recording patient feedback (for later transcription), and a video camera so that the session can be shown to appropriate groups from your health care organization. If you use this approach, make sure to obtain participants' consent in advance using a release form. This type of facility may also have a one-way mirror on one of the walls, allowing for inconspicuous viewing of the meeting process by appropriate representatives of your organization. Patients should be informed ahead of time that they are being observed and that the mirror is used to minimize the amount of distraction. Seeing patients comment (or complain) firsthand about your service has a much higher personal impact than reading comments on a survey form.

If you decide to conduct focus group research in a hotel meeting room, the same procedures may be used as in a research facility. The main difference, of course, is that you won't find a one-way mirror available for inconspicuous viewing or videotaping. If the video camera is apparent, it may inhibit patient responses somewhat due to self-consciousness. In the author's experience, this factor is minimized by an experienced moderator who keeps the group focused on the task(s) at hand—they soon forget that the camera is present. Only the moderator and the patients should be in the room during the focus group because patients tend to open up more slowly and be less frank if they are talking directly to a group of representatives from the company they are being asked to assess.

An on-site meeting room offers the least expensive option for conducting focus group research. The main problem with this setting, though, is the potential for interruptions. Also, participating patients may feel less talkative when the meeting is held on the health care organization's territory. By preparing your organization for the importance of these meetings in advance, you can ensure that no interruptions will occur and that the door can remain closed throughout the meeting. Furthermore, the "territory" issue can be minimized by holding the discussion in a meeting room or classroom that is viewed as completely separate (even in the same building) from the clinical facilities.

In order to get the most from your focus group research, Greenbaum (1993) recommended that a variety of steps be taken before, during, and after the actual meetings. The following guidelines* reflect these recommendations:

- Begin planning the details of your focus group research the moment you decide to use this mechanism for obtaining patient feedback. These details include such things as
  1. establishing the focus group research objectives
  2. retaining a moderator if you are not using in-house personnel
  3. deciding on the number of groups to be used in the research series
  4. determining the geographic location of the groups
  5. identifying the time of the focus group meetings (7:30 AM or 6 PM or 8 PM are most common)
- Brief the moderator with sufficient information so that he or she can function as a partner in the research effort rather than as an outsider. The effectiveness of the focus group is often contingent on the quality of information provided during the briefing.
- Develop a moderator's guide. This is basically an outline of the discussion to be held during the focus group session. It should include the following sections:
  1. *Introduction:* In this section, the moderator introduces him- or herself, explains the purpose of the session, and allows all par-

*Source: Reprinted from T.L. Greenbaum, *The Handbook for Focus Group Research,* p. 35, © 1993 by Sage Publications, Inc. Reprinted by Permission of Sage Publications, Inc.

ticipants to introduce themselves. Also, if audio- or videotaping or one-way mirror observation is taking place, patients should be informed of this.

2. *Warm-up:* In this section, general issues related to the main topic are discussed. This is used to discuss basic information about the patient's health care experiences.
3. *Details:* This section includes all key points to be covered throughout the discussion.
4. *Key content:* This section identifies areas that the moderator should probe during the session in order to ensure that the discussion of the topic is thorough.
5. *Summary:* This section provides participating patients with the opportunity to share any information about the topic they may have forgotten or otherwise omitted. Often, this is elicited by asking participants to give "advice for the chief executive officer (or president)" of your health care organization.

- *Provide food for the participants:* Although opinions vary, it is generally preferred to feed the participants before they enter the focus group room or session. This reduces the clutter, and therefore distractions, during the actual discussion.
- *Manage the noise level:* Insist that it remain quiet in the vicinity of the meeting.
- *Provide name tags for the participants:* Use only first names (the "most commonly used name" that the participant prefers to be addressed by), without any titles, keeping the atmosphere less formal and therefore more relaxing and conducive to participation. You should also make sure to write each person's name on both sides of the name tag so the moderator can see the name from all over the room.
- *Decide on the optimal number of participants for the session:* The rule of thumb is 10 for a full group and 5–6 for a mini-group.
- *Select the most desirable people to participate:* Consider the following:
  1. Choose the patients who best meet the recruitment criteria— the more homogeneous the group, the better the participants will relate to each other in the discussion.
  2. Eliminate patients who appear unlikely to contribute meaningfully to the discussion, considering such factors as:
     –attitude problems toward the group or the topic
     –excessive shyness
     –language problems
     –hearing problems
     –extremely poor eyesight

- *Ensure that the room is set up properly:* Consider easel placement, writing supplies (each participant should have a pad and pencil in front of him or her), and room temperature (comfortable for participants).
- *Conduct a postgroup discussion between the moderator and appropriate representatives of your health care organization after all participants have left the room:* Identify any particular problems encountered, unexpected insights gained, or potential biases introduced into the research.

At Friendly Hills HealthCare Network, focus group research was used to gain an understanding of the relative importance of various elements and service indicators that make up the PMRC. Full-sized groups of 10 participants were recruited with the following criteria:

- age groups of 20–44, 45–64, and 65+
- individuals who visited a Friendly Hills HealthCare Network health care center within the past 12 months
- individuals with access to transportation to and from the Friendly Hills HealthCare Network's Education and Research Center in LaHabra, California

Computer-based keypad response technology was used to process rankings and comparisons efficiently. This afforded the capability of obtaining considerable quantitative information by using a research methodology that traditionally yields qualitative information alone. Next, participation incentives in the form of gift certificates were determined and obtained. For the patients in the 65+ age group, these consisted of gift certificates for buffet dinners valued at $10 each. For those selected for the remaining two age groups, the incentive needed to be somewhat higher due to the greater inconvenience for these age groups to attend our sessions. Therefore, each participant in the 20–44 and 45–64 age groups was provided with a $25 gift certificate to a local retail clothing store.

In order to recruit participants meeting the identified criteria, the assistance of the Friendly Hills HealthCare Network's MIS department was required. They provided a list of names and telephone numbers of all patients within the listed age groups who had visited a Friendly Hills HealthCare Network health care center within the past 12 months. Then, numbers were assigned to each letter of the alphabet, and a table of random numbers was consulted to establish a random sequence of alphabet letters from which to choose participants by their last name. This provided an equal opportunity for participants with last names beginning with all letters of the alphabet to be selected. Next, participants and "backup participants" were randomly selected in the respective age groups. Participants were contacted and provided with a brief background of the research effort; if they met all criteria, they were scheduled for the designated discussion times. Those who accepted the invitation received a follow-up confirmation letter with specific directions to the location of the research facility.

Next, a detailed *Focus Group Moderator's Guide* (Appendix A) was developed. This contained an outline of activities to be undertaken during the session (Exhibit 6–5), the objectives of our focus group research, the service indicators for each service element within each service category, and specific instructions for the facilitator.

Exhibit 6–5 Focus Group Outline of Activities

Section	Activities To Be Completed
Welcome to the focus group meeting	1. Greeting to meeting room—provide a name tag (preprinted).
	2. Provide participants with food and beverages.
	3. Interact with participants (small talk).
Introduction	4. Introduce moderators: Patrick Shelton and Eric Olson.
	5. Introduce any additional FHHN personnel present.
	6. Briefly explain the purpose of the session.
	– "To better understand what is important to you in determining your satisfaction with services provided by Friendly Hills HealthCare Network
	– To help Friendly Hills improve services for members"
	7. Clarify that this is NOT designed to measure their current level of satisfaction (this will be measured using another technique later).
	8. Alert participants to the audiotape and/or video recorders that are recording the session (emphasize that these are used only for ensuring accuracy of our research; obtain consents).

continues

Exhibit 6–5 continued

Section	Activities To Be Completed
	9. Inform participants that they will be using key-pads during the session and that they will receive instructions for using them.
	10. Ensure confidentiality: – Participant names are NOT shared with any providers – The combined information is for research purposes (and may be published at a later date)
	11. Participants introduce themselves. – First name only – How long they have been a member of FHHN
Warm-up	12. "When you think of excellent health care, what comes to mind?" – Have a scribe record these on a flipchart. – Use our service categories to get the discussion going.
Research details provided to participants	13. Show the six service categories (i.e., all at once) that we will be working with one at a time.
	14. Explain that there are various elements of service within each category – For example, under "access to care," several elements would include: – ease of scheduling appointments by telephone – ease of scheduling appointments in person – length of time you waited between the preferred appointment day and the day of your visit
	15. Explain that for members to be satisfied with each element of services at FHHN, our providers or employees need to do a variety of things – For example, under "ease of scheduling appointments by telephone": – telephone needs to be answered promptly – you prefer speaking to a person (vs. a machine) – no long periods of time on "hold" etc. – These things are called "service indicators" for purposes of this research

continues

Exhibit 6–5 continued

Section	Activities To Be Completed
	16. Explain how the research will be conducted:
	– We will concentrate on one service category at a time (access to care, convenience, communication, personal caring, perceived quality of care, facilities)
	– Within each service category, we will ask you, as a group, to do two things:
	1. Rank the relative importance to you of the various service elements in determining your satisfaction with FHHN.
	2. Rank the relative importance of the various service indicators within each element.
	– First you will view the list of service elements, then discuss which elements are most important to you.
	– Use your keypad to individually rank the elements and then indicators according to their importance to you.

The objectives for this focus group research were as follows:

- Determine the relative importance (weighted contribution to their satisfaction) that each participant assigned to each of the identified satisfaction elements within the six main service categories.
- Determine the relative importance that each participant assigned to each of the identified service indicators.
- Identify any additional service elements or indicators that contribute to the collective participants' mental report card (perceptions of satisfaction with Friendly Hills HealthCare Network services).
- Determine the relative importance of any newly identified service indicators.

Throughout the research process, it was critically important to emphasize that the research was not designed to measure the participants' current level of satisfaction, but rather to better understand what is most important to them in determining their satisfaction with services provided by Friendly Hills HealthCare Network. Each focus group was conducted over a 3-hour period of time with refreshments provided to the 65+ age group conducted during the day, and light dinners provided to the other focus groups, which were scheduled in the early evening after normal business hours.

The data from all three focus group sessions resulting from the use of keypad response technology were reported in the form of bar charts indicating the relative importance of each service indicator within each service element within each main service category of member/patient satisfaction. This provided visual evidence of differences in relative importance of various elements between the studied age groups. Additionally, based on a 100-point scale, the relative importance ascribed to each element was tabulated (Figures 6–2, 6–3, 6–4, 6–5, 6–6, and 6–7). This afforded a quantitative representation of the

Category: Access
Element: Ease of Scheduling Appointments by Phone
INDICATORS

	IMPORTANCE (by Age Group)			
	20 to 44	45 to 64	65 and up	Total
Number of rings of phone	50.0	64.1	48.2	54.1
Speak with live person	80.4	93.8	98.2	90.8
Minimal "on hold" time	80.4	89.1	85.7	85.0
Staff helpfulness on phone	89.3	79.7	80.4	83.1
Multiple day/time offers	69.6	70.3	80.4	73.4
Total time required to make appt.	64.3	65.6	69.6	66.5
AVERAGE:	72.3	77.1	77.1	75.5

Figure 6–2 Tabulation of Relative Importance of "Ease of Scheduling Appointments by Phone." *Source:* Adapted from P.J. Shelton, The Straight-A's Program: A Systematic Approach to Measuring and Enhancing Patient/Member Satisfaction in an Ambulatory Managed Care Setting, in *Making Capitation Work: Clinical Operations in an Integrated Delivery System, Supplement #2,* G.G. Mayer, A.E. Barnett, and N.P. Brown, eds., © 1997, Aspen Publishers, Inc.

Category: Access
Element: Ease of Scheduling Appointments in Person
INDICATORS

	IMPORTANCE (by Age Group)			
	20 to 44	45 to 64	65 and up	Total
Convenient location of scheduler	58.9	65.6	76.8	67.1
Minimal wait to speak with scheduler	62.5	71.9	76.8	70.4
Total time spent with scheduler	46.4	59.4	58.9	54.9
Written verification of appt. time	53.6	76.6	78.6	69.6
AVERAGE:	55.4	68.4	72.8	65.5

Figure 6–3 Tabulation of Relative Importance of "Ease of Scheduling Appointments in Person." *Source:* Adapted from P.J. Shelton, The Straight-A's Program: A Systematic Approach to Measuring and Enhancing Patient/Member Satisfaction in an Ambulatory Managed Care Setting, in *Making Capitation Work: Clinical Operations in an Integrated Delivery System, Supplement #2,* G.G. Mayer, A.E. Barnett, and N.P. Brown, eds., © 1997, Aspen Publishers, Inc.

Category: Access
Element: Wait Between Preferred Day & Visit
INDICATORS

	IMPORTANCE (by Age Group)			
	20 to 44	45 to 64	65 and up	Total
Availability of preferred day	82.1	75.0	64.3	73.8
Nature of your visit	62.5	78.1	85.7	75.4
Availability of preferred time	85.7	75.0	71.4	77.4
Responsiveness to expressed urgency	100.0	96.9	96.4	97.8
AVERAGE:	82.6	81.3	79.5	81.1

Figure 6–4 Tabulation of Relative Importance of "Wait Between Preferred Day and Visit." *Source:* Adapted from P.J. Shelton, The Straight-A's Program: A Systematic Approach to Measuring and Enhancing Patient/Member Satisfaction in an Ambulatory Managed Care Setting, in *Making Capitation Work: Clinical Operations in an Integrated Delivery System, Supplement #2,* G.G. Mayer, A.E. Barnett, and N.P. Brown, eds., © 1997, Aspen Publishers, Inc.

Category: Access
Element: Time Waiting in Reception Room
INDICATORS

	IMPORTANCE (by Age Group)			
	20 to 44	45 to 64	65 and up	Total
Explanations provided for extended wait	57.1	92.2	85.7	78.3
Total wait time in reception room	83.9	95.3	71.4	83.6
AVERAGE:	70.5	93.8	78.6	81.0

Figure 6–5 Tabulation of Relative Importance of "Time Waiting in Reception Room." *Source:* Adapted from P.J. Shelton, The Straight-A's Program: A Systematic Approach to Measuring and Enhancing Patient/Member Satisfaction in an Ambulatory Managed Care Setting, in *Making Capitation Work: Clinical Operations in an Integrated Delivery System, Supplement #2,* G.G. Mayer, A.E. Barnett, and N.P. Brown, eds., © 1997, Aspen Publishers, Inc.

relative importance of each element to each age group studied. These *relative* numbers were termed the relative importance index (RII). In Chapter 7, dealing with data management, we will see how the RII was used for each of the 41 involved health care centers.

USING A "MYSTERY SHOPPER" FUNCTION IN YOUR HEALTH CARE ORGANIZATION

Another supplemental mechanism for taking the pulse of various SPs and MOTs that make up the PMRC is the use of a "mystery shop-

Category: Access Element: Time Waiting in Exam Room INDICATORS				
	IMPORTANCE (by Age Group)			
	20 to 44	45 to 64	65 and up	Total
Explanations provided for extended wait	60.7	90.6	80.4	77.2
Total wait time in exam room	82.1	89.1	71.4	80.9
AVERAGE:	71.4	89.8	75.9	79.1

Figure 6–6 Tabulation of Relative Importance of "Time Waiting in Exam Room." *Source:* Adapted from P.J. Shelton, The Straight-A's Program: A Systematic Approach to Measuring and Enhancing Patient/Member Satisfaction in an Ambulatory Managed Care Setting, in *Making Capitation Work: Clinical Operations in an Integrated Delivery System, Supplement #2,* G.G. Mayer, A.E. Barnett, and N.P. Brown, eds., © 1997, Aspen Publishers, Inc.

Category: Access Element: Acess to Emergency Medical Care INDICATORS				
	IMPORTANCE (by Age Group)			
	20 to 44	45 to 64	65 and up	Total
Ease of reaching care by phone	87.5	87.5	96.4	90.5
Directions provided for getting care	78.6	82.8	87.5	83.0
Transportation to emergency services	71.4	68.8	87.5	75.9
AVERAGE:	79.2	79.7	90.5	83.1

Figure 6–7 Tabulation of Relative Importance of "Access to Emergency Medical Care." *Source:* Adapted from P.J. Shelton, The Straight-A's Program: A Systematic Approach to Measuring and Enhancing Patient/Member Satisfaction in an Ambulatory Managed Care Setting, in *Making Capitation Work: Clinical Operations in an Integrated Delivery System, Supplement #2,* G.G. Mayer, A.E. Barnett, and N.P. Brown, eds., © 1997, Aspen Publishers, Inc.

per." These individuals are commissioned by the health care organization to visit various health care centers or departments anonymously and evaluate them on the parameters contained on the PMRC. These people are trained observers who are aware of optimum and nonoptimum SP and MOT management so they can rationally "grade" those things they experience and observe on a *Mystery Shopper's Report Card* (Appendix 6–A). Many organizations use this approach to monitor the extent to which established service quality standards are being implemented on a daily basis.

Chapter 7 will focus on collecting, processing, and communicating the data that result from measuring patient satisfaction.

CONCLUSION

Seeking and responding to patient feedback regarding patients' perceptions of service quality is one of the most essential nonclinical endeavors a health care organization can undertake as we approach the new millennium and beyond. By measuring patients' degree of satisfaction with the way all MOTs and SPs are currently being managed, you can determine your organization's current grades on those patients' mental report cards. This then forms the foundation for you to identify specific action(s) needed to increase patients' satisfaction and loyalty.

There are a variety of mechanisms available for obtaining feedback that reflects patient satisfaction. These include, but are not limited to, the following: postappointment telephone surveys, open-ended questionnaires, objective survey questionnaires, an internet web site, dedicated computer kiosks, lay advisory panels, patient focus groups, and complaint/grievance analysis. A survey is the most commonly used method of gathering quantitative patient satisfaction data. Whether you choose to "build your own" survey instrument, purchase an "off-the-shelf" version, or have a consultant develop one, the more you know about the overall development, sampling, administration, and data collection processes, the better equipped you will be to make educated choices along the way. After all, what you really want "at the end of the day" is reliable, valid, and credible data on which to base your improvement efforts.

Although formal research constitutes the foundation of quantitative patient satisfaction measurement, it is important to maintain an ongoing "frontline" view of how various MOTs and SPs are being managed. One helpful approach to this is with the use of a well-prepared "mystery shopper" using a detailed mystery shopper's report card similar to that provided in Appendix 6–A. This can be used to monitor the extent to which established service quality standards are being implemented on a daily basis.

ACTION STEPS

1. List the mechanisms your health care organization currently has in place for gathering satisfaction feedback from patients. Then answer the following questions: If enough mechanisms are in place, are you getting the stream of information you

need to remain in touch with patient perceptions? If not, why not? Should you have other means of capturing patient feedback? If so, what would you recommend?

2. Using information from this chapter, prepare a checklist of those aspects of patient satisfaction survey research that you would want carefully evaluated if a consultant proposed to perform this research for you.

3. Brainstorm a list of technology(ies) or communication channels that are currently in place for clinical and/or administrative use that you might also use to gather patient feedback.

4. Have a variety of direct patient contact people in your organization use Appendix 6–A, the "mystery shopper's report card," to assess current service quality strengths and weaknesses as they see them.

REFERENCES

Alreck, P.L., & Settle, R.B. (1985). *The survey research handbook*. Homewood, IL: Irwin.

Atlantic Information Services. (1996). *A guide to patient satisfaction survey instruments: Profiles of patient satisfaction measurement instruments and their use by health plans, employers, hospitals, and insurers*. Washington, DC: Author.

Crouch, S., & Housden, M. (1998). *Marketing research for managers* (2nd ed.). Oxford, England: Butterworth-Heinemann.

Dillon, W.R., Madden, T.J., & Firtle, N.H. (1990). *Marketing research in a marketing environment* (2nd ed.). Homewood, IL: Irwin Publishing.

Greenbaum, T.L. (1993). *The handbook for focus group research*. New York: Lexington Books.

Jobe, J., & Mingay, D. (1988, August). Cognitive research improves questionnaires. *American Journal of Public Health*.

Leedy, P.D. (1993). *Practical research planning and design* (5th ed.). New York: Macmillan.

Osborne, D., & Gaebler, T. (1994). *Reinventing government: How the entrepreneurial spirit is transforming the public sector*. London: Penguin Books.

Phipps, R., & Simmons, C. (1998). *Understanding customers 1998–99: CIM workbook*. Oxford, England: Butterworth-Heinemann.

Smith, J.A., Scammon, & Beck. (1995). Using patient focus groups for new patient services. *Journal on Quality Improvement, 21*(1), 23–31.

SUGGESTED READING

Al-Asaaf, A.F., & Schmele, J.A. (1993). *The textbook of total quality in health care*. Delray Beach, FL: St. Lucie Press.

Albrecht, K. (1992). *The only thing that matters*. New York: Harper Business.

Albrecht, K., & Bradford, L.J. (1990). *The service advantage: How to identify and fulfill customer needs.* Homewood, IL: Dow Jones-Irwin.

Allen, H.M. (1995). Toward the intelligent use of health care consumer surveys. *Managed Care Quarterly, 3*(4), 10–21.

American Health Consultants. (1998, January). Can you give your patients the ideal visit? *Patient Satisfaction & Outcomes Management,* 8–9.

Arnetz, J.E., & Arnetz, B.B. (1996). The development and application of a patient satisfaction measurement system for hospital-wide quality improvement. *International Journal for Quality in Health Care, 8*(6), 555–566.

Bader, G.E., Bloom, A., & Chang, R. (1994). *Measuring team performance: A practical guide to measuring team success.* Irvine, CA: Richard Chang Associates.

Barsky, J.D. (1995). *World-class customer satisfaction.* New York: Irwin Professional.

Baum, N., & Henkel, G. (1992). *Marketing your clinical practice.* Gaithersburg, MD: Aspen.

Bell, C.R., & Zemke, R. (1992). *Managing knock your socks off service.* New York: AMACOM.

Breen, G., & Blankenship, A.B. (1982). *Do-it-yourself marketing research* (2nd ed.). London: McGraw-Hill.

Broad, M.L., & Newstrom, J.W. (1992). *Transfer of training: Action-packed strategies to ensure high payoff from training investments.* New York: Addison-Wesley.

Brown, S.A. (1992). *Total quality service: How organizations use it to create a competitive advantage.* Scarborough, Ontario: Prentice Hall Canada.

Brown, S.A. (1997). *Breakthrough customer service: Best practices of leaders in customer support.* Toronto, Canada: John Wiley & Sons Canada.

Buell, V.P. (Ed.). (1986). *Handbook of modern marketing* (2nd ed.). New York: McGraw-Hill.

Business Research Lab. (1996–1998). *Customer satisfaction surveys—Relationship versus transaction measurement* [On-line]. Available: www.corporate@netropolis.net

Business Research Lab. (1997). When should changes be made to a customer satisfaction tracking questionnaire? [On-line]. Available: www.corporate@netropolis.net

Capezio, P., & Morehouse, D. (1992). *Total quality management: The road of continuous improvement.* Shawnee Mission, KS: National Press.

Chang, R.Y., & Kelly, P.K. (1994). *Satisfy internal customers first!: A practical guide to improving internal and external customer satisfaction.* Irvine, CA: Richard Chang Associates.

Disend, J.E. (1991). *How to provide excellent service in any organization: A blueprint for making all the theories work.* Radnor, PA: Chilton Book.

Flocke, S.A. (1997, July). Measuring attributes of primary care: Development of a new instrument. *Journal of Family Practice, 45*(1), 64(11).

Genovich-Richards, J. (1995). Member satisfaction surveys: The next frontier. *Managed Care Quarterly, 4*(4), 1–9.

Gopalakrishna, P., & Mummalaneni, V. (1992). Examination of the role of social class as a predictor of satisfaction received: A model and empirical test. *Journal of Ambulatory Care Marketing, 5*(1), 35–48.

Hall, M.F. (1995). Patient satisfaction or acquiescence? Comparing mail & telephone survey results. *Journal of Healthcare Marketing, 15*(1), 54(8).

Harvard Business Review. (1994). *Command performance: The art of delivering service quality.* Boston: Harvard Business School.

Hayes, B.E. (1992). *Measuring customer satisfaction: Development and use of questionnaires.* Milwaukee, WI: ASQC Quality Press.

Hayes, J., & Dredge, F. (1998). *Managing customer service.* Hampshire, England: Gower.

Hinton, T., & Schaeffer, W. (1994). *Customer-focused quality: What to do on Monday morning.* Englewood Cliffs, NJ: Prentice Hall.

Khayat, K., & Salter, B. (1994). Patient satisfaction surveys as a market research tool for general practices. *British Journal of General Practice, 44,* 215–219.

Lancaster, W., & Lancaster, J. (1992). Tracking patient satisfaction at an academic medical center. *Journal of Ambulatory Care Marketing, 5*(1), 27–33.

Leebov, W. (1988). *Service excellence: The customer relations strategy for health care.* Chicago: American Hospital.

Leebov, W., Vergare, M., & Scott, G. (1990). *Patient satisfaction: A guide to practice enhancement.* Oradell, NJ: Medical Economics Books.

Leland, K., & Bailey, K. (1995). *Customer service for dummies.* Chicago: IDG Books Worldwide.

Mayer, G.G., Barnett, A., & Brown, N. (1997). *Making capitation work: Clinical operations in an integrated delivery system.* Gaithersburg, MD: Aspen.

McKinley, R.K., Manka-Scott, T., Hastings, A., French, D., & Baker, R. (1997). Reliability & validity of a new measure of patient satisfaction with out of hours primary medical care in the United Kingdom: Development of a patient questionnaire. *British Medical Journal, 314*(7075), 193(6).

Mears, P. (1995). *Quality improvement tools & techniques.* New York: McGraw-Hill.

Nelson, A.M. et al. (1997). *Improving patient satisfaction now: How to earn patient and payer loyalty.* Gaithersburg, MD: Aspen.

Ostasiewski, P., & Fugate, D.L. (1994). Implementing the patient circle: Call on patients to help improve perceptions of health care quality. *Journal of Health Care Marketing, 14*(4), 20(7).

Prager, L.O. (1995). New survey seeks to improve science of satisfaction. *American Medical News, 38*(31), 7.

Prager, L.O. (1996). Latest *Consumer Reports* rates managed care plans. *American Medical News, 39*(31), 4(2).

Rubenzer, B.E. (1995, Winter). The AHRA patient satisfaction survey. *Radiology Management, 18*(5), 33–35.

Sachs, L. (1986). *Do-it-yourself marketing for the professional practice.* Englewood Cliffs, NJ: Prentice Hall.

Serb, C. (1997). If you liked the food, press ! *Hospitals & Health Networks, 71*(7), 99.

Singh, J., Wood, V., & Goolsby, J. (1990). Consumers' satisfaction with health care delivery: Issues of management, issues of research design. *Journal of Ambulatory Care Marketing, 4*(1), 105–115.

Stanger, J. (1995). Custom versus standardized patient satisfaction surveys: A Pacific Telesis case study. *Managed Care Quarterly, 3*(4), 41–44.

Terry, K. (1996). How to get the best reading of patient satisfaction. *Medical Economics, 73*(13), 101(8).

Wellington, P. (1995). *Kaizen strategies for customer care: How to create a powerful customer care program—and make it work.* London: Pitman.

Whiteley, R.C. (1991). *The customer driven company: Moving from talk to action.* Menlo Park, CA: Addison-Wesley.

Zeithaml, V.A., & Bitner, M.J. (1996). *Services marketing.* London: McGraw-Hill.

Mystery Shopper's Report Card

MOT or SP To Be Observed	Specific Attribute	A	B	C	D	F	NA
Print media promotion	Professional design/layout						
	Claims substantiated						
	Benefit-oriented						
Patient calls HCC on telephone	Answered promptly						
(normal business hours;	Answered appropriately						
general impression)	Speak w/ "live" person						
	Clear & understandable						
	Pleasant voice tone						
	Staff seem unrushed						
	Ask before place on "hold"						
	Minimum "on-hold" time						
	Music/info. while "on-hold"						
	Efficient call transfer						
Patient calls HCC on telephone	Staff helpfulness						
(purpose: to make an appointment)	Resp. to expressed urgency						
	Multiple day/time offers						
	How soon appt. available						
	Preferred date available						
	Preferred time available						
	Preferred provider available						
	Minimum time required						
Patient informed of HCC location	Convenient to home						
	Convenient to work						
Patient informed of HCC hours	Convenient provider hours						
	Convenient staff hours						

MOT or SP To Be Observed	Specific Attribute	A	B	C	D	F	NA
	Early morning hours offered						
	Evening hours available						
	Weekend hours available						
Patient calls HCC on telephone	Speak w/ "live" person						
(nonbusiness hours;	Able to contact provider						
non-emergency)	Getting telephone advice						
Patient calls HCC on telephone	Responsive to caller needs						
(nonbusiness hours; emergency)	Arranges for getting care						
	Arranges for transporting						
Patient travels to HCC	Clear directions provided						
	Main thoroughfare access						
	Public transportation access						
Patient views HCC exterior signage	Easily visible from street						
	Appearance of signage						
Patient parks vehicle for HCC visit	Parking provided at N/C						
	Ease of finding space						
	Closeness to HCC entrance						
	"Disabled" spaces available						
	Lighted during evening hours						
	Security personnel on site						
Patient views HCC facility	Appearance—decor						
from exterior	Appearance—cleanliness						
	Appearance—maintenance						
Patient views receptionist's	Openness (vs. small/						
"window"	frosted)						
Greeting of patient by receptionist	Patient soon acknowledged						
	Patient greeted by name						
	Receptionist's tone cheerful						
Patient views receptionist's	Well-organized						
work area	Cleanliness of area						
	Modern equipment						
Patient views reception room	Decor—nicely decorated						
	Color-coordinated						
	Neatness of room						
	Cleanliness of room						
Patient sits down	Enough seating available						
	Comfort of seating						
	Cleanliness of seating						
	Condition of seating						

MOT or SP To Be Observed	Specific Attribute	A	B	C	D	F	NA
Patient notices temperature in	Comfortable level						
reception room	maintained						
Patient asked to complete	Requested courteously						
information forms							
Patient views information forms	Print quality						
provided	Print size (12–14 point)						
	Neatly organized						
	Logically arranged						
	Easy to read						
	Easy to understand						
Patient looks over reading	Accessible						
materials in reception room	Up-to-date						
	Appropriate						
	Sufficient variety						
	Health-related						
Patient waiting time in reception	Apology made						
room	Patient informed of wait						
	Explanation(s) provided						
	Delay changes updated						
	Total waiting time minimal						
Patient's name is called by nurse/	Staff smiles, greeting						
medical assistant	patient						
	Name pronounced correctly						
	Name enunciated clearly						
Nurse/medical assistant speaks	Friendly						
with patient	Treated as welcome visitor						
	Staff—pleasant tone of voice						
	Staff—listens attentively						
	Respectful to patient						
	Personal concern evident						
Patient views staff appearance	Professional/uniformed						
	Clothing clean & neat						
	Grooming clean & neat						
	Minimal jewelry worn by staff						
Patient views carpeting	Spotlessly clean						
	In good condition						
Patient views photographs,	Appropriateness						
paintings, etc. on wall	Oriented to patient population						

MOT or SP To Be Observed	Specific Attribute	A	B	C	D	F	NA
Patient hears noise level throughout office	Quiet (acceptable noises only)						
Patient views treatment room	Cleanliness of everything						
	No signs of previous pt.						
Patient views equipment	Modern, "state-of-the-art"						
	Cleanliness of equipment						
	Mechanical operation						
Patient waits to be seen in treatment room	Patient informed of wait						
	Explanation(s) provided						
	Waiting for nurse to enter						
	Waiting for tx "set-up"						
	Total waiting time minimal						
Patient speaks with staff nurse/assistant	Friendly staff						
	Knowledgable staff						
	Staff prepares pt for visit						
Patient notices air quality in treatment room	Fresh, no "clinical odors"						
Patient observes appearance of provider	Professional appearance						
	Clothing clean & neat						
	Grooming clean & neat						
Patient greeted by provider	Greets patient by name						
	Smiles when greeting patient						
	Makes patient feel welcome						
Patient observes provider working w/staff	Communication						
	Teamwork						
Patient observes provider willingness to listen	Eye contact maintained						
	Prov. clarifies understanding						
	Provider appears unrushed						
Patient experiences rapport-building	Relationship dimension emphasized						
	Conversation focused on patient						
	Cultural sensitivity						
	Provider professional attitude						
	Pleasant tone of voice						
	Timely return of calls						
Provider obtains history of main complaint	Detailed history taken						
	Considers overall health						

MOT or SP To Be Observed	Specific Attribute	A	B	C	D	F	NA
Patient views provider's personal concern	Empathy demonstrated to patient						
	Caring attitude displayed						
	Exhibits interest in problem						
Nursing staff communicates with provider	No need to "repeat story"						
Patient observes provider's humanistic side	Minimize patient discomfort						
	Sensitive to patient pain						
	Patient confidentiality respected						
Patient notes thoroughness of examination	Sufficient time spent with patient						
	Provider focuses on problem						
Provider recommends diagnostic testing/x-rays	Rationale explained to patient						
	Results impact on treatment						
	What to expect during test						
	Logistics of getting test done						
	Prompt results available						
	Convenient lab location						
	Convenient lab hours						
	Minimum waiting in lab						
Provider explains diagnosed problem to patient	Understandable terminology						
	Visual aids used						
	Patient's questions answered						
	Adequate time spent						
	Written information given						
	References for education						
Provider explains treatment options	Consequences—no treatment						
	Conservative option offered						
	Understandable terminology						
	Treatment success likelihood						
	Supp. treatment measures						
	Adequate time to explain						
	Patient's questions answered						
	Empathy re: treatment concern						

MOT or SP To Be Observed	Specific Attribute	A	B	C	D	F	NA
Process of patient receiving	Immediate treatment						
treatment	Provider's hands washed						
	Explained during process						
	Sensitive to patient pain						
	Dressings carefully placed						
Process of patient receiving	Dressings neatly applied						
treatment	Referral given if needed						
Provider gives patient prescription	Rationale explained to						
for drug(s)	patient						
	Understandable terminology						
	Proper use of medication						
	Possible side effects						
	Possible adverse reactions						
	Problem of not taking drug						
	Problem—incorrect drug use						
	Cost to patient, if applicable						
	Patient questions answered						
	Written instructions provided						
Patient getting prescribed	Conven. pharmacy location						
medication	Conven. pharmacy hours						
	Rx filled quickly						
Patient gives educated consent	Anatomical context						
for surgery	explained						
	Likely outcome of surgery						
	Explained risks of surgery						
	Likely outcome if no surgery						
	Alternative procedures						
	Anesthesia (L/G/R) to be used						
	Where surgery to be done						
	Possible out-of-pocket costs						
	What to bring to surgery						
	Directions to surgery location						
	What people they'll encounter						
	Accurate discomfort estimate						
	Accurate disability estimate						
Outcome or result following	Obtained desired result						
treatment	Printed post-tx instructions						
	Any complication(s) explained						
	Complication managed well						

MOT or SP To Be Observed	Specific Attribute	A	B	C	D	F	NA
Patient schedules follow-up appt. w/ receptionist	Conven. scheduler location						
	Min. wait to see scheduler						
	Multiple day/time offers						
	How soon appt. available						
	Preferred date available						
	Preferred time available						
	Preferred provider avaiable						
	Written appt. received						
	Minimum time required						
	Informed what will be done						
Patient sees receptionist's friendliness	Greets patient by name						
	Smiles when greeting patient						
	Treats patient as guest						
Patient sees receptionist's courtesy	Pleasant tone of voice						
	Professional attitude						
	Listens attentively						
Patient feels respected by receptionist	Privacy & confidentiality						
	Respect shown to patient						
	Tactful handling of financial issues						
	Cultural sensitivity						
Receptionist personally concerned	Empathy demonstrated to patient						
	Caring attitude displayed						
	Exhibit true interest in patient						
Patient informed of laboratory results	Prompt results available						
	Patient privacy respected						
	Compassionate communication						
Reminders for upcoming scheduled visit	Telephone reminder						
	Written reminder						
Preventive care acquisition	Telephone reminder						
	Written reminder						
	Printed educational materials						
	Available education references						

CHAPTER 7

Patient Satisfaction Data Collection, Processing, and Communication

During the planning stages of your patient satisfaction measurement and improvement project, the logistics for collecting data should have been clearly mapped out. The real work begins with the receipt of your first completed survey questionnaires from participating patients. This is when the process of counting the number of patients who respond to each question in each way begins. The overall purpose of data processing is to put meaning into the data that you have collected. In turn, this provides summary figures so that the results are easily grasped and understood. Only after decision makers fully understand the gathered data can appropriate improvement planning take place.

This chapter will provide an overview of the characteristics of data. Then, the sequential "handling" of completed questionnaires, from initial receipt and inspection through editing, coding, data transfer ("entry"), and tabulation, will be presented. Next, several common methods of data display will be reviewed, followed by a discussion of data analysis—where the true meaning of the collected information is determined. Finally, the all-important process of communicating the patient satisfaction study findings throughout your organization as well as to outside stakeholders will be discussed.

CHARACTERISTICS OF DATA

Each piece of data you collect from your returned survey questionnaires is called an "observation." Each observation, in turn, has a "value" assigned to it, which may either be numerical or non-numerical. The observations you collect during the course of your patient satisfaction research are called a "data set." Data that have not been altered in any way (i.e., unchanged from when they were collected) are termed "raw data." For our purposes, the raw data you collect will be in the form of pages of numbers that, alone, are fairly meaningless. Before raw data can be interpreted, they need to be summarized in the form of a table, graph, or statistic.

Essentially, data can be classified in four different ways: the kind of data, the scale of measurement of the data, the number or groups from which data arise, and the quantity of variables in the data. All data have certain clearly recognized characteristics that, in turn, determine the statistical technique(s) that can be used in data analysis. Table 7–1 provides a detailed breakdown of data classification.

MANAGING RAW DATA FROM COMPLETED QUESTIONNAIRES

It is important for the researcher to monitor the collection of data very carefully. The quality of the mailing list (and reliability of the firm providing it) can, for example, be assessed by carefully observing the "nondeliverable" returned surveys. If there are many nondeliverables or "no such address" notations, this indicates that the list is inaccurate. Furthermore, the anticipated quality and accuracy of your survey results— degree to which the surveyed sample will be representative of your patient population—will be adversely affected by an inaccurate mailing list.

Alreck and Settle provided considerable guidance in the handling of completed survey questionnaires (1985, p. 255). The following discussion is based on their recommendations. Completed questionnaires are referred to as "source documents" because they are the source of the raw data. Very early in the data collection process, it will become apparent that you are gathering a tremendous physical volume of data. As you might imagine, these data are considered extremely valuable. Therefore, it is essential that you devise a system for handling source documents and use that system consistently throughout the time completed surveys are being received. The following sequence may be used as a guideline that will help you manage your source documents:

- Open mail surveys and discard (or file) any extraneous items such as cover letters, envelopes, and so forth.
- Record consecutive numbers at the end of the questionnaire as they are received. This unique number can be recorded later in the

Table 7–1 Classification of Survey Questionnaire Data

Classification Basis	Classes	Description	Example
Kind of data	Discrete	Categorical; exists independently of each other	Male/female? First visit: yes/no?
	Continuous	Together form a continuum	Chronological age
Scale of measurement of data	Nominal	Assigned a descriptive name	ABC health care center patient
	Ordinal	Assigned an order of sequence	Day of the week (Mon–Sun)
	Interval	Measured in terms of difference in standard equidistant units; Likert scale	Patrick is 3 years younger than Fred; income
	Ratio	Numerical comparison of one item to another item	Percentage of visits to a nonphysician provider; age; weight
Number of groups from which data arise	One-group	From a single group of subjects	Pretest of a questionnaire item
	Two-group	Study of two groups (experimental)	"Control" and "experimental"
	Many-group	Multigroup populations in which contrasting variables are studied against several varying group contexts	Various patient age groups who visited ABC or DEF health center
Variables	Univariate	Only one variable within the population	Age only, NP/EstPt only, etc.
	Bivariate	Contain two variables	Measure relative satisfaction in two areas for each individual within the population studied
	Multivariate	Contain a variety of variables	Measure relative satisfaction in multiple areas for each individual within the population studied

Source: PRACTICAL RESEARCH, PLANNING, AND DESIGN, by Leedy, © 1997. Adapted by permission of Prentice-Hall, Inc., Upper Saddle River, NJ.

data file, together with the data, so that you can refer back to the source document (survey) at any time to make corrections or to simply inspect it, if necessary. This can be accomplished either by hand or with the use of a consecutive number stamp. This is particularly important if more than one person is accountable for data handling.

• Sight edit each completed questionnaire to determine if it is acceptable for processing and to make any corrections or notations that may be necessary. The first aspect to be examined is completeness. Some questionnaires may not be filled in at all (especially true with mail surveys), or there may be a handwritten comment provided by the "respondent"; this should be recorded so as to gain an understanding of reasons for failure to cooperate. Aside from that, these surveys can be eliminated from those to be processed, or tallied.

Each questionnaire that appears to be complete at a glance should be inspected carefully. Each page and section should be checked to see that the respondent followed instructions and recorded responses in the proper place. Criteria should be established as to when a particular survey questionnaire is to be considered "acceptable." This is particularly important if more than one person is sight editing because you do not wish to introduce the variability of individual judgments.

You may wish to form three general "stacks" of returned surveys: those that are obvious rejects, those that present with questionable acceptability, and those that are clearly acceptable. This affords the researcher with the opportunity to examine the questionable surveys and make an informed decision whether or not to use those source documents.

Some data may be missing from survey to survey; this should not be cause for rejection. On the other hand, if entire sections are left blank, or the respondent has completed only the beginning portion, such surveys must be rejected.

If a respondent has mistakenly recorded answers where there should not be any, the superfluous data should be marked out by the sight editor.

• Postcode all of your source documents. This consists of assigning a code value to any response that does not already have such a code. For example, a particular question may offer multiple response categories, followed by an "other" category and a note to specify what other response. Because the variety of possible other responses could not be anticipated and precoded, each such response must be postcoded so they can be transferred to the data file for processing.

Often, postcoding can be performed at the same time as the sight editing. A separate postcoding notebook should be maintained to enter all new codes for the answers that have none, along with the actual response and the assigned code value. There must be a code list for each survey item that may require postcoding.

If a survey question asks, "What city do you live in: [1] Anaheim, [2] Sutton Coldfield, [3] London, [4] Brea, and [5] other?, there may be an instruction to specify what other is included with the item. Then, when the sight editor sees the "other" checked and "Villa Park" written in, the editor would check the code notebook for that item to see if that city had already been encountered and recorded with a code on the code list. If not, the editor would assign the next code value, in sequence, to that answer and record the value and the words "Villa Park."

The objective of the coding process is to provide a *unique* code for each acceptable answer. Failure to list a new code and category in the code notebook is the most common and detrimental error made when postcoding new questionnaires.

- Transfer the questionnaire data to a file to be tabulated and/or processed. This consists of reading the codes for each item and then either hand tabulating or computer processing the data. If the information is to be hand tabulated, then the codes on the questionnaires must be recorded on specially designed summary sheets before the actual tabulation process can begin.

On the other hand, if a computer is to be used, the data need to be transferred from the source documents to the computer file using your preferred (and predetermined) recording format. This recording format can vary in sophistication depending on the computer application being used. Several common applications include, but are not limited to, the following:

1. *Spreadsheet program, such as Microsoft's EXCEL or Lotus 1 2 3:* Setup for this approach requires that a separate spreadsheet cell be assigned to each questionnaire item of every completed survey. Transfer of source document data is best accomplished by establishing a separately numbered column for each survey with a separately numbered row for each survey item. Then, using the computer keyboard's numeric keypad, each survey item's numeric "value" can be entered followed by depression of the "enter" key. This automatically places the cursor in the cell assigned

to the next survey item, ready for data entry. Average "scores" can easily be computed for each survey item of all the surveys recorded. Then, this can be used as the basis of any desired frequency tables or graphic presentation of the data, such as pie charts or bar graphs needed to communicate information during the reporting process.

2. *Manual input into a statistical software program, such as SPSS from SPSS, Inc. or SAS, which is a statistical analysis system:* The accuracy of manually keyed-in data can be "verified" by having them keyed in twice. The second entry is done to compare with the first—making sure they are identical. This process assumes that data entry personnel will rarely make precisely the same mistake in precisely the same place in the file. Because this almost doubles the cost and time requirements for data entry, it is typically reserved for those instances when there is a serious need for a high degree of accuracy. A more cost-efficient means of checking accuracy is to "spot check" several source documents randomly against the data entered in the file. If few or no errors are detected, there is no need to alter the file. If, however, many errors are noted, it would be best to verify the file or create a new one using more accurate data entry personnel.

3. *Computer input via scanning technology automates the data entry process:* This may be in the form of *optical character recognition* (OCR), *optical mark recognition,* or *intelligent character recognition* (ICR). In this case, the questionnaire is usually precoded, and the appropriate codes are marked by the respondent. The completed questionnaire pages are fed directly into an electronic scanner that "reads" the codes directly from the questionnaire and stores them in the computer. When this methodology is anticipated during the questionnaire design phase, "alignment marks" need to be printed in various margin locations throughout the questionnaire to ensure accuracy of document position during scanning.

When an outside agency is charged with data transfer, tabulation, and reporting, it is essential that you indicate specifically how this is to be done.

METHODS OF SUMMARIZING AND DISPLAYING DATA

The raw data that are collected are typically in the form of pages of numbers or questionnaire responses. This, in itself, is fairly meaningless. It is how you display the data that affects the ease of highlighting your organization's service quality strengths and weaknesses. In order for data to be interpreted, they must first be summarized. The three main methods used to describe and present summarized data are tables, graphics, and statistics.

Tables are commonly used in patient satisfaction survey research to report the absolute (actual number) or relative (percentage) quantity of respondents who respond to specific survey questionnaire items in a defined way. Table 7–2 shows an example of a relative frequency table depicting specific response items on the patient satisfaction survey conducted at Friendly Hills HealthCare Network in 1996.

When tables are used within the context of a research report, they should be edited/condensed versions of those generated by computations. Only the relevant values and entries should be included. In order to develop clear, easily comprehensible tables, several guidelines were developed by Alreck and Settle (1985, p. 371).

Table 7–2 Relative (%) Frequency Table—Patient Satisfaction Survey Responses

Attribute Measured	Staff Member Referenced	% Responding "Good," "Very Good," "Excellent"
Friendliness and courtesy	Health care provider	92.5
	Nursing staff	91.8
	Receptionist	87.7
Respect shown to you by . . .	Health care provider	93.1
	Nursing staff	92.6
	Receptionist	88.3
Personal concern shown by . . .	Health care provider	90.7
	Nursing staff	89.9
	Receptionist	83.1
Explanation of medical problem	Health care provider	88.0
Explanation of required procedures/lab tests	Health care provider	88.9
Explanation of prescribed medications	Health care provider	89.0
Communication with staff	Health care provider	88.9
Willingness to listen	Health care provider	88.3

- Name each table with a consecutive number or letter, preferably not with Roman numerals.
- Title each table with a brief description of exactly what is contained in the body of the table.
- Label rows, columns, and sections with meaningful words, rather than codes that are labeled below.
- Use a standard format when possible, so that many tables are quickly recognized once the first is understood.
- Use space and distance effectively to show relationships or provide identification.
- Keep similar content in the same columns, rows, or sections, using space to separate distinct content.
- Allow sufficient "white space" and do not contain too much information in one table or make it too dense.
- Use vertical, rather than horizontal, pages whenever possible, even if more tables are needed.
- Remember, each table should virtually "stand alone," so that it is meaningful without reference to text.
- Always try to keep it clean and simple.

Several common formats are used to represent data summaries graphically. If you wish to demonstrate how a total quantity is divided into different categories, the best type of diagram is a *pie chart* (Figure 7–1). In a pie chart, each category is represented by a wedge in the pie.

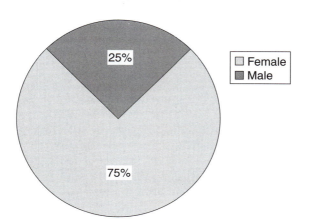

Figure 7–1 Relative Frequency of Male/Female Survey Respondents

The angular size of each wedge is proportional to the fraction of the total that belongs to that category. That is, each sector will vary according to the relative frequency of each category. For example, if 25% of the data falls into a particular category (say male respondents), then 25% of the pie chart should be marked accordingly. Think of the pie graph as a circle with 360°; the respective segment of the pie graph should measure 90° (25% of 360°). Relative frequencies are found by dividing the actual frequency by the total of the frequencies.

If you wish to demonstrate a comparison of the size of one category with that of each of the others, then a bar chart is the best choice. More specifically, a bar chart should be used when

- You have many categories or discontinuous x values to present (i.e., responses to multiple choice questions) where the profile or distribution of your x values is of interest. For example, responses to a multiple-choice question may range from "very good" to "very bad," with three or more categories in between. The distribution of these responses can be seen most readily from a bar chart.
- You need to show a lot of information on one chart. Stacked and multiple bar charts are used for this purpose.
- The data to be presented are relatively straightforward.

Figure 7–2 demonstrates the use of a bar chart to compare survey responses to a variety of provider job satisfaction categories.

An extensive bar chart (Figure 7–3) was used to display the composite Friendly Hills HealthCare Network patient satisfaction scores. This chart represents all satisfaction perception items contained on the survey conducted in 1996. Due to the massive amount of data represented, a separate key was developed for interpretation (Exhibit 7–1).

DATA ANALYSIS

Analysis of data involves the transformation of raw data into a form that will make these data easy to understand and to interpret. It is the rearranging, ordering, and manipulation of the data to provide descriptive information. Describing responses or observations is usually the initial stage of analysis. The process of data analysis can range from examining percentage changes to applying sophisticated statistical techniques. The reasons for the analysis and the interests of the intended audience both play an important role in selecting the analysis method. Most audiences will have little difficulty understanding goals that include increasing the percentage of "excellent" ratings received

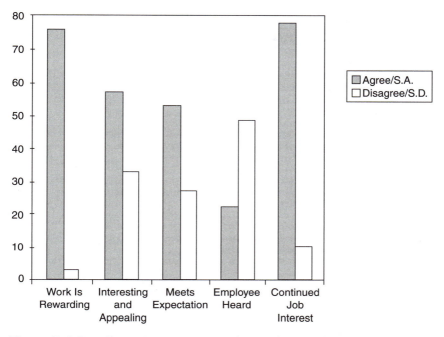

Figure 7–2 Bar Chart Comparing Satisfaction/Dissatisfaction with Five Attributes of Employee Satisfaction. Courtesy of Friendly Hills HealthCare Network.

on the "overall satisfaction" component of patient satisfaction surveys. Management, on the other hand, requires much more "actionable data," containing a high degree of specificity that can serve to drive future improvement efforts.

Hinton and Schaeffer discussed several "red flags" in analyzing data (1994, p. 52).

- *You can't make the data answer a question that you didn't ask:* Don't make assumptions about patient satisfaction perceptions based on responses to survey questions that are unrelated to what you decide after the fact you would like to know.
- *Don't "force fit" data or stretch research results to prove a point:* Tell the story the way the data tell it. Once you begin tampering with the integrity of the information you transmit, all the information you transmit is at risk, as well as your integrity as the researcher.

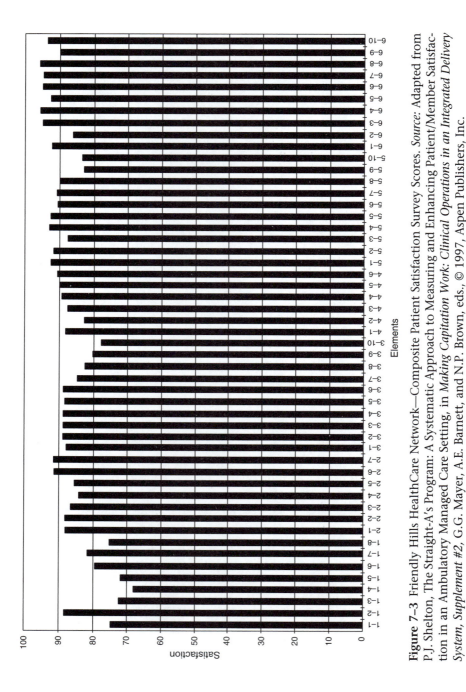

Figure 7–3 Friendly Hills HealthCare Network—Composite Patient Satisfaction Survey Scores. *Source:* Adapted from P.J. Shelton, The Straight-A's Program: A Systematic Approach to Measuring and Enhancing Patient/Member Satisfaction in an Ambulatory Managed Care Setting, in *Making Capitation Work: Clinical Operations in an Integrated Delivery System, Supplement #2*, G.G. Mayer, A.E. Barnett, and N.P. Brown, eds., © 1997, Aspen Publishers, Inc.

Exhibit 7–1 Patient Satisfaction Elements: Key to Figure 7–3

Friendly Hills HealthCare Network
Patient Satisfaction Survey
Chart Titles: Elements

Access: Arranging For & Getting Health Care
1-1   Ease of scheduling appointments by phone
1-2   Ease of scheduling appointments in person
1-3   Length of time you waited before you could see your health care provider
1-4   Amount of time waiting in reception room
1-5   Amount of time waiting in exam room before seeing your health care provider
1-6   Access to medical care in an emergency
1-7   Ease of seeing health care provider of your choice
1-8   Ease of getting medical information using the telephone advice system

Convenience
2-1   Location of the health care center you visited
2-2   Hours of the health care center you visited
2-3   Parking at the health care center
2-4   Services for getting prescriptions filled
2-5   Getting prescriptions refilled
2-6   Getting laboratory work done when ordered by your provider
2-7   Getting X-rays that your provider ordered

Communication
3-1   Health care provider's explanation of your medical problem
3-2   Health care provider's explanation of required medical procedures and/or lab tests
3-3   Explanation of prescribed medicine(s)
3-4   Communication between provider and staff
3-5   Willingness of the health care provider to listen
3-6   Explanation of any required consents
3-7   Education about ways to manage your current health problem
3-8   Education about ways to avoid illness
3-9   Availability of educational programs that teach healthier living
3-10 Reminders to use preventive services

Quality of Health Care You Received
4-1   Thoroughness of the health care provider's exam
4-2   Amount of time health care provider spent with you

continues

Exhibit 7–1 continued

4-3   Thoroughness of medical treatment received
4-4   How well health care provider and nursing staff work as a team to serve your health needs
4-5   Overall quality of care from health care provider
4-6   Overall quality of care from nursing staff

Personal Caring
5-1   Friendliness and courtesy shown by health care provider
5-2   Friendliness and courtesy shown by nursing staff
5-3   Friendliness and courtesy shown by receptionist
5-4   Respect shown to you by health care provider
5-5   Respect shown to you by nursing staff
5-6   Respect shown to you by receptionist
5-7   Personal concern shown by health care provider
5-8   Personal concern shown by the nursing staff
5-9   Personal concern shown by receptionist
5-10 Telephone courtesy when calling health center

Friendly Hills HealthCare Center Facility
6-1   Overall outside appearance of the health center
6-2   Appearance of signs on the outside of the building
6-3   Cleanliness of the reception area
6-4   Cleanliness of the treatment area
6-5   Comfort of the indoor temperature
6-6   Neatness of the reception room
6-7   Neatness of the receptionist's work area
6-8   Neatness of the treatment area
6-9   Noise level (quietness) in the office
6-10 Air quality (freshness) in the health care center

Courtesy of Friendly Hills HealthCare Network.

- *Be sure that the person who uses or attempts to use sophisticated analysis techniques understands the power and limitations of those techniques:* If your organization does not have in-house capabilities for the application of statistical analytic techniques, enlist the services of a research firm or skilled consultant for this portion of your research.
- *Don't view the research on a "stand-alone" basis only. Blend it with other information:* The patient satisfaction survey results represent a

"snapshot" of patient perceptions of service quality at a given point in time. Defection data direct our attention to "fatal flaws," whereas complaint data supplement our understanding of dissatisfaction sources. But, the input of those who deal with patients on a daily basis is critically important. This helps record an ongoing "videotape" of patient expectations and perceptions of satisfaction or dissatisfaction. This dynamic information must be used in conjunction with more formalized survey research results.

When patient satisfaction survey questionnaires are designed to evaluate various operating units and various positions within those units, several analysis types can be considered. First, evaluate a particular operating unit, such as one of many departments or health care centers. Next, compare this to the "average scores" for similar operating units, departments, or health care facilities located within the same region. More specifically, a position category (i.e., receptionist, nursing staff, health care provider) within a particular department or health care center can be assessed, with the objective in mind of developing highly tailored improvement efforts that address unique local improvement needs. Second, comparisons in time allow for documentation of incremental improvements. Finally, there is the opportunity for comparing the performance of your organization to competitors' or similar noncompeting health care organizations.

The use of consultants who use standardized patient satisfaction survey instruments and consult with many health care organizations allows you to make accurate performance comparisons.

Correlation analysis can be used to determine the performance attributes that have the greatest influence on overall patient satisfaction, as discussed in Chapter 4 in the context of our relative importance index. Calculating a correlation coefficient is an option in most statistical analysis software packages (such as SAS or SPSS). The correlation coefficient is a number between +1 and -1 that indicates the degree of linear association between two variables. Large numerical values suggest a strong association. A correlation coefficient of +1 indicates a perfect positive correlation. A correlation coefficient near 0 implies little linear relationship between variables.

A positive correlation between a particular satisfaction attribute, say "health care provider's explanation of your medical condition" and "overall satisfaction," emphasizes the importance patients place on provider explanations in determining their satisfaction with your health care organization.

Generally speaking, performance attributes involving human inter-actions tend to be highly correlated with overall satisfaction. Perfor-mance attributes with lower correlations are more related to mechani-cal or "systems" aspects of the experience than to human interactions. If this proves to be true in your organization, then improvements in the human-interaction attributes should have the greatest impact on overall satisfaction.

COMMUNICATING SURVEY RESULTS THROUGHOUT THE ORGANIZATION

One of the biggest challenges facing the patient satisfaction re-searcher is converting a complex set of data to a form that can be read and understood quickly by executives, managers, and other employees who will make decisions based on the research. The goal is to commu-nicate information clearly to the right people in a timely fashion. Among considerations are the following: Who gets this information? How will they use it? When users feel confident that they understand the data, they are far more likely to apply it appropriately.

In smaller health care organizations, managers may be in constant contact with patients, thereby gaining firsthand knowledge of patient expectations and perceptions. But, in larger organizations, this is often not the case. The larger a health care organization is, the more difficult it will be for managers to interact directly with the patient, and the least firsthand information they will have about patient expectations. Therefore, they must rely on data derived directly from patients, such as the patient satisfaction survey.

Whether the patient satisfaction research was conducted in-house or by a third party, it is very important that the data are made known as soon as they are analyzed and available. Transmitting the informa-tion to those who can act on it in a timely, appropriate manner is critical. Make sure that departments or geographic areas that have done particularly well get recognition. Remember that this is patient *satisfaction*, not *dissatisfaction*. Be sure that management is aware of the jobs that have been done well and recognize those people who have done the work.

With regard to areas of dissatisfaction, discussions should be held with responsible managers as soon as possible. Ultimately, it is very important that you have all the backup data with regard to key prob-lems that have surfaced. Be sure that the responsible managers have a complete understanding of an issue prior to any "open forum" presentation of the information. They will want time to think and respond with plans for corrective action.

The skills required for communicating survey results effectively are almost as delicate and sophisticated as those involved in conducting the patient satisfaction research itself. Yet, the communication process may be no different than other types of communication in business or professional settings. Regardless of the message, the audience, or the media, a few general principles should be kept in mind.

- *The communication should be timely:* In most cases, survey results should be communicated as soon as they have been summarized and analyzed for meaning. From a practical standpoint, it may be best to delay a communication slightly until a convenient time, such as the next edition of the organization's newsletter or the next general management meeting. Several questions about the timing must be answered. Is the audience ready for the information in view of other things that may be happening within the organization? Are they expecting it? When is the best time to have the maximum impact on the audience?
- *The communication should be targeted to specific audiences:* The communication will be more efficient when it is designed for a particular group. The message can be specifically tailored to the interests, needs, and expectations of the group.
- *The media should be carefully selected:* For particular groups, some media may be more effective than others. Face-to-face meetings may be better than special bulletins. A memo to top management may be more effective than the health care organization's newspaper. The proper selection of a communication method can help improve the effectiveness of the process.

One of the most important target audiences is top management. These individuals are responsible for the allocation of resources for patient satisfaction improvement efforts such as training, systems reengineering, and facilities remodeling. At Friendly Hills HealthCare network, we used the existing format of a monthly leadership meeting to disseminate patient satisfaction survey results—this involved managers, directors, vice-presidents, and senior vice-presidents, along with the chief operating officer and chief executive officer (CEO). This monthly meeting was a cultural tradition throughout the organization and was held in a large auditorium and videoconferenced out to five separate locations representing the various Southern California regions where multiple health care centers were located. The information depicting networkwide patient satisfaction levels was copresented by the CEO, Albert Barnett, and myself. We chose to approach the presentation to leadership as a measurement of organizational alignment with the Friendly Hills HealthCare Network mission: "To provide comprehensive, quality health care in a spirit of personal caring." The following overhead transparencies (Figures 7–4, 7–5, 7–6, 7–7, and 7–8) were among those used for the presentation.

Assuming that your health care organization has defined values and a mission statement in place that the staff (both professional and ancillary) are familiar with, presenting your findings in this context is worth considering. This way, you are essentially asking and answering the question, "How are we doing in the eyes of our patients?" If the entire organization is aware of and aligned with your mission, this offers a familiar foundation on which to build plans for future improvement.

The next step in communicating Friendly Hills HealthCare Network's composite survey results involved publishing key results in the organization's newsletter for review by employees at all levels. The

"QUALITY OF HEALTH CARE YOU RECEIVED"*

Thoroughness of HC provider's exam	88.2%
Amount of time HC provider spent with you	82.8%
Thoroughness of medical treatment received	87.8%
How well HC provider & nursing staff work as a team to serve your health care needs	89.3%
Overall quality of care from health care provider	90.0%
Overall quality of care from nursing staff	90.7%

* % responding "good," "very good" or "excellent"

Figure 7–4 Friendly Hills HealthCare Network 1996 Patient Satisfaction Survey Results. *Source:* Adapted from P.J. Shelton, The Straight-A's Program: A Systematic Approach to Measuring and Enhancing Patient/Member Satisfaction in an Ambulatory Managed Care Setting, in *Making Capitation Work: Clinical Operations in an Integrated Delivery System, Supplement #2,* G.G. Mayer, A.E. Barnett, and N.P. Brown, eds., © 1997, Aspen Publishers, Inc.

"PERSONAL CARING"*

Friendliness & courtesy shown by:	• Health care provider	92.5%
	• Nursing staff	91.8%
	• Receptionist	87.7%
Respect shown to you by:	• Health care provider	93.1%
	• Nursing staff	92.6%
	• Receptionist	88.3%
Personal concern shown by:	• Health care provider	90.7%
	• Nursing staff	89.9%
	• Receptionist	83.1%

* % responding "good," "very good" or "excellent"

Figure 7–5 Friendly Hills HealthCare Network 1996 Patient Satisfaction Survey Results. *Source:* Adapted from P.J. Shelton, The Straight-A's Program: A Systematic Approach to Measuring and Enhancing Patient/Member Satisfaction in an Ambulatory Managed Care Setting, in *Making Capitation Work: Clinical Operations in an Integrated Delivery System, Supplement #2,* G.G. Mayer, A.E. Barnett, and N.P. Brown, eds., © 1997, Aspen Publishers, Inc.

"OVERALL SATISFACTION WITH F.H.H.N."

"SATISFIED"	• Completely satisfied	22.2%
	• Very satisfied	45.0%
	• Somewhat satisfied	19.7%
"NEITHER SATISFIED OR DISSATISFIED"		3.0%
"DISSATISFIED"	• Somewhat dissatisfied	6.3%
	• Very dissatisfied	2.6%
	• Completely dissatisfied	1.2%

Figure 7–6 Friendly Hills HealthCare Network 1996 Patient Satisfaction Survey Results. *Source:* Adapted from P.J. Shelton, The Straight-A's Program: A Systematic Approach to Measuring and Enhancing Patient/Member Satisfaction in an Ambulatory Managed Care Setting, in *Making Capitation Work: Clinical Operations in an Integrated Delivery System, Supplement #2,* G.G. Mayer, A.E. Barnett, and N.P. Brown, eds., © 1997, Aspen Publishers, Inc.

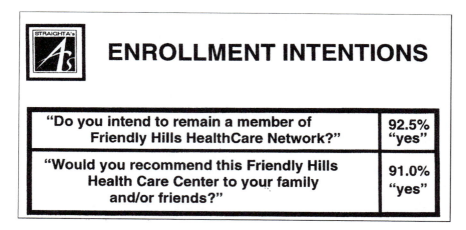

Figure 7–7 Friendly Hills HealthCare Network 1996 Patient Satisfaction Survey Results. *Source:* Adapted from P.J. Shelton, The Straight-A's Program: A Systematic Approach to Measuring and Enhancing Patient/Member Satisfaction in an Ambulatory Managed Care Setting, in *Making Capitation Work: Clinical Operations in an Integrated Delivery System, Supplement #2*, G.G. Mayer, A.E. Barnett, and N.P. Brown, eds., © 1997, Aspen Publishers, Inc.

NETWORK IMPROVEMENT PRIORITIES

1. **Access to emergency medical care**
2. **Preventive service reminders**
3. **Waiting time in exam room**
4. **Education to avoid illness**
5. **Waiting time in reception room**

Figure 7–8 Friendly Hills HealthCare Network Composite Improvement Priorities—1996. *Source:* Adapted from P.J. Shelton, The Straight-A's Program: A Systematic Approach to Measuring and Enhancing Patient/Member Satisfaction in an Ambulatory Managed Care Setting, in *Making Capitation Work: Clinical Operations in an Integrated Delivery System, Supplement #2*, G.G. Mayer, A.E. Barnett, and N.P. Brown, eds., © 1997, Aspen Publishers, Inc.

entire survey process was explained so readers could appreciate the origin of our data. This was also an ideal opportunity to inform them that data specific to their health care center or department would be forthcoming to respective regional directors and health care center supervisors. This was important because there were significant differences in patient satisfaction levels (and therefore improvement priorities) at each health care center. Thus, outstanding performance could be recognized and improvements relating to weaknesses in areas important to patients could be planned for.

All health-care-center-specific data were then provided as outlined above and local leadership was asked to combine this information with their own observations and develop a plan for improving areas identified as "weak" at their facility. Because the patient satisfaction survey instrument was designed to be department-specific, position-specific, and even provider-specific, the process of identifying "opportunities for improvement" was supported.

The results of your organization's patient satisfaction surveys (in-house or contracted out) should be communicated to third-party payers on a regular basis. This is important because they are already probably monitoring patient satisfaction on their own. If contractual payment levels are in any way correlated with the ratings on patient satisfaction surveys, it can be helpful to challenge their data with your own credibly obtained, valid, and reliable data—particularly if you can demonstrate significant rating improvements.

The next chapter will examine the processes involved with identifying, categorizing, and prioritizing service quality improvements in your organization.

CONCLUSION

The collection of patient satisfaction survey data begins with the sequential "handling" of completed questionnaires ("source documents"), from initial receipt and inspection through editing, coding, and data transfer ("entry"), and ends with tabulation, which provides summary figures. Tabulation can be done manually onto specially designed summary sheets, partially automated by inputting the information directly into a spreadsheet or statistical software program, or wholly automated by using OCR or ICR scanning technology.

These figures—the so-called "raw data"—then need to be described and summarized using tables, graphics, and statistics. This process is extremely important because the manner in which you display data affects the ease of highlighting your organization's service quality strengths and weaknesses. One of the biggest challenges facing the patient satisfaction researcher is converting a complex set of data to a form that can be read and understood quickly by executives, managers, and others who will make decisions based on the research. Analysis of these data involves rearranging, ordering, and manipulating to provide descriptive information. This process can range from examining percentage changes to applying sophisticated statistical techniques—all aimed at making the data "actionable" rather than "dust-collecting."

Communication of this information organizationwide needs to be timely and targeted to specific organizational audiences, using the most appropriate media. One helpful approach involves the arrangement of information so that it functions as a measurement of alignment with the organization's established vision, values, and mission. This is particularly valuable if these are solidly embedded within the culture of the organization. This offers a familiar foundation on which to build plans for improvement.

ACTION STEPS

1. For each patient feedback mechanism you currently have in place, list the sequential steps by which the resulting data are being managed.
2. List the methods your organization uses to display patient satisfaction research data. Assess each method in terms of "ease of understanding," "value for making improvement decisions," and "ability to reflect current patient perceptions."
3. Summarize how patient satisfaction data are analyzed in your organization. What, if any, mechanisms are in place to make sure that the analyzed data convert to action? How would you develop or improve this to produce more rapid improvement?
4. List the ways that patient satisfaction feedback data are communicated throughout your organization.

REFERENCES

Alreck, P.L., & Settle, R.B. (1985). *The survey research handbook*. Homewood, IL: Irwin.

Hinton, T., & Schaeffer, W. (1994). *Customer-focused quality: What to do on Monday morning*. Englewood Cliffs, NJ: Prentice Hall.

SUGGESTED READING

Albrecht, K., & Bradford, L.J. (1990). *The service advantage: How to identify and fulfill customer needs.* Homewood, IL: Dow Jones-Irwin.

Breen, G., & Blankenship, A.B. (1982). *Do-it-yourself marketing research* (2nd ed.). London: McGraw-Hill.

Buell, V.P. (Ed.). (1986). *Handbook of modern marketing* (2nd ed.). New York: McGraw-Hill.

Chang, R.Y. (1994). *Building a dynamic team: A practical guide to maximizing team performance.* Irvine, CA: Richard Chang Associates.

Costello, S.J. (1994). *Managing change in the workplace.* New York: Irwin Professional.

Crouch, S., & Housden, M. (1998). *Marketing research for managers* (2nd ed.). Oxford, England: Butterworth-Heinemann.

Dillon, W.R., Madden, T.J., & Firtle, N. (1990). *Marketing research in a marketing environment* (2nd ed.). Homewood, IL: Irwin.

Dutka, A. (1994). *AMA handbook for customer satisfaction: A complete guide to research, planning & implementation.* Lincolnwood, IL: NTC Business Books.

George, S., & Weimerskirch, A. (1994). *Total quality management: Strategies and techniques proven at today's most successful companies.* New York: John Wiley & Sons.

Leedy, P.D. (1993). *Practical research planning and design* (5th ed.). New York: Macmillan.

Martin, P., & Pierce, R. (1994). *Practical statistics for the health sciences.* South Melbourne, Australia: Nelson.

Mayer, G.G., Barnett, A., & Brown, N. (1997). *Making capitation work: Clinical operations in an integrated delivery system.* Gaithersburg, MD: Aspen.

Phillips, J.J. (1991). *Handbook of training evaluation and measurement methods* (2nd ed.). Houston, TX: Gulf.

Phipps, R., & Simmons, C. (1998). *Understanding customers 1998–99: CIM workbook.* Oxford, England: Butterworth-Heinemann.

Stamatis, D.H. (1996). *Total quality service: Principles, practices, and implementation.* Delray Beach, FL: St. Lucie Press.

Thomas, J.R., & Nelson, J.K. (1990). *Research methods in physical activity* (2nd ed.). Champaign, IL: Human Kinetics.

Woodruff, R.B., & Gardial, S.F. (1996). *Know your customer: New approaches to understanding customer value and satisfaction.* Oxford, England: Blackwell.

Zeithaml, V.A., & Bitner, M.J. (1996). *Services marketing.* London: McGraw-Hill.

CHAPTER 8

Identifying and Prioritizing Service Quality Improvement Needs

Improving service quality in ways that increase patient satisfaction and loyalty is the primary objective of satisfaction/loyalty research in any health care organization. Recognized gaps in service delivery between patient expectations and actual experience set the stage for dissatisfaction. The gap may be related to a "sick" system or process, substandard staff performance, or the failure of senior management to allocate sufficient resources to keep equipment and facilities well maintained. Regardless of cause, appropriate measures for closing the gap must be given priority if a health care organization is to survive in today's competitive marketplace.

GATHERING INPUT FROM EXTERNAL AND INTERNAL CUSTOMERS

Service quality improvement involves such activities as resolving performance problems, reengineering service delivery systems/processes, renewing senior management commitment to service excellence, and providing frontline employee vigilance for performance improvement opportunities. The success of improvement efforts is contingent on having mechanisms in place for obtaining (and responding to) both external and internal customer input. External "customers" provide important insights that assist with the identification and prioritization of improvement needs. These include, but are not limited to, the following:

- *Patients:* These people provide satisfaction survey responses, they may complain when things go wrong, and they tend to use the health care organization's grievance procedures when they feel they have been "victimized" by the system. The ultimate patient feedback consists of determining the nature of so-called "fatal flaws" that lead to their defection or disenrollment from your health care organization—they "vote with their feet."

- *Family members of patients:* Often, these people are in a much better (i.e., more objective) overall position to observe various aspects of the patient's health care experience. They form impressions, opinions, and attitudes that, in turn, influence the perceptions of the patient they are accompanying as well as drive their own future behaviors.
- *Third-party payers:* Because their competitive survival relies on satisfied customers, you can bet that these people will be gathering patient satisfaction data of their own. In their quest to sustain favorable relationships with contracted providers and organizations, they will surely share identified service quality strengths and weaknesses with you.
- *Employers contracting for employee health care benefits:* Proactive employers regularly monitor employee satisfaction. A reputation for providing high-quality health care as part of the compensation package can both heighten employee morale and strengthen organizational recruitment capability.
- *Accrediting agencies:* As discussed in Chapter 1, both the National Committee for Quality Assurance (NCQA) and the Joint Commission on Accreditation of Healthcare Organizations (Joint Commission) require health care organizations to measure and sustain acceptable levels of patient satisfaction. Providing accreditation applicants with a standardized patient satisfaction survey instrument is quite helpful. This forms a framework for performance improvement that can facilitate the continuous improvement efforts of any health care organization.
- *Regulatory agencies:* With an ever-increasing elderly population in the United States, the federal government pays close attention to the quality of care provided to Medicare recipients. On the state level, such departments as the Department of Corporations want assurance that appropriate grievance procedures and other operational activities serve all components of the respective geographic population. Therefore, providing special service modifications for the elderly and the indigent has become the norm.

In addition to the extremely important input of external customers, it is vital that health care organizations turn to their internal customers to help identify opportunities for improvement. These are the folks who encounter patients firsthand on a daily basis, including both medical and "nonmedical" personnel. Medical internal customers would include, but are not limited to, the following:

- *Health care providers:* These include physicians (MDs, DOs, DPMs), nurse practitioners, physician assistants, and nonphysician providers (such as optometrists, chiropractors, physical therapists, etc.). Today's health care consumer is more likely to voice his or her opinion of an organizational service quality deficit to the provider.
- *Nursing staff:* These include registered nurses (RNs) and licensed vocational ("practical"—midwest/eastern United States) nurses (LVNs or LPNs).
- *Medical assistants:* These are people who perform a variety of direct patient contact activities that are commonly delegated to them by providers and/or nurses. As such, they are in a position to hear of the special service quality concerns of patients firsthand. In an ambulatory setting, medical assistants are often viewed by patients as part of the nursing team.
- *Specialty services:* These are people who patients come in contact with, including laboratory personnel (e.g., phlebotomists), radiology technicians, pharmacists, and ancillary pharmacy personnel. All of these supportive services see patients in special circumstances that complement and support their clinical treatment. When patients encounter difficulty in accessing (finding or scheduling) these services, they are likely to share their frustration with the staff member. These people, in turn, can be a valuable resource for feedback related to patient perceptions of their special service.
- *Member services or customer relations managers:* These individuals receive direct patient feedback on a daily basis. Regularly gathering feedback from both frontline employees and supervisors can be a valuable source of up-to-the-minute satisfaction information.

Nonmedical internal customers who are in contact with patients on a daily basis, and therefore are in a position to spot opportunities for improved service quality, include, but are not limited to, the following:

- *Frontline personnel:* Receptionists, appointment secretaries, and volunteers are frequently in a position to have patients talk freely with them about their concerns, interests, and needs. Because patients are far less likely to be intimidated by these people, they may hear patient concerns that are not expressed in the presence of other medical or nonmedical personnel.

- *Management:* Many organizations insist that managers, directors, regional directors, and senior management alike spend a minimum number of hours per month in direct patient contact to remain in touch with their special needs and concerns. If your organization does not currently do this, it would be worthwhile to consider it. No amount of secondhand information in any format can replace the observational value of firsthand patient contact.

This chapter will present a framework within which the reader can identify and prioritize patient satisfaction enhancement activities. First, the all-important patient input in the form of survey responses (calculating the "dissatisfaction index" [DI] and "improvement priority index" [IPI]), complaints, grievances filed, and "defections" will be discussed. Then, improvement feedback available from patient family members, third-party payers, and contracted employers will be presented. Next, attention will be directed toward the improvement influences of accrediting agencies. And finally, the valuable input provided by internal customers such as frontline medical, nonmedical, and management personnel will be presented.

Patient Input for Determining Improvement Needs

Niles and colleagues emphasized the use of patient satisfaction data to improve the quality of patient care (1996). The lessons learned in this research include the following:

- Industry-based management principles of customer-centeredness can be adapted to the health care environment as a quality improvement strategy.
- Health care providers and other workers react positively to patient feedback data clearly connected to a patient experience in which they are involved.
- Linking a patient-based quality measurement tool to the process of care increases its usefulness in diagnosing quality problems, motivating staff, and focusing improvement efforts while limiting its value for benchmarking (because the process may differ between organizations).

Furthermore, it was felt that, by mapping the process of care from the patient's viewpoint, a more complete "diagnosis" of the source of quality problem can be made, "enabling substantially more focused improvement efforts."

The Quantitative Approach (Survey-Based) to Improvement Prioritization

Recall from Chapter 4 that one of the data types derived from the patient satisfaction survey response is the so-called DI. This is derived by calculating the percentage of respondents who expressed dissatisfaction (Likert-scaled responses of "fair" or "poor" in a quality-rating item, "disagree" or "strongly disagree" in a positively phrased statement, "agree" or "strongly agree" in a negatively phrased survey item) on a given survey item. Note that this is not simply the arithmetic difference between "100" and the percentage of survey responses to a given item indicating satisfaction (Likert-scaled responses of "very good" or "excellent," etc.). This is an important distinction because a number of respondents may have selected a neutral response such as "neutral," "no opinion," or "not applicable."

Furthermore, based on our focus group research using response-keypad technology, we were able to determine the relative importance of the various determinants of patient satisfaction in three distinct age groups. This afforded the development of a unique age-adjusted relative importance index (RII) for each health care center facility, whereby the elements of satisfaction within each satisfaction category (access, convenience, communication, perceived quality of health care received, personal caring, and health care facilities/equipment) could be ranked according to their relative importance to patients in determining their satisfaction. In Figures 8–1 through 8–8 (reprints of Figures 4–1 through 4–6 and Figures 6–2 through 6–7), we can see that differences in relative importance among satisfaction elements and among indicators of each element do occur between the three age groups.

From the data in Figure 8–1, we can see that the order of most to least important overall, based on the average of the three age groups for the satisfaction element "ease of scheduling appointments by phone," is as follows:

- 90.8 = "speak with live person"
- 85.0 = "minimal 'on hold' time"
- 83.1 = "staff helpfulness on phone"
- 73.4 = "multiple day/time offers"
- 66.5 = "total time required to make appointment"
- 54.1 = "number of rings of phone"

This is with an *overall importance score* within the satisfaction category of "access" of 75.5.

Category: Access
Element: Ease of Scheduling Appointments by Phone
INDICATORS

	IMPORTANCE (by Age Group)			
	20 to 44	45 to 64	65 and up	Total
Number of rings of phone	50.0	64.1	48.2	54.1
Speak with live person	80.4	93.8	98.2	90.8
Minimal "on hold" time	80.4	89.1	85.7	85.0
Staff helpfulness on phone	89.3	79.7	80.4	83.1
Multiple day/time offers	69.6	70.3	80.4	73.4
Total time required to make appt.	64.3	65.6	69.6	66.5
AVERAGE:	72.3	77.1	77.1	75.5

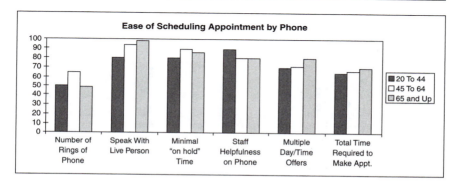

Figure 8–1 Relative Importance of Various Indicators of the "Ease of Scheduling Appointments by Phone" Patient Satisfaction Element. *Source:* Adapted from P.J. Shelton, The Straight-A's Program: A Systematic Approach to Measuring and Enhancing Patient/Member Satisfaction in an Ambulatory Managed Care Setting, in *Making Capitation Work: Clinical Operations in an Integrated Delivery System, Supplement #2,* G.G. Mayer, A.E. Barnett, and N.P. Brown, eds., © 1997, Aspen Publishers, Inc.

The order of most to least important overall, based on the average of the three age groups for the satisfaction element "ease of scheduling appointments in person," is as follows:

- 70.4 = "minimal wait to speak with scheduler"
- 69.6 = "written verification of appointment time"
- 67.1 = "convenient location of scheduler"
- 54.9 = "total time spent with scheduler"

This is with an *overall importance score* within the satisfaction category of "access" of 65.5.

Category: Access
Element: Ease of Scheduling Appointments in Person
INDICATORS

	IMPORTANCE (by Age Group)			
	20 to 44	45 to 64	65 and up	Total
Convenient location of scheduler	58.9	65.6	76.8	67.1
Minimal wait to speak with scheduler	62.5	71.9	76.8	70.4
Total time spent with scheduler	46.4	59.4	58.9	54.9
Written verification of appt. time	53.6	76.6	78.6	69.6
AVERAGE:	55.4	68.4	72.8	65.5

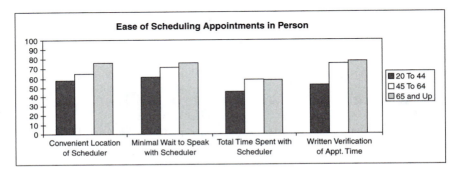

Figure 8–2 Relative Importance of Various Indicators of the "Ease of Scheduling Appointments in Person" Patient Satisfaction Element. *Source:* Adapted from P.J. Shelton, The Straight-A's Program: A Systematic Approach to Measuring and Enhancing Patient/Member Satisfaction in an Ambulatory Managed Care Setting, in *Making Capitation Work: Clinical Operations in an Integrated Delivery System, Supplement #2*, G.G. Mayer, A.E. Barnett, and N.P. Brown, eds., © 1997, Aspen Publishers, Inc.

The order of most to least important overall, based on the average of the three age groups for the satisfaction element "wait between preferred day and visit," is as follows:

- 97.8 = "responsiveness to expressed urgency"
- 77.4 = "availability of preferred time"
- 75.4 = "nature of your visit"
- 73.8 = "availability of preferred day"

This is with an *overall importance score* within the satisfaction category of "access" of 81.1.

The order of most to least important overall, based on the average of the three age groups for the satisfaction element "time waiting in reception room," is as follows:

Category: Access
Element: Wait Between Preferred Day & Visit
INDICATORS

	IMPORTANCE (by Age Group)			
INDICATORS	20 to 44	45 to 64	65 and up	Total
Availability of preferred day	82.1	75.0	64.3	73.8
Nature of your visit	62.5	78.1	85.7	75.4
Availability of preferred time	85.7	75.0	71.4	77.4
Responsiveness to expressed urgency	100.0	96.9	96.4	97.8
AVERAGE:	82.6	81.3	79.5	81.1

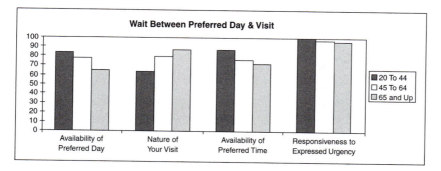

Figure 8–3 Relative Importance of Various Indicators of the "Wait Between Preferred Day and Visit" Patient Satisfaction Element. *Source:* Adapted from P.J. Shelton, The Straight-A's Program: A Systematic Approach to Measuring and Enhancing Patient/Member Satisfaction in an Ambulatory Managed Care Setting, in *Making Capitation Work: Clinical Operations in an Integrated Delivery System, Supplement #2,* G.G. Mayer, A.E. Barnett, and N.P. Brown, eds., © 1997, Aspen Publishers, Inc.

- 83.6 = "total wait time in reception room"
- 78.3 = "explanations provided for extended wait"

This is with an *overall importance score* within the satisfaction category of "access" of 81.0.

The order of most to least important overall, based on the average of the three age groups for the satisfaction element "time waiting in exam room," is as follows:

- 80.9 = "total wait time in exam room"
- 77.2 = "explanations provided for extended wait"

This is with an *overall importance score* within the satisfaction category of "access" of 79.1.

Category: Access
Element: Time Waiting in Reception Room
INDICATORS

	IMPORTANCE (by Age Group)			
	20 to 44	45 to 64	65 and up	Total
Explanations provided for extended wait	57.1	92.2	85.7	78.3
Total wait time in reception room	83.9	95.3	71.4	83.6
AVERAGE:	70.5	93.8	78.6	81.0

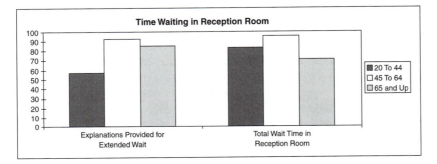

Figure 8–4 Relative Importance of Various Indicators of the "Time Waiting in Reception Room" Patient Satisfaction Element. *Source:* Adapted from P.J. Shelton, The Straight-A's Program: A Systematic Approach to Measuring and Enhancing Patient/Member Satisfaction in an Ambulatory Managed Care Setting, in *Making Capitation Work: Clinical Operations in an Integrated Delivery System, Supplement #2,* G.G. Mayer, A.E. Barnett, and N.P. Brown, eds., © 1997, Aspen Publishers, Inc.

The order of most to least important overall, based on the average of the three age groups for the satisfaction element "access to emergency medical care," is as follows:

- 90.5 = "ease of reaching care by phone"
- 83.0 = "directions provided for getting care"
- 75.9 = "transportation to emergency services"

This is with an *overall importance score* within the satisfaction category of "access" of 83.1.

The order of most to least important overall, based on the average of the three age groups for the satisfaction element "ease of seeing provider of choice," is as follows:

- 93.0 = "ability to see preferred provider type"
- 92.4 = "ability to see specific provider"

Category: Access
Element: Time Waiting in Exam Room
INDICATORS

	IMPORTANCE (by Age Group)			
	20 to 44	45 to 64	65 and up	Total
Explanations provided for extended wait	60.7	90.6	80.4	77.2
Total wait time in exam room	82.1	89.1	71.4	80.9
AVERAGE:	71.4	89.8	75.9	79.1

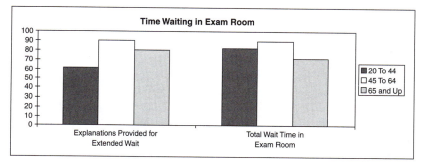

Figure 8–5 Relative Importance of Various Indicators of the "Time Waiting in Exam Room" Patient Satisfaction Element. *Source:* Adapted from P.J. Shelton, *The Straight-A's Program: A Systematic Approach to Measuring and Enhancing Patient/Member Satisfaction in an Ambulatory Managed Care Setting,* in *Making Capitation Work: Clinical Operations in an Integrated Delivery System, Supplement #2,* G.G. Mayer, A.E. Barnett, and N.P. Brown, eds., © 1997, Aspen Publishers, Inc.

This is with an *overall importance score* within the satisfaction category of "access" of 92.7.

The order of most to least important overall, based on the average of the three age groups for the satisfaction element "ease of using telephone advice system," is as follows:

- 90.8 = "knowledge level of phone nurse"
- 74.4 = "time spent on hold"
- 61.0 = "number of phone rings"

This is with an *overall importance score* within the satisfaction category of "access" of 75.4.

Now, combining all of the above information within the patient satisfaction category of "access," we can determine the RII of each named element for the combined age groups to be as follows:

- 92.7 = "ease of seeing provider of choice"
- 83.1 = "access to emergency medical care"

Category: Access
Element: Access to Emergency Medical Care
INDICATORS

	IMPORTANCE (by Age Group)			
	20 to 44	45 to 64	65 and up	Total
Ease of reaching care by phone	87.5	87.5	96.4	90.5
Directions provided for getting care	78.6	82.8	87.5	83.0
Transportation to emergency services	71.4	68.8	87.5	75.9
AVERAGE:	79.2	79.7	90.5	83.1

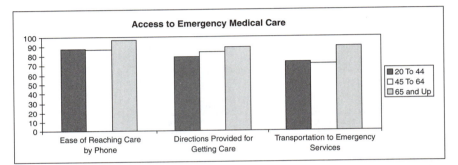

Figure 8–6 Relative Importance of Various Indicators of the "Access to Emergency Medical Care" Patient Satisfaction Element. *Source:* Adapted from P.J. Shelton, The Straight-A's Program: A Systematic Approach to Measuring and Enhancing Patient/Member Satisfaction in an Ambulatory Managed Care Setting, in *Making Capitation Work: Clinical Operations in an Integrated Delivery System, Supplement #2,* G.G. Mayer, A.E. Barnett, and N.P. Brown, eds., © 1997, Aspen Publishers, Inc.

- 81.1 = "wait between preferred day and visit"
- 81.0 = "time waiting in reception room"
- 79.1 = "time waiting in exam room"
- 75.5 = "ease of scheduling appointments by phone"
- 75.4 = "ease of using telephone advice system"
- 65.5 = "ease of scheduling appointments in person"

The next step in using your RII data consists of combining it with your DI for each item within the patient satisfaction survey category of "access." In order for you to appreciate the value of this process in determining your survey-based improvement priorities, we will take a step-by-step approach using theoretical survey data to derive our various DIs.

- Step 1. Determine the relative importance of each element of the satisfaction category "access."

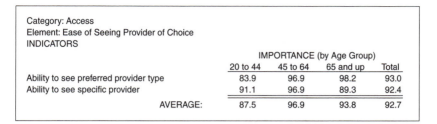

Category: Access				
Element: Ease of Seeing Provider of Choice				
INDICATORS				
	IMPORTANCE (by Age Group)			
	20 to 44	45 to 64	65 and up	Total
Ability to see preferred provider type	83.9	96.9	98.2	93.0
Ability to see specific provider	91.1	96.9	89.3	92.4
AVERAGE:	87.5	96.9	93.8	92.7

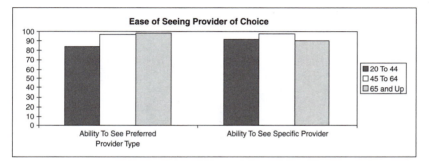

Figure 8–7 Relative Importance of Various Indicators of the "Ease of Seeing Provider of Choice" Patient Satisfaction Element. *Source:* Adapted from P.J. Shelton, The Straight-A's Program: A Systematic Approach to Measuring and Enhancing Patient/Member Satisfaction in an Ambulatory Managed Care Setting, in *Making Capitation Work: Clinical Operations in an Integrated Delivery System, Supplement #2*, G.G. Mayer, A.E. Barnett, and N.P. Brown, eds., © 1997, Aspen Publishers, Inc.

You may use any of a number of patient-centered techniques to determine this. See Chapter 4 for a detailed description of the quantitative focus group process used at Friendly Hills HealthCare Network. It is necessary to convert each importance ranking into an arbitrary number such that the highest rank (i.e., considered most important) is the largest number.

• Step 2. Define "dissatisfaction" for the purposes of your organization's patient satisfaction survey research.

If the patient satisfaction survey response format you are using is based on a Likert scale (excellent...very good...good...fair...poor...does not apply or strongly agree...agree...neutral...disagree...strongly disagree), then you may choose the "bottom two boxes" to represent "dissatisfied" so that the DI for each item of your survey is calculated by adding the total number of "fair" responses to the total number of "poor" responses and dividing

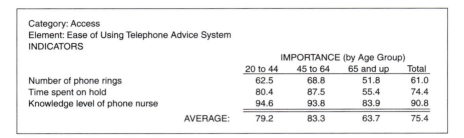

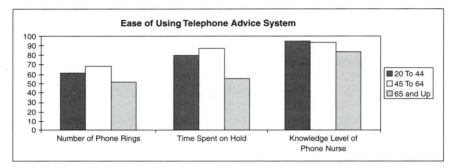

Figure 8–8 Relative Importance of Various Indicators of the "Ease of Using Telephone Advice System" Patient Satisfaction Element. *Source:* Adapted from P.J. Shelton, The Straight-A's Program: A Systematic Approach to Measuring and Enhancing Patient/Member Satisfaction in an Ambulatory Managed Care Setting, in *Making Capitation Work: Clinical Operations in an Integrated Delivery System, Supplement #2,* G.G. Mayer, A.E. Barnett, and N.P. Brown, eds., © 1997, Aspen Publishers, Inc.

the result by the total number of survey responses received for that survey item. This, then, represents the relative quantity (percentage) of patients dissatisfied with whatever is presented in that survey item—your DI for the current survey research.

- Step 3. For each survey questionnaire item, multiply your RII by your DI to obtain your IPI.

For example, assume that your DIs for the survey items covering the element category of "access" are as follows:

- "ease of seeing provider of choice" = 9.5%
- "access to emergency medical care" = 3.2%
- "wait between preferred day and visit" = 11.6%
- "time waiting in reception room" = 13.2%
- "time waiting in exam room" = 6.4%
- "ease of scheduling appointments by phone" = 7.4%

- "ease of using telephone advice system" = 14%
- "ease of scheduling appointments in person" = 10.2%

Then, multiplying the two sets of figures together (RI × DI) for each item, we would get the following IPIs:

- "ease of seeing provider of choice" (DI = 9.5%) × (RII= 92.7) = IPI = 8.81
- "access to emergency medical care"(DI = 3.2%) × (RII = 83.1) = IPI = 2.66
- "wait between preferred day and visit"(DI = 11.6%) × (RII = 81.1) = IPI = 9.41
- "time waiting in reception room"(DI = 13.2%) × (RII = 81.0) = IPI = 10.69
- "time waiting in exam room"(DI = 6.4%) × (RII = 79.1) = IPI = 5.06
- "ease of scheduling appointments by phone"(DI = 7.4%) × (RII = 75.5) = IPI = 5.59
- "ease of using telephone advice system"(DI = 14%) × (RII = 75.4) = IPI = 10.56
- "ease of scheduling appointments in person"(DI = 10.2%) × (RII = 65.5) = IPI = 6.68
- Step 4. Place your calculated IPIs in declining order to obtain the priority ranking of improvement efforts within this satisfaction category.

1. "time waiting in reception room"	10.69
2. "ease of using telephone advice system"	10.56
3. "wait between preferred day and visit"	9.41
4. "ease of seeing provider of choice"	8.81
5. "ease of scheduling appointments in person"	6.68
6. "ease of scheduling appointments by phone"	5.59
7. "time waiting in exam room"	5.06
8. "access to emergency medical care"	2.66

Patient Complaint and Grievance Data

The next source of patient input in determining your improvement priorities lies with patient complaints. In essence, a complaint is a patient's statement about expectations that have not been met. More importantly, it is an opportunity for your health care organization to satisfy a dissatisfied patient by solving a service breakdown. Barlow and Moller refer to a complaint as "the biggest bargain in market research" (1996, p. 19). The message is simple: "A complaint is a gift customers give to a business.... When organizations listen to customers with open minds and more flexible points of view, they can experience complaints as gifts." Patient complaints tell a health care organization how to improve services; they are the most efficient and least costly way of getting information from patients and understanding their expectations about the services you offer. The way your health care organization handles patient complaints has a significant impact on patient satisfaction and loyalty.

According to John Goodman (1986), president of Technical Assistance Research Programs (TARP), a Washington, DC research and consulting organization specializing in customer service research, studies conducted across numerous industries over a 5-year period found that the loyalty and repurchase intentions of customers whose problems were handled and resolved satisfactorily are "within a few percentage points" of the same indices for customers who had experienced no service failure. In a series of studies conducted by Berry, Zeithaml, and Parasuraman (1993), over a 10-year period, it was consistently found that "the best satisfaction scores come from customers who have experienced no problems, the second best from those who have had problems resolved satisfactorily, and the worst from customers whose problems go unresolved" (p. 465).

According to Leonard Berry, professor of marketing and director, Center of Retailing Studies at Texas A&M University, and one of the leading service quality researchers in the United States, "The message from our research is pretty clear: Do it right the first time. If you don't, you'd better be darned sure you do it right the second time. If you fail, you've not met the customer's expectations twice—that's about all the room he'll give you." Furthermore, data from TARP's research confirm that although as many as 96% of unhappy customers won't complain to the offending business, they *will* tell, on average, 9–10 friends, acquaintances, and colleagues how bad your service is. In the context of our efforts to ensure patient satisfaction (and loyalty), it would behoove us to take serious notice of complaint patterns when determining improvement priorities.

Researcher Arthur Dolinsky (1995) conducted multistate research on health care complaints, examining 422 completed surveys. Dolinsky developed the so-called "complaint intensity outcome framework" (CIOF), a model for helping health care providers address patient complaints more effectively. Basically, this is depicted in a two-dimensional grid (Figure 8–9), wherein complaint intensity (CI) is plotted on the grid's y axis and consumer satisfaction with the complaint outcome (CO) is plotted on the x axis.

A *complaint intensity* score is defined as the frequency of patient complaints about a specific service attribute weighted by the mean importance rating that those who have complained about the attribute attach to their complaint. An *outcome satisfaction* score is defined as the

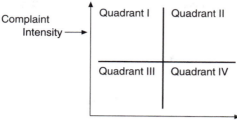

Figure 8–9 Complaint Intensity Outcome Framework. *Source:* Reprinted with permission from *Journal of Health Care Marketing,* published by the American Marketing Association, A. Dolinsky, 1995, Vol. 15, No. 2, p. 42.

patient's mean satisfaction rating of the outcome of his or her complaint about the attribute in question. A service's position on the complaint intensity outcome grid provides a health care organization with information about how much attention should be given to that attribute.

The relative position of the attributes in the framework's two-dimensional grid places them in one of four quadrants. Each quadrant prescribes a different strategy. Primary attention is needed for attributes lying in quadrant I. This stems from the attribute's undesirable outcome satisfaction and CI scores. Thus, an immediate-focus strategy is prescribed. A health care organization might pursue two types of approaches in implementing this strategy:

1. Improve the actual and/or perceived performance for the attributes in question. This would help ensure that the frequency and attached importance of such related attribute complaints are minimized in the future.
2. Improve mechanisms for resolving complaints, particularly when dealing with their most critical clients. This would help ensure that patients view their complaint outcome more favorably for the attributes in question.

Much less focus is needed for the attributes in quadrants II and III. This stems from the desirable outcome satisfaction scores in quadrant II and the desirable complaint intensity scores in quadrant III. Some actions, however, might be contemplated for these attributes because of the unfavorably high intensity and dissatisfaction scores that characterize the attributes in quadrants II and III, respectively. Health care organizations should consider a possible attribute-upgrade strategy for attributes that fall in quadrant II, and a possible complaint-mechanism upgrade strategy for attributes that fall in quadrant III.

The patient satisfaction elements ("attributes") that fall in quadrant IV require no corrective action. This stems from their highly acceptable scores on both dimensions of the framework. To whatever extent possible, health care organizations should identify those favorable actions they are currently taking with respect to this quadrant's satisfaction elements. This can be of assistance in guiding future strategy adjustments for the attributes in other quadrants.

Dolinsky's research (1995) revealed that 17% of the respondents indicated that at some point, typically in the last 2 years, they complained about some aspect of their visit to a physician's office. This figure is similar to the incidence of complaints reported in other studies conducted in health care settings. However, it is quite low in comparison to the 25% to 75% incident rate reported in other product or service areas.

The most frequently reported complaints were about physician quality, which accounted for 47% of total complaints. In contrast, the least frequently reported complaints pertained to the quality of administrative personnel, which accounted for 8% of all complaints. Regarding the importance attached to complaints, respondents assigned the highest importance to complaints about physician quality, and the lowest importance to complaints about the quality of administrative personnel. In order to apply this CIOF grid properly, health care organizations initially must ensure that they possess appropriate complaint information (e.g., information about complaint importance, satisfaction with complaint resolution, etc.).

For optimal health care, a sense of trust between both parties in a patient-provider dispute is essential. Therefore, health providers (and health care organizations) should establish in-house mechanisms to solicit and resolve complaints openly. Health care organizations can take several steps to solicit complaints from dissatisfied patients, including enclosing information sheets describing complaint procedures with their clients' bills (in a complete or partial fee-for-service environment), posting complaint procedures in provider health care facilities, and establishing a toll-free number for receiving patient comments and complaints.

Such a mechanism must be in place if a health care organization is serious about improving patient satisfaction. The cost associated with establishing meaningful complaint resolution mechanisms might be of concern to many health care organizations. Nonetheless, the cost of setting up these mechanisms may be far overshadowed by the cost of not establishing them, which includes fallout from negative word-of-mouth and a potential loss of repeat business.

Improved patient satisfaction can be facilitated by improving complaint-handling mechanisms. However, health care organizations should recognize that if their performance is satisfactory, no complaints will occur in the first place. Health care organizations must not forget that they can ensure patient satisfaction directly by offering quality service. Good complaint resolution can help patient satisfaction via indirect means, by offering a backup to patients who perceive that quality service is lacking.

Grievances differ from complaints in that grievances are formal complaints demanding formal resolution by the health care organization. Complaints that are not resolved to the satisfaction of the patient may evolve into formal grievances. There are greater legal implications and patient satisfaction issues involved with grievances.

The resolution of grievances is distinctly formal. State and federal regulations require health maintenance organizations (HMOs) to have clearly delineated member grievance procedures, to inform members of those procedures, and to abide by them. Clearly defined grievance and appeals procedures are usually required in insurance and self-funded plans as well. As a general rule, members may be contractually prohibited from filing a lawsuit over benefits denial until they have gone through the plan's grievance procedure. Conversely, if a plan fails to inform a member of grievance rights or fails to abide by the grievance procedure, the plan has a real potential for liability.

State regulations (and federal regulations for federally qualified HMOs and competitive medical plans) often spell out the minimum requirements for the grievance procedure. Such requirements might include such issues as

- timeliness of response
- who will review the grievance
- what recourse the member has
- limitation on how long the member has to file a grievance

Each health care organization must review applicable state and federal regulations to develop its grievance procedure. The procedure should be reviewed by legal counsel to evaluate its utility as a risk management function. Kongstvedt offered a general outline of a suggested grievance procedure (1996, p. 485).*

---

*Source: Reprinted from P. Kongstvedt, *The Managed Health Care Handbook,* 3d. ed., pp. 485–487, © 1996, Aspen Publishers, Inc.

- *Filing of formal grievance:* Assuming that the plan has been unable to resolve a member complaint satisfactorily, the member must be informed of and afforded the opportunity to file a formal grievance. This is typically done on a form that asks for essential identification information and a narrative of the problem.
- *Investigation of grievance:* This step takes place from the time the completed grievance form is received and ends when the plan responds. This may include further interviews with the member, interviews with or written responses from other parties, and any other pertinent information. The time period may be set by law or may be set by the plan, but it should not exceed some reasonable period (i.e., 60 days). At the end of that time period, the plan responds to the member with its findings and resolution. The response includes the requirements for the member to respond back to the plan if the resolution is not satisfactory.
- *Appeal:* If a member's grievance is not resolved to his or her satisfaction, the member has the right to appeal. This appeal may involve having the case reviewed by a senior officer of the company or by an outside reviewer. This first appeal is typically done without any formal hearings or testimony, but rather is based on the material submitted for review by both the plan and the member. Again, the plan usually sets a reasonable time period for requesting the appeal (such as 30 days) and a reasonable time period for the review to occur (such as 30 days).
- *Formal hearing:* If the response is still not satisfactory, your health care organization may wish to provide the right to request a formal hearing within 15 working days. The plan must then respond within 15 working days, with an indication of when and where the hearing will take place. The purpose of the formal hearing is to afford the member a chance to present his or her case in person to an unbiased individual or a panel of unbiased individuals. A resolution of the grievance is rarely given to the member at the close of the hearing. The resolution is communicated to the member (usually within 15 working days) and any other pertinent parties, along with the statement that the member has the right of further appeal to arbitration or the government agency, as appropriate.
- *Arbitration:* In those states where arbitration is allowed, the plan would comply with the regulations regarding arbitration terms of selection of the arbitrator(s) and the form of the hearing.
- *Appeal to government agencies:* In all cases, if the member is not satisfied with the results of the formal hearing, he or she has the right to appeal to the appropriate government agency. For commercial members, the state insurance department has jurisdiction. In cases

where the grievance involves quality of care, the health department may have jurisdiction.

- *Lawsuit:* Although not part of a plan's grievance procedure, the last legal remedy for a disgruntled member is legal action.

Whereas in an ideal world, no patient/member would ever have to file a grievance, the reality of the matter is that not all perceived patient problems can be solved readily to the patient's satisfaction—even with the best of complaint management procedures in place. As an indicator for needed organizational improvements, grievance data including trend analysis can be quite helpful in a continuous quest for improved patient satisfaction.

The "Fatal Flaws" of Patient Disenrollment or Defection

Reichheld (1996) emphasized the importance of studying customer defections in any organization:

> One of the most illuminating units of failure in business is customer defection, because it sheds light on two critical flows of value. First, a customer defection is the clearest possible sign of a deteriorating stream of value from the company to its customer. Second, increasing defection rates diminish cash flow from customers to the company—as a result of reduced customer duration. For companies with the desire and capacity to learn, moreover, losing a customer is a fine opportunity to search for the root causes of the departure, to uncover business practices that need fixing, and sometimes to win the customer back and reestablish the relationship on firmer ground. (p. 192)

Keeping a watchful eye on those patients who have left your organization and, even better, spotting those who are about to leave, can be quite enlightening. The most important reason for getting patient feedback is the insight it provides. Only your patients know what you need to improve to meet their expectations. And ex-patients can give you *specific* reasons for their leaving—a view of your health care organization you can't get anywhere else! Defectors also provide an early warning system. What caused one person to leave may also be annoying to other patients, and you can use that information to improve and prevent future problems.

In a study of HMOs in Miami and Los Angeles ("Voting with Their Feet," 1997), there was a tenfold difference in annual disenrollment rates. Kaiser Permanente in Los Angeles, with a 4% rate, retained the most members, and Foundation Health Plan topped the chart with 42% disenrollment. According to the study, "this may be more reliable than some other satisfaction measures—such as surveys—because disenrollment data do not depend on beneficiary recollection" ("Voting with Their Feet," 1997, p. 16).

Another revealing measure is the portion of enrollees who leave a health care organization within 4 months of signing on. Once again, Kaiser Permanente fared best, with a 5% dropout rate. Miami's CareFlorida and Los Angeles' United Health Plan shared the worst showing, with short-term disenrollment rates of 30% and 29% respectively.

If your health care organization is going to learn from defectors, then you must first define what "defection" means to you. It may mean that a patient has disenrolled from your integrated health care network. Or it may mean that, in a private medical practice, the patient has requested his or her medical records to be transferred to another provider...followed by no further visits to your facility.

The first step toward identifying "defectors" from your health care organization is defining your "customers." Although not all of your customers are actual end users of your services (i.e., patients), they likely have either a direct or an indirect influence over whether certain patients continue to use your services. For example, additional customers would include third-party payers and/or employers contracting for employee health care. The loss of either of the latter two customers could have serious market share and financial consequences.

The second defector identification step is to develop a system that carefully tracks all of your customers on an ongoing basis—immediately detecting those who meet your definition of defection. This requires special vigilance because individual patient "open-enrollment" sign-ups and employer, HMO, or third-party payer contracts may come up for renewal at any time throughout the year.

Once you have determined that one of your "customers" has defected or is about to defect, the next step is to telephone them for a brief but well-designed structured interview. The goal of this telephone interview is to bring you specific, relevant information. Questions should not threaten, manipulate, or put patients (or other "customers") on the defensive. Remember, you are attempting to identify opportunities for improvement.

Input from Family Members of Patients

As we mentioned at the beginning of this chapter, family members of patients are often in a position to objectively observe (and comment on) their loved one's health care experiences. Hickey and colleagues (1996) interviewed a number of patient family members to identify problems with the discharge process. The following excerpts from two of these interviews illustrate the value of input from patient family members:

> It was a cold, raw day in February. My 73-year-old mother was going to be discharged some time during the day, but no one could give me the approximate time of her discharge in advance. So I took the day off work and sat by the phone waiting to hear from the hospital. When I did not hear anything by noon, I went to the hospital and waited with my mother. She was finally discharged at 2 PM. Before I could bring her home, I needed to stop at the HMO and pick up her medications. She was too weak to wait in line at the HMO, so I left her in the car (with the car running so she would stay warm) and proceeded to wait 45 minutes in line for her medications. By the time we finally got home it was 4:30.... Then I needed to help her get settled and make dinner. We ate dinner around 8:00.... I had to go to work the next day but stayed up late to make sure she would have everything she needed while I was at work.... I wonder if all this was necessary, a whole day (and night) spent getting my mother home and settled?

> My wife was finally cleared to leave the hospital at 1 PM. She couldn't walk to the lobby, so the nurse called the escort to bring a wheelchair. When the escort finally arrived, I was told they couldn't take my wife *and* her flowers—I would need to bring the flowers to the car myself and he would come back to take my wife to the lobby once we were ready. So I made three trips to the car with my wife's flowers and gifts. By the time I waited for the elevators and walked the block to my car, an hour went by.... In hotels (when you're not sick) you can get someone to help you with your luggage.... Why can't you get the same service in the hospital? (p. 340)

Although these examples took place in a hospital setting, the value of obtaining such feedback in an ambulatory care setting is clear. Patients are often dependent on family members to get them to and from their appointments. When problems occur, it is often the relative who is inconvenienced as much or more than the patient.

Employer and Third-Party Payer Input

The patient service quality concerns of these external customers will most likely originate either from individual complaints or from the results of satisfaction surveys they conduct themselves. The weight of this source of improvement input depends on the number of patients represented. If, for example, a high-ranking executive of a contracting employer has a substantive complaint against your health care organization, the entire contract may be at risk—representing a loss of hundreds (if not thousands) of other patients. On the other hand, when survey results are used, there should be little in the way of surprises if you are conducting (and responding to) your own patient satisfaction surveys. This would put you in a position of responding with your plans for improvement in the area of concern. This may at least placate them until such time as they gather further satisfaction data—proving or disproving the effectiveness of your improvement efforts.

Accrediting Agency Input

The Joint Commission has established standards for quality assessment and improvement (Exhibit 8–1). Although these are written in general terms, they can serve as guidelines in assessing your health care organization's opportunities for improvement.

As discussed in Chapter 1, but bears repeating, NCQA, the accrediting agency for managed care organizations, uses the Health Plan Employer Data and Information Set (HEDIS) to measure, among other things, member (patient) satisfaction. This forms the basis for employers to make "apples-to-apples" comparisons of one health care organization to another when making contracting decisions. By monitoring and constantly improving the same sorts of satisfaction issues, your organization is more likely to compare favorably to competitors who don't go to the trouble to do so.

General Employee Input—Suggestions re: Improvement Opportunities

Employees are among the richest resources for identifying opportunities to serve patients better. The only way to capture this virtual "gold mine" of information systematically is to have a "safe" and non-threatening mechanism in place. Employee ideas for improvement should be solicited and rewarded on a regular basis so as to support a continuous improvement organizational culture.

In a traditional U.S. suggestion scheme, the primary focus of the organization is economic gains directly resulting from the suggestion. An employee submits an idea, most probably concerning his or her own work using a specially designed form. Then, the completed form is submitted to a committee that screens suggestions carefully for the

Exhibit 8–1 New Joint Commission Standards for Quality Assessment and Improvement

1. The organization's leaders set expectations, develop plans, and implement procedures to assess and improve the quality of the organization's governance, management, clinical, and support processes.
2. The leaders undertake education concerning the approach and method of continuous quality improvement.
3. The leaders set priorities for organizationwide quality improvement activities that are designed to improve patient outcomes.
4. The leaders allocate adequate resources for assessment and improvement of the organization's governance, managerial, clinical, and support processes through:
   a. The assignment of personnel, as needed, to participate in quality improvement activities.
   b. The provision of adequate time for personnel to participate in quality improvement activities.
   c. Information systems and appropriate data management processes to facilitate the collection, management, and analysis of data needed for quality improvement.
5. The leaders ensure that the organization staff are trained in assessing and improving processes that contribute to improved patient outcomes.
6. The leaders individually and jointly develop and participate in mechanisms to foster communication among individuals and among components of the organization, and to coordinate internal activities.
7. The leaders analyze and evaluate the effectiveness of their contributions to improving quality.

Source: Data from Payer-Hospital Collaboration to Improve Patient-Satisfaction with Hospital Discharge, Joint Commission Journal on Quality Improvement, Vol. 22, No. 5, pp. 336–344, © 1996.

big winners. The committee members will likely assess the idea's viability, the costs of implementing it, and any consequent savings to the organization.

The committee of assessors will decide whether the idea should be taken further. Ideas that have merit might then be implemented either without further refinement or following more development by the originator and/or others. Employees who offer suggestions that do not pass the screening go unrewarded, even unacknowledged. The process is slow, few individuals ever actually get recognized, and many hard feelings are generated because the majority of suggestions are rejected. The system creates winners and losers, stifles creativity, and generally loses its momentum over time.

Wellington (1995) emphasized the differences in suggestion systems used in the Japanese culture. The term "Kaizen" means "Kai"(change) + "Zen"(good) = improvement. This is the basis of a continuously improving organization.*

> An employee who has an improvement idea concerning any part of their company will first present it to his or her own work-team. They will assess the idea, brainstorming refinements and discussing its potential benefits, with the originator participating fully throughout. But from this early stage the idea passes from individual to team ownership, though the originator will not be disregarded as he or she could be asked by the team to lead the planning project which will evolve from an idea the team agrees has merit.

> The work-team will be responsible for preparing a business/ implementation proposal, using as necessary advice from other work-teams and individual employees with specialist knowledge or skills. The proposal will include a cost-benefit analysis clearly indicating *how the idea will improve customer satisfaction.* Once the proposal is ready it will be presented to the team's leader and then the leaders of any other teams whose work would be affected if the idea were implemented. The team leader(s) will then decide whether to present the idea to their immediate managers who, in turn, will discuss the idea's merit and, if appropriate, seek a release of funds from senior management for a trial of the idea.

> It will be the team's responsibility to manage the trial and, if it is successful, see it through to full adoption. A key question during the idea's consensus assessment is, does it lead to a new performance standard? If all it amounts to is a different methodology it is not an improvement, nothing will have changed and customers will not be served any better than before. An idea must create a new performance standard (i.e., lower waste, lower cost, greater speed etc.).

> Not only will the originator(s)—the work-team(s)—of an implemented idea be rewarded with morale-boosting recogni-

---

Source: Reprinted with permission from P. Wellington, Kaizen Strategies for Customer Care, p. 15, © 1995, Pearson Education.

tion, the originators of failed ideas will also be rewarded, for in Kaizen it is important to acknowledge the effort behind *every* suggested idea whether or not it ever sees the light of day. In fact, each team's and team leader's performance is judged partly on the sheer number of improvement suggestions generated in a given period. That only a comparatively few of the contributed ideas are implemented does not matter; the point is, everyone should participate in their company's life. Kaizen's team-based ethos is obvious in the way its suggestion system operates, as are the awareness and competencies of all employees generally who can identify a potential improvement even within functions beyond their own. (p. 41)

According to Wellington (1995, p. 42), in the 1980s, suggestions in Japanese companies averaged close to 20 per worker per year, with 75% being adopted. In 1986, 48 million total suggestions were generated in Japan.

This form of suggestion system is broken down into three stages and is based on the premises of starting with quantity and improving quality (economic impact) in the second phase. Stage one stresses participation and involvement. Stage two involves education and the development of workers in better problem-solving and team skills. In stage three, more emphasis is placed on the economic impact of suggestions. The first stage breaks traditional barriers and makes improvement a normal part of the job. As skills improve, better ideas with greater impact are generated. This approach recognizes that the major difference between humans and other animals is the ability to think and generate new ideas. To deny workers the opportunity to create and change their work environment is to deny their humanity!

Behavioral psychologists have long demonstrated that in order to change behavior, one must reward and recognize the new, desired behavior. LeBoeuf (1985) emphasized this principle succinctly: "Behavior that gets rewarded gets repeated." The key questions for management then become, "What is the behavior we want to change?" And then, "How are we going to reward, recognize, and encourage the new behavior?" (p. 9)

Although medical personnel are primarily focused on clinical matters during their encounters with patients, other issues related to activities leading to (or limiting) the actual visit are commonly mentioned by patients. When this occurs, only those who are constantly on the lookout for ways to serve patients better will translate a seemingly simple comment into an improvement idea. This holds true for health care providers, nursing staff, and specialty services alike.

One example of using input from nursing employees to improve patient satisfaction occurred at Deaconess Hospital, a 590-bed facility located in Evansville, Indiana (Zimmerman, Zimmerman, & Lund, 1996). It seems that patients were upset with the noise levels during their hospitalizations. This noise was associated with nursing staff activities. The hospital was in Press-Ganey's (a patient satisfaction measurement organization) 59th percentile for hospital noise levels. Therefore, a team of employees was charged with the responsibility to "reduce the impact of noise level on nursing units as measured by patient satisfaction surveys." The team brainstormed to generate a list of possible causes of excessive noise. This list included "night shift activities, nurses' stations, and construction" as the top three sources of potential excessive noise. The identified opportunities for improvement included "employees at nurses' stations, patient visitation, and night noise." Based on these opportunities, the team developed the following opportunity statement:

> An improvement opportunity exists in reducing the noise level generated at the nurses station during the late evening and night time hours. This causes dissatisfaction among patients as reflected on patient surveys. Reduction of the noise level should result in increased patient satisfaction. (p. 180)

Employee input was solicited to help identify potential sources of excessive noise as well as to determine what they had been told by patients regarding noise levels. This concluded that the top five reasons for excessive noise were

1. talking and laughing by employees, visitors, and other patients
2. noise associated with nursing shift changes
3. night shift nursing activities
4. evening shift nursing activities
5. day shift nursing activities

The employee team came up with a number of possible approaches to noise reduction. The top three solutions that emerged by consensus were: glassing in the nurses' stations, using soundproofing materials/ insulation on nursing unit areas, and providing headsets for patients. Once all factors (cost, time, etc.) were considered, it was decided that the nurses' stations would be enclosed in glass. When the project was completed, Deaconess Hospital concluded that it was "a positive way to reduce noise and protect patient confidentiality" (Zimmerman et al., 1996, p. 180).

In 1996, the Imaging Services Department of St. Jude Medical Center in Fullerton, California, identified "explanations of tests and treatments" as an opportunity for improvement (Press Ganey, 1995, p. 5). They formed an APPLE Quality Team, which represented all modalities within the imaging services department, and set out to achieve a 5% increase in raw score or reach the 85th percentile in the percentile ranking in the specific area of "explanations of tests and treatments." They worked toward their goals by making three commitments:

1. Use obstacles to our advantage. Example: The team capitalized on the flexibility of not being given a structured program format—this allowed relevant issues to be addressed immediately.
2. Turn every negative into a positive. Example: Unforeseen delays were treated as an opportunity to 'make it right' for the patient.
3. Leave such a positive impression on the patient that they will want to respond to the survey. Example: The staff was uncomfortable mentioning the survey to the patient at the time of their service and had better results concentrating on providing exceptional, memorable service. (p. 5)

With these commitments in place, the APPLE team met weekly to brainstorm and make recommendations. Education inservice materials were combined with promotions and motivational activities, and games were initiated as a way to motivate employees and acknowledge those providers who deliver quality care. The APPLE project officially concluded with the end of the fiscal year 1996. The results continue to have a positive impact on the staff and patients of St. Jude Medical Center. This is evidenced by the following:

- continued high scores on Press-Ganey surveys and quarterly reports
- application of successful strategies to next fiscal year goals
- nomination of eight imaging services employees for St. Jude Medical Center "values in action" annual services awards (more than the previous 3 years combined)

Frontline nonmedical personnel such as receptionists, appointment secretaries, and so forth are, as mentioned earlier in this chapter, in an ideal position to have patients talk freely with them about their concerns, interests, and needs.

These people should be encouraged to pass on patient viewpoints. It is important not to blame the messenger for the message. It can be hard to listen to critical comments relayed by staff, especially if you think the patient has a faulty impression, but if you don't learn to listen without interrupting and without getting defensive or critical of the staff member, this source of feedback will dry up.

If a frontline employee relays a patient service story that suggests that the employee did not handle the patient very well, then it is more helpful to explore the different ways the employee could have handled the situation better. This will have a more positive effect on the employee's future behavior than simply shouting at him or her or cutting him or her off in mid-story. Your objective should be to coach your staff to do better next time—to learn from their experience. If this is done in an unpleasant fashion, then the next time they handle something badly, they will try to keep that fact hidden from you, and they may never improve their performance as a result. Furthermore, they will be less likely to even consider making suggestions for improving patient service.

Health care facility managers must also provide input when it comes to identifying opportunities for patient satisfaction improvements. They have already been provided with the list of improvement priorities based on the patient satisfaction survey research (recall $RII \times DI = IPI$). This represents a "snapshot" recorded in an instant in time when the survey research was conducted. Managers need to factor in their own direct observations of staff interacting with patients on the job. Then, improvement considerations should be evaluated on the basis of

- specific patient satisfaction elements
- high success likelihood, given the logistics of implementation
- affordability
- mechanism(s) for evaluating the success of the improvement implementation

Senior management must also play a key role in providing patient satisfaction improvement considerations. These leaders must demonstrate throughout the organization that patient satisfaction is important. This can be done in several ways.

- Acknowledge areas where the health care organization needs to improve patient satisfaction.

- Involve management and employees in the development of plans for patient satisfaction improvement.
- Link management bonuses to patient satisfaction scores.
- Provide clear and frequent communication about what is being done to improve patient satisfaction.

Linking patient satisfaction scores with employee and management monetary incentives is just a case of having management put its money where its mouth is. Monetary incentives for improving patient satisfaction scores should reach all levels of the health care organization, from top management to frontline employees. Incentive programs can be structured so that all employees in a department can receive compensation if the department's patient satisfaction goals are met. Additionally, exemplary service on the part of individual employees can be rewarded on an ad-hoc basis. Management incentives do not have to result in incremental expenditures; a reallocation of current incentives will suffice.

Senior management's commitment to patient satisfaction must be communicated to every employee. The expectation that each employee will contribute to improving patient satisfaction should be understood clearly by every employee. Training, communication of expectations, and feedback on accomplishments are critical in closing the gap between the perceptions of senior management and those of other employees.

Health care organization leaders must create a "service vision" that is an ideal and unique image of the future. Experts agree that vision is a prerequisite for service excellence. According to service quality guru, Ron Zemke, organizations with concise, understandable, and actionable service strategies are four times as likely to receive superior service ratings from the customers as those without them (Zemke & Schaaf, 1990). Then, promoting commitment to the service vision is critical if leaders are to translate service vision into specific actions.

CATEGORIZING IMPROVEMENTS BY CHANGE MECHANISM

It is important to recognize that the processes involved with improving various elements of patient satisfaction vary considerably. The organization's grades on a patient's mental report card are determined by a variety of moments of truth and surrogate perceptions. There are three basic types of patient satisfaction improvements:

- behavior-based improvements
- systems-based improvements
- administration-based improvements

The real difference between these three lies in the mechanism by which each is brought about. Behavior-based changes are best facilitated with appropriate training and education. As the name implies, the objective of behavior-based change is to bridge the gap in employee behavior between what is currently occurring to that which is most desirable by patients. Systems-based improvements require initial education in systems and process thinking. Then, real substantive improvements must be "designed" by teams working to "rethink" and redesign how patient-related tasks get performed on a routine basis. Finally, administration-based improvements are initiated by gaining senior management's commitment and support to those changes requiring significant financial investment. For example, if surveys (and/or complaint or grievance data) indicate that patients are dissatisfied with the poor maintenance, appearance, or cleanliness of a health care facility, financial resources need to be allocated to bring about the necessary changes. No amount of employee training or systems reengineering will make a difference in this area of future patient satisfaction surveys.

The next three chapters will focus on the details of addressing an organization's behavior-based, systems-based, and administrative-based patient satisfaction improvement priorities. This represents the next overall step toward developing a systematic and effective plan for you to improve patient satisfaction continuously.

CONCLUSION

The process of identifying and prioritizing service quality improvement needs is multifaceted. Input must be gathered from internal as well as external customers of your health care organization. The external customers include patients, family members of patients, third-party payers, employers contracting for employee health care benefits, accrediting agencies, and regulatory agencies. Internal customers include health care providers, nursing staff, medical assistants, specialty services and frontline personnel, and all levels of management.

The quantitative component of the prioritization process involves both the patient satisfaction survey data (see Chapter 6) and the RII (see Chapter 4). Specifically, by multiplying the DI (percentage of patient satisfaction survey respondents rating a given survey item as "fair" or "poor") by the RII, you get the IPI. Mathematically, this is expressed in the following formula: IPI = DI × RII.

It is strongly recommended that you combine the IPI with input gathered from internal and current and past external organizational customers. Although the IPI quantitatively reflects improvement priorities at the instant in time when the survey research was conducted, ongoing input from organizational customers will reflect continually changing patient expectations. This ensures that your organization's patient satisfaction improvement efforts will remain focused on those areas that are most meaningful to patients. These, in turn, need to be divided into three categories according to change mechanism: behavior-based, systems/process-based, and administration-based. The next three chapters will address each of these improvement types in order.

ACTION STEPS

1. Make a list of your organization's "external customer" sources that are used to prioritize patient satisfaction improvement efforts. If you feel that additional external customer groups should be added to this list, name them.
2. Make a list of your organization's "internal customer" sources that are used to prioritize patient satisfaction improvement efforts. If you feel that additional internal customer groups should be added to this list, name them.
3. If your organization has relatively current (less than 1 year old) patient satisfaction survey research data available, identify the primary areas of "dissatisfaction." If not already done, perform a correlation analysis to see what areas your patients consider to be most important. Then, rank order the areas of improvement by combining "dissatisfaction" data with "importance" data, as discussed in this chapter.
4. Divide current areas of needed improvement into the three recommended categories: behavior-based, systems/process-based, and administration-based.

REFERENCES

Barlow, J., & Moller, C. (1996). *A complaint is a gift: Using customer feedback as a strategic tool.* San Francisco: Berrett-Koehler.

Berry, L.L., Zeithaml, V., & Parasuraman, A. (1993). Service quality: A profit strategy for financial institutions. In E. Scheuing & W. Christopher (Eds.), *The service quality handbook*. Homewood, IL: Dow Jones Irwin.

Dolinsky, A. (1995). Complaint intensity and health care services: A framework to establish priorities for quality improvements can be used to improve patient satisfaction. *Journal of Health Care Marketing, 15*(2), 42(6).

Goodman, J. (1986). Don't fix the product, fix the customer. *The Quality Review, 2*(3), 6–11.

Hickey, K., et al. (1996, May). Payer-hospital collaboration to improve patient satisfaction with hospital discharges. *The Journal of the Joint Commission, 22*(5), 336.

Kongstvedt, P.R. (1996). *The managed care health care handbook* (3rd ed.). Gaithersburg, MD.

LeBoeuf, M. (1985). *The greatest management principle in the world*. New York: Berkley Books.

Niles, et. al. (1996, May). Using qualitative & quantitative patient satisfaction data to improve the quality of cardiac care. *Journal of Quality Improvement*.

Press-Ganey. (1995). *Press-Ganey success stories*.

Reichheld, F.F. (1996). *The loyalty effect: The hidden force behind growth, profits, and lasting value*. Boston: Harvard Business School Press.

Voting with their feet: Medicare-risk (dis)enrolees. (1997). *Business and Health, 15*(2), 16(1).

Wellington, P. (1995). *Kaizen strategies for customer care: How to create a powerful customer care program—and make it work*. London: Pitman.

Zemke, R., & Schaaf, D. (1990). *The service edge: 101 companies that profit from customer care*. Ontario: Penguin.

Zimmerman, D., Zimmerman, P., & Lund, C. (1996). *Healthcare customer revolution*. Chicago: Irwin, 177–180.

SUGGESTED READING

Albrecht, K., & Bradford, L.J. (1990). *The service advantage: How to identify and fulfill customer needs*. Homewood, IL: Dow Jones-Irwin.

Brown, S.A. (1992). *Total quality service: How organizations use it to create a competitive advantage*. Scarborough, Ontario: Prentice Hall Canada.

Brown, S.A. (1997). *Breakthrough customer service: Best practices of leaders in customer support*. Toronto, Canada: John Wiley & Sons Canada.

Business Research Lab. (1998). *Don't let research results sit on the shelf* [On-line]. Available: www.corporrate@netropolis.net.

Cannie, J.K. (1994). *Turning lost customers into gold:...and the art of achieving zero defections*. New York: AMACOM.

Davis, S.L., & Adams-Greenly, M. (1994). Integrating patient satisfaction with a quality improvement program. *Journal of Nursing Administration, 24*(12), 28–31.

Drummond, M.E. (1993). *Fearless and flawless public speaking with power, polish and pizazz*. San Diego: Pfeiffer and Company.

Dube, L.M., Belanger, M., & Trudeau, E. (1996). The role of emotions in health care satisfaction. *Journal of Healthcare Marketing, 16*(2), 45(7).

Dunckel, J., & Taylor, B. (1988). *The business guide to profitable customer relations: Today's techniques for success.* Seattle, WA: Self-Counsel Press.

Dutka, A. (1994). *AMA handbook for customer satisfaction: A complete guide to research, planning & implementation.* Lincolnwood, IL: NTC Business Books.

Hayes, J., & Dredge, F. (1998). *Managing customer service.* Hampshire, England: Gower.

Hinton, T., & Schaeffer, W. (1994). *Customer-focused quality: What to do on Monday morning.* Englewood Cliffs, NJ: Prentice Hall.

Hradesky, J.L. (1995). *Total quality management handbook.* New York: McGraw-Hill.

Katz, J.M., & Green, E. (1997). *Managing quality: A guide to system-wide performance management in health care* (2nd ed.). St. Louis, MO: Mosby-Year Book.

Lancaster, W., & Lancaster, J. (1992). Tracking patient satisfaction at an academic medical center. *Journal of Ambulatory Care Marketing, 5*(1), 27–33.

Scheuing, E.E., & Christopher, W.F. (Eds.). (1993). *The service quality handbook.* New York: AMACOM.

Zeithaml, V.A., & Bitner, M.J. (1996). *Services marketing.* London: McGraw-Hill.

Zeithaml, V.A., Parasuraman, A., & Berry, L.L. (1990). *Delivering quality service: Balancing customer perceptions and expectations.* New York: The Free Press.

CHAPTER 9

Addressing Behavior-Based Improvement Priorities

Patient perceptions of health care service quality are, in large part, formed by observing various behaviors of the providers and staff with whom they interact. In turn, the "grades" that patients give a health care organization on their mental report cards are generally reflective of the quality of those interpersonal contacts. Previous chapters presented a variety of mechanisms for soliciting, recording, and responding to patient feedback, including patient satisfaction surveys. In order to continuously improve patient satisfaction, special attention must be given to those behaviors associated with the management of each moment of truth (MOT).

In this chapter, we will discuss several important considerations related to changing (and maintaining) the behavior of employees and/or providers. We will begin with some of the basic principles of influencing human behavior because this behavior is a key aspect of organizational performance. Then, we will discuss the clear delineation of behavioral expectations—the establishment of performance standards. Next, we will carefully examine the principles and techniques of effective training. This will include a variety of related issues, such as the following:

- introduction to training—what it can (and cannot) accomplish
- understanding the adult learner
- identifying training needs
- developing measurable training objectives
- elements of adult instruction
- training techniques/methods
- learning materials

256

Then, methods for the development of targeted patient satisfaction improvement (PSI) training programs for your health care organization will be addressed. These programs will focus on health care providers as well as staff, with facility/department-specific training for staff. The setting will vary from new employee orientation to established employee reorientation and distinct stand-alone workshops. In each instance, the overriding objective is to deliver effective patient satisfaction training within the framework of normal organizational operations.

This chapter will also present various logistical challenges such as scheduling and space allocation. Then, you will be provided with guidelines for effective training presentation and for ensuring the "transfer of training" to the workplace. Of course, if you wish to improve the quality of training continuously, then a means of systematically evaluating the effectiveness of each training session needs to be in place. The Kirkpatrick (1994) four-level evaluation model forms the foundation on which I recommend you approach the process of training evaluation.

INFLUENCING BEHAVIOR—THE KEY TO PERFORMANCE MANAGEMENT

Generally speaking, people do what they do because of what happens to them when they do it. Indeed, all behavior is a function of its consequences. LeBouef (1985) alluded to this fact in his phrase, "Behavior that gets rewarded gets repeated." In a broader sense, it must be recognized that everything we do produces some consequence for us. Psychologists refer to behavioral consequences as "those things and events that follow a behavior and change the probability that the behavior will be repeated in the future."

Changing the consequences of a behavior can alter the rate or frequency of that behavior. Although this seems somewhat complex at first glance, the simple fact is that there are only four behavioral consequences. Two function to increase behavior and two function to decrease it. *Positive reinforcement* and *negative reinforcement* increase behavior; *punishment* and *extinction* decrease behavior.

- *Positive reinforcement* causes a behavior to increase because a desired, meaningful consequence follows the behavior.
- *Negative reinforcement* causes a behavior to increase in order to escape or avoid some unpleasant consequence.

- *Punishment,* like positive reinforcement, is defined by its effect—an action is punishing only when the behavior you don't want stops.
- *Extinction,* on the other hand, decreases a particular behavior as a result of the withdrawal of positive reinforcement—the employee does something and it is ignored.

During the course of a normal workday, an employee engages in hundreds of behaviors, each of which is followed by a consequence that will either strengthen or weaken that behavior. Some consequences occur naturally without the involvement of other people, such as unlocking a door lock with the proper key or turning the room lights on by flicking the light switch. Typically, little conscious thought is given to these behaviors. However, as soon as other people are involved in producing consequences, conscious consideration is often given to the interaction. The "other person" may be a fellow employee, a patient, a manager, or a supervisor. Ideally, consequences in a health care organization should increase the behaviors that facilitate patient satisfaction and decrease those behaviors (i.e., rudeness, disrespect, indifference, etc.) that diminish patient satisfaction.

Daniels (1994), president of Precision Learning Systems, emphasized the organizational value of carefully designing consequences: "All we have to do to get the performance we want is to identify behaviors that are producing the poor outcome and arrange consequences that will stop them. Then identify the behaviors that will produce the desirable outcomes and arrange consequences that will positively reinforce them" (p. 27). The characteristics of the performance that is generated by positive or negative reinforcement are very different. Negative reinforcement will generate just enough behavior to escape or avoid punishment—the classic "minimum necessary to get by." Positive reinforcement produces *discretionary effort* that far exceeds the minimum required. The latter is essential in creating a culture that consistently strives to exceed patient expectations.

It is important to recognize that the effect of a consequence is not determined by the intention of the manager or supervisor. Rather, the employee (performing the behavior) defines whether a consequence is positive or negative. A common management myth is that people do not need positive reinforcement—"They get paid to do that.... I shouldn't have to pat them on the back for it." Therefore, nothing is said about good performance. This sets the stage for either extinction of the desired behavior or a less desirable behavior replacing it and, unfortunately, getting positively reinforced. If an employee takes the initiative to go above and beyond what is required to be courteous to a patient, then those behaviors, if they lack a favorable consequence, will at some point stop. Therefore, management's action or inaction can influence employee behavior.

The next attribute of consequences is so-called "shelf life." A delay between the action and its consequence will significantly decrease the impact the consequence has on behavior. This is called—*impact erosion.* The more immediate and certain the consequence, the more effective it is in changing behavior. One of the most common causes of poor performance among employees is associated with a lack of timely feedback. This is why formal "summative" performance appraisals conducted every 6 months or year, which only summarize the quality of performance during the previous period, are relatively ineffective in modifying day-to-day performance. However, feedback provided on a frequent and informal daily basis—"formative appraisal"—has much more effect on the behavior.

Another semantic distinction must be made between the terms *reinforcer* and *reward.* This is made on the basis of the immediacy factor. Typically, a reward is something that is received at some time in the future with some degree of uncertainty associated with it. An employee may not qualify for the reward, the reward requirements may change, and so forth. Therefore, employees will respond much more predictably to small, immediate, certain consequences than they will to a large, future, uncertain one. Thus, the consequences that cause people to do their best every day occur every day. Incentives, such as bonuses, profit sharing, and retirement benefits are necessary, but they are not sufficient to maximize employee performance on a daily basis.

The consequence implications for bringing about behavioral changes that improve patient satisfaction are enormous. A commonly held belief is that people generally resist change. Deming disagreed with this when he stated that "people don't resist change... they resist being changed" (Scholtes, 1988, p. 21). This shifts the emphasis to whatever force is controlling the change. However, it seems more appropriate to place the emphasis on the consequences associated with the change. If a particular change (new behavior), such as how patients are greeted when they arrive at the health care facility, is immediately followed by a positive consequence, then little resistance for adopting the new behavior could be anticipated. Much of this chapter is devoted to providing guidelines for modifying provider and employee behaviors so as to better meet patients' needs or perceived needs. Such changes can only be long term (i.e., "institutionalized") if the organizational environment consistently supports them.

Daniels developed the "ABCs of performance management," wherein he placed emphasis not only on the consequence of peoples' behavior, but on the antecedents that set the stage for behavior to begin (1994, p. 35). Thus, the antecedents lead to behavior beginning, and the consequences cause the behavior to continue. Daniels created a model for systematically analyzing the antecedents and consequences influencing a behavior. In an ABC analysis, consequences are classified on three dimensions (Exhibit 9–1).

1. *Positive or negative:* This answers the question, "Is the consequence positive or negative from the perspective of the employee?"
2. *Immediate or future:* In other words, "Does the consequence occur as the behavior is happening (immediate) or some time later (future)?"
3. *Certain or uncertain:* This relates to the probability that the employee will actually experience the consequence.

When a problem behavior is identified, especially if it has been demonstrated to detract from patient satisfaction, you will likely find that the consequences are positive, immediate, and certain in support of the behavior. At the same time, the consequences provided for the behavior that is desired (i.e., contributing to patient satisfaction) are negative, immediate, and certain. The key to changing behavior lies with rearranging consequences so they are more favorable for the desired behavior.

Exhibit 9–1 Antecedent-Behavior-Consequence Analysis

		Consequences		
Antecedents	**Behavior**	**P/N**	**I/F**	**C/U**
Setting event	Performance	Positive or negative consequence	Immediate or future consequence	Certain or uncertain consequence

Source: Adapted with permission from A. Daniels, *Bringing Out the Best in People*, p. 36, © 1994, The McGraw-Hill Companies.

Geary, Rummler, and Brache (1995) identified a number of interrelated factors that affect human performance.

- Performance specifications: Do performance standards exist? Do performers consider the standards attainable?
- Task support: Can the task be done without interference from other tasks? Are adequate resources available for performance?
- Consequences: Are consequences aligned to support desired performance? Are consequences meaningful from the viewpoint of the performer? Are consequences timely?
- Feedback: Do performers receive information about their performance? Is the information they receive relevant, accurate, timely, specific, and easy to understand?
- Skills/knowledge: Do the performers have the necessary skills and knowledge to perform? Do the performers know why the desired performance is important?
- Individual capacity: Are the performers physically, mentally, and emotionally able to perform?

Although this list appears to ignore the importance of employee motivation, the authors contend that if capable (*individual capacity*), well-trained (*skills/knowledge*) people are placed in a setting with clear expectations (*performance specifications*), sufficient time and resources (*task support*), and reinforcing consequences (*consequences*), and given appropriate feedback (*feedback*), then they will be motivated! Because all performance begins with clear performance expectations, we will now focus our attention on the development of performance standards that contribute to patient satisfaction.

ESTABLISHING PATIENT SATISFACTION PERFORMANCE STANDARDS

The first step in becoming a truly patient-focused health care organization known for exceptional service is to define exactly what "exceptional service" means. In a study of 307 service organizations, Shetty reported that most employees could not define the concept of quality service. Concern for quality was evident in policy statements and quality improvement, but it had not reached the employee level. According to Martin (1989), there are several important benefits to the establishment of patient satisfaction performance standards. These standards help to

- *Establish a target:* Written standards of patient service establish a goal toward which all health care providers and employees can direct their efforts. They provide a clear sense of what to strive for. Furthermore, they establish a sense of purpose and direction for employees.
- *Communicate expectations:* Clearly defined standards communicate to all employees exactly what is expected in terms of behavior when dealing with patients. This ensures that all providers and staff alike are "singing from the same song sheet" in this regard. Consistently reinforcing these patient-driven standards makes them common knowledge; there are no surprises about what is expected.
- *Create a valuable management tool:* A complete list of patient service standards can assist with employee recruitment, hiring decisions, job descriptions, and performance appraisals. New employee orientation, existing employee reorientation, and stand-alone training workshops provide natural forums for introducing and/or emphasizing established standards of behavioral performance.

The first step toward establishing patient-defined service standards involves delineating your health care organization's existing or desired service encounter sequences. Refer back to Chapter 5 and recall that patients experience a sequence of MOTs and surrogate perceptions (SPs) (outlined in Appendix 5–A) that make up their mental report card. Next, map out the major chronological steps that make up each patient encounter. Your existing patient-based research, as discussed in Chapters 6 and 8, must then be used to determine service expectations. From this, abstract patient expectations and requirements must be translated into concrete, specific behaviors and actions associated with each patient encounter in the service encounter sequence. Abstract requirements (e.g., personal caring) can call for a different behavior or action in each patient service encounter.

The next step toward establishing patient-defined service standards involves selecting specific behaviors and actions to be incorporated into standards. Several important criteria should be adhered to when developing standards.

- *Patient service standards should be based on behaviors and actions that are very important to patients.* This is critically important because improvements in adherence to standards that are unrelated to patient satisfaction will have no measurable impact on PSI efforts.
- *Patient service standards should cover provider and staff behavior that needs to be improved or maintained.* Health care organizations get

the highest leverage or biggest impact from focusing on behaviors and actions that need to be improved (as determined via the mechanisms discussed in Chapter 8).

- *Patient service standards should cover behaviors and actions that providers and employees can actually improve.* People's behavior can only match standards consistently if people understand, accept, and have control over the behaviors and actions specified in the standards. Thus, standards should cover controllable aspects of employees' work.
- *Patient service standards should be developed in cooperation with the providers and employees who are expected to adhere to them.* This will ensure that providers and employees accept them. Imposing standards on unwilling employees often leads to resistance, resentment, absenteeism, or even turnover—generally declining employee morale.
- *Patient service standards should be predictive rather than simply reactive.* Although patient complaint and satisfaction survey data identify current weaknesses, current and future patient expectations should be considered in designing behaviors that improve patient satisfaction.
- *Patient service standards should be challenging but realistic.* If standards are not challenging, employees get little reinforcement for mastering them. On the other hand, unrealistically high standards leave an employee feeling dissatisfied with performance and frustrated by not being able to attain the behavioral goal.

Standards should be developed for the important satisfaction elements of each of the six categories of patient satisfaction defined in Chapter 3 (access, convenience, communication, perceived quality of health care received, personal caring, and health care facilities/equipment). Several basic characteristics should be present in effective patient service standards.

- *Specific:* The standards should tell employees exactly what behavior is expected of them. There should be no need to guess about or interpret expectations.
- *Concise:* No long explanation of the service quality philosophy behind the standards is required or even desirable. Rather, the standards should get right to the point and spell out who should do what when and how.
- *Measurable:* In order to be specific, the standards must be observable and objective, which makes them capable of being measured.

In Exhibit 9–2, notice how generalized service quality behaviors should be converted to specific measurable standards. Note that the measurable aspect of each standard should be highlighted (bold, italics, or otherwise).

- *Based on patient requirements:* Your research should clearly indicate what patients expect as a minimum, as well as what would most likely delight them by exceeding their expectations. Whenever realistic, the target should be to exceed expectations—"experience enhancers." In areas determined to be less important (see relative importance index), simply meeting those expectation may be perfectly acceptable.
- *Written into job descriptions and performance reviews:* This process effectively converts performance standards from lofty "wish lists" to credible management tools that employees respect.
- *Fairly enforced:* Patient satisfaction performance standards that are enforced with some employees and not with others (or in some instances, but not in others) quickly erode. Organizationwide health care standards require that everybody, including senior management, conform to them. Facility-specific or department-

---

Exhibit 9–2 Converting Service Quality Behaviors to Service Standards

General Service Quality Behaviors	Specific Service Standards
Answer the telephone promptly.	Answer the phone within three rings.
Return patient phone calls in a timely fashion.	Return all patient phone calls within 24 hours.
Be attentive to patients.	Make eye contact with the patient within 5 seconds of his or her approaching you.
Be empathetic with an upset patient.	Always apologize if a patient is upset.
Take personal responsibility for helping the patient.	Always give the patient your name, phone number, and extension.
Assist patients in finding their way in your health care facility.	Always take the time to clearly show the way to or escort patients to their destination within your health care facility.

specific standards apply to everyone within that facility or department, including management.

Friendly Hills HealthCare Network developed a set of network service standards (1994a) that defined critical success factors and key strategies for telephone, in-person, and written communications. Exhibit 9–3 presents several of the telephone service standard critical success factors and their respective key strategies.

Exhibit 9–3 Friendly Hills HealthCare Network Telephone Service Standards

Critical Success Factor	Key Strategies
Response time	• Answer all calls within *three rings*.
Returning calls	• Return all calls before the end of your shift/work day.
	• Try to get specifics—what time is best to reach them, what numbers, etc.
	• Let the caller know when you expect to return the call.
	• Document your return calls so you have a record.
Greeting/listening	• Identify your area/department, give your name, and ask, "How may I help you?"
	• Give the caller an opportunity to state concerns.
	• Let the caller know you listened and understood by confirming what was said.
	• Offer assistance (i.e., offer to transfer the call, give them the proper extension and name of the department, have a supervisor come to the phone, or take a thorough message and have a supervisor return the call).
Greeting information	• Be cheerful.
	• Empathize—understand the caller's emotions/point of view.
	• Request specific information to pinpoint the caller's needs (who is your doctor, who did you see, when were your tests conducted, etc.).
Hold/Transfer	• Always let the caller respond before you place him or her on hold.

continues

Exhibit 9–3 continued

Critical Success Factor	Key Strategies
	• Offer an explanation as to why the caller is being placed on hold and for how long. Or offer the caller a choice, asking, "Do you want to hold or can we return your call shortly?"
	• Check with all calls on hold at least every minute and a half.
	• If a caller has been on hold for several minutes, offer a "choice" again.
	• If you must transfer a call, let the caller know why you are transferring him or her, to whom, and to what department/extension—wait for the receiving party to whom you are transferring to answer and give them relevant information so the caller will not have to repeat it.
	• If you connect with voice mail, give the caller the option to get off the line before connecting.
Confidentiality	• Speak clearly, but in a low tone of voice, to avoid being overheard.
	• Be aware of who is around you before speaking.
	• Be sensitive to the caller's feelings; if necessary, move to a more private location to discuss sensitive issues.
Scheduling appointments by telephone	• Try to make an appointment for the caller without transferring the call whenever possible.
	• Ask the person for preferences—a.m., p.m., day of the week, etc.
	• Clarify the reason for the appointment.
	• Ask for specifics when necessary—age, etc.
	• Offer appointment choices.
	• Confirm the date, time, and location of the appointment.
Ending telephone conversations	• Confirm what was discussed.
	• Ask for any further questions.
	• Use the caller's name and say "goodbye."
	• Wait for the caller to hang up before you hang up.

Courtesy of Friendly Hills HealthCare Network.

As we have mentioned repeatedly, the grades your health care organization will receive on each patient's mental report card (PMRC) are determined by patients' perceptions of their experiences (and observations) while interacting with your providers and employees. Exhibit 9–4 presents several of the Friendly Hills HealthCare Network personal interaction standards (1994b).

Exhibit 9–4 Friendly Hills HealthCare Network Personal Interaction Standards

Critical Success Factor	Key Strategies
Verbal communication	• Be positive and friendly.
	• Greet each patient with, "Hello. How are you?" Express a personal interest.
	• Establish eye contact when speaking and/or acknowledging the (patient).
	• Ask politely for the person's name, reason for appointment, who they are seeing that day—using his or her name.
	• Give explanations for delays.
	• Acknowledge mistakes, even if they are not yours, and try to correct them; do not place the problem on the individual or place blame on another person or department.
	• Offer assistance (have a supervisor meet with the patient, if necessary, to resolve any issue).
	• Ask for feedback, clarification, and/or understanding.
Nonverbal communication	• Smile.
	• Make and maintain eye contact.
	• Let people know you are listening by nodding your head etc.
	• Make sure your physical appearance presents a professional image.
	• Do not chew gum while on duty.
	• Whenever possible, lead or take people where they need to go rather than directing them.
Appearance	• Wear your name badge with picture side showing/not covered up.
	• Clothing should be neat, clean, and well-pressed.

continues

Exhibit 9–4 continued

Critical Success Factor	Key Strategies
	• Hair should be neat, clean, and combed.
	• FHHN and department dress codes should be followed at all times.
Environment	• Your working area and all public working areas should be kept neat, clean, and orderly.
	• All equipment/furniture should be kept in good condition. Report equipment/furniture in poor condition to your supervisor.
	• Atmosphere should be professional at all times.
	• Proper lighting should be maintained.
	• Current literature should be displayed in waiting areas if appropriate.
	• Personal items such as cartoons and jokes should not be posted in public areas.
Waiting/delays	• Acknowledge any wait immediately upon the person's arrival.
	• Apologize for waits and, if possible, offer options.
	• Keep people informed—if an appointment is running late, tell them; update individuals every 5–10 minutes, in person, so they know they haven't been forgotten.
Confidentiality	• Speak quietly; go directly to the person with whom you need to speak, rather than speak loudly across the room or in front of others.
	• Do not discuss confidential matters within earshot of others.
	• Provide privacy by moving to a private area.
Customer relations	• Go the extra mile.
	• Listen.
	• Try to handle any problems—on the spot.
	• Display confidence and interest.
	• If someone complains, do not place blame; absorb the blame and make it right.
	• Be positive in all interactions; never argue.
	• Give people options; allow them to retain control.

Courtesy of Friendly Hills HealthCare Network.

Well-developed standards provide a qualitative measure of fit between a health care organization's abstract corporate values and actions at even the most basic level of detail. If consistent excellent performance is to be achieved, a culture of commitment to the standards must permeate the health care organization.

PRINCIPLES OF EFFECTIVE TRAINING—A FOUNDATION FOR PERFORMANCE IMPROVEMENT

Training plays an important role in developing a productive, patient-centered work force. Training represents one major approach to helping employees control or manage change. This happens because training is designed to lead the trainee to master new knowledge, attitudes, and skills. Training is a way of organizing information and experience so that an employee can behave differently on the job—to his or her own and the patient's benefit.

Effective training instructors, coaches, and facilitators focus on one or a combination of learner performance needs: attitude, skills, or knowledge. In some cases, a change of attitude (affective learning) is needed to improve specific areas of patient satisfaction (i.e., managing a myriad of MOTs). Although some improvement might occur with knowledge and skills training, negative patient perceptions won't cease until an employee's attitude improves. Coaching and facilitating skills are critical in these situations.

Training or coaching that is skill-based (physical or psychomotor learning) is particularly helpful with new employee orientation or when changes in job descriptions or technology require learning new skills. "Retraining" can also assist an employee who has not quite mastered a required skill yet. Determining a need for this type of training can be relatively straightforward when standards of performance are in place—comparing actual to expected performance on the job. Skills training usually involves demonstration, practice, and feedback from the facilitator or other expert.

Training that needs to impart knowledge (cognitive learning) to adults can be particularly challenging because this reminds adults of "school days" in the "content-push" environment of traditional formal education. Because training is often perceived as "dull" from the outset, retention rates may be somewhat low. Nevertheless, certain concepts, facts, procedures, policies, and so forth are required for successful job performance. Therefore, the provision of practical, necessary knowledge may require a creative approach to bring the material "alive" in order to maintain the learner's interest.

Thomas (1992) stated that there is confusion, even in the training profession, as to the precise nature of training. In his attempts to identify what the "real definition of training is," several common suggestions are listed (p. 71).

- Training is the process of equipping people with the specific attitudes, skills, and knowledge needed to carry out their responsibilities.
- Training is not education—education seeks to maximize the differences between people, whereas training aims to standardize individual performance to required levels.
- Training is a process of integrating personal and organizational goals.
- Training is the process by which we attempt to close the gap between an individual's present performance levels and his or her desired performance levels.
- Training is about helping people learn and develop; it should be centered on the learner and it should be fun.

Tracey, president of Human Resources Enterprises of Cape Cod, defined training and development as "all the learning experiences provided to employees to bring about changes in behavior that promote the attainment of the goals and objectives of the organization" (1992, p. 40). Included in this broad definition are all enterprise-conducted, -sponsored, and -supported activities and programs designed to:

- Develop the group and team skills needed to achieve organization goals and objectives
- Develop in individual employees the knowledge and skills needed to perform the jobs, duties, and tasks found in the organization
- Develop new skills in current employees to enable them to remain productive despite changes in technology, equipment, procedures, techniques, products, or markets
- Prepare selected employees to assume supervisory, managerial, and executive positions in the organization (management succession or regeneration)
- Improve the productivity of both individuals and work teams
- Encourage employee self-development and involvement in a program of lifelong learning

When considering the definition(s) and organizational performance implications of training, it is important to acknowledge that a variety of performance issues cannot be altered by training. In fact, these issues may prevent existing training from being effective, thereby appearing to fail in justifying the expense. Several causes or reasons for poor performance may require other organizational development interventions. These causes of poor performance include, but are not limited to, the following:

- *Lack of feedback:* Without feedback, employees assume that they are doing the job right, whether they are or not. Without positive feedback, even the most conscientious employee's performance may deteriorate over time.
- *Task interference:* An inefficient process or procedure, unclear directions, work overload, or conflicting priorities can interfere with behaviors that were recommended during training. If an employee can't do a job well because there are stumbling blocks in the way, management must get rid of the impediments before expecting training to alter performance.
- *Lack of practice:* How often is the employee expected to exhibit the desired behavior? If it is infrequent, perhaps a job aid would be appropriate. A checklist might, for example, remind an employee of the procedures for requesting a highly specialized laboratory or radiographic test.
- *Punishing performance:* Is the employee punished for doing the job well, whereas poor performers suffer no negative consequence? Is the person exhibiting the desired performance behaviors given extra work because he or she performs well?
- *Rewarding nonperformance:* Does the employee receive some advantage for not performing the desired behaviors? This is the classic case of an employee with a reputation for poor performance being given less to do.

Understanding the Adult Learner—A Prerequisite for Effective Training

Knowles, former Boston University Professor and author of 17 books and more than 170 articles, popularized the term "andragogy" referring to "the art and science of helping adults learn" (1987, p. 169). Initially, all formal educational institutions were established exclusively for the education of children and youth. There was only one model of assumptions about learners and learning—the "pedagogical model." Pedagogy literally means "the art and science of teaching children." Pedagogy assigns full responsibility for making all decisions about what should be learned, how it should be learned, when it should be learned, and if it has been learned, to the teacher. The role of students is to be submissive recipients of the directions and transmitted content of the teacher. In the first quarter of the twentieth century, when the concept of adult education was being organized, pedagogy was the only model teachers or trainers of adults had to go on. As a result, adults were taught as if they were children, and problems such as high dropout rates (where attendance was voluntary), low motivation, and poor performance were common.

Based on research conducted by Knowles and others, several assumptions about adults as learners have been formulated:*

- *Adults have a need to know why they should learn something.* Adults will expend considerable time and energy exploring what the benefits of their learning something will be and what the costs of their not learning it will be before they will be willing to invest time and energy in learning it.
- *Adults have a deep need to be self-directing.* The psychological definition of "adult" is one who has achieved a self-concept of being in charge of his or her own life and of being responsible for making his or her own decisions and living with the consequences. As a result, adults have a deep psychological need to be seen and treated by others as being capable of taking responsibility for themselves. Imposing the "other-directed" pedagogical model on adults in a training situation places them in a dependent role that conflicts with their need for self-directing independence.
- *Adults have a greater volume and different quality of experience than youth.* Generally speaking, the longer we live, the more experience and more varied experience we accumulate. This affects learning in several ways.
  1. Adults' background of experience is, in itself, a rich resource for many kinds of learning for themselves and for others.
  2. Adults have a broader base of experience to which to attach new ideas and skills and give them richer meaning.
  3. One can rest assured that a group of adults, especially if there is an age mix, will have a wider range of differences in back-

---

*Source: Reprinted with permission from M.S. Knowles, *Training and Development Handbook*, p. 168, © 1987, The McGraw-Hill Companies.

ground, interests, ability, and learning styles than is true of any group of youth.

4. The wealth of adults' previous experiences functions as somewhat of a resistant force because it tends to cause people to develop habits of thought and biases, to make presuppositions, and to be less open to new ideas.

- *Adults become ready to learn when they experience in their life situation a need to know or be able to do something in order to perform more effectively and satisfyingly.* We learn best when we choose voluntarily to make a commitment to learn. Adults experience "being told" as infringing on their adultness—their need to be self-directing—and tend to react with resentment, defensiveness, and resistance.
- *Adults enter into a learning experience with a task-centered (or problem-centered or life-centered) orientation to learning.* As a result, it is best for trainers to arrange programs around tasks, problems, and life situations.
- *Adults are motivated to learn by both extrinsic and intrinsic motivators.* Extrinsic motivators such as wage raises, promotions, better working conditions, and the like will move adults to learn up to the point that these needs are reasonably well satisfied. By far, the more potent and persistent drivers are such intrinsic motivators as the need for self-esteem, broadened responsibilities, power, and achievement. Thus, training should ideally appeal to both the desire for job advancement and life enrichment.

Assumptions associated with pedagogy versus andragogy have a number of implications for what we do in training. One basic implication is the importance of making a clear distinction between a *content plan* and a *process design*. The pedagog thinks in terms of drafting a content plan that answers the following questions:

- What content needs to be covered?
- How can this content be organized into manageable units?
- How can these content units be transmitted in a logical sequence?
- What would be the most effective means of transmitting this content?

The andragog, on the other hand, when planning an educational activity, sees the task as twofold. First and primary, to design and manage a process for facilitating the acquisition of content by the learners. Second, the educator is to serve as one content resource, recognizing that many other resources exist. It is not a matter of the pedagog being concerned with content and the andragog not being concerned. Rather, the pedagog is concerned with transmitting the content and the andragog is concerned with facilitating the acquisition of the content by the learners. The familiar adage that comes to mind to emphasize this point is that the adult trainer should be the "guide on the side...not the sage on the stage." Table 9–1 summarizes contrasting pedagogical versus andragogical assumptions about learners.

At this point, it should be obvious that in an adult training setting, special consideration needs to be given to the principles of andragogy. One would think that, given this body of knowledge pertaining to optimum conditions for adults to learn, all contemporary training would be appropriately designed to reflect this information. This is not the case! Every day, thousands of adults are subjected to training programs that are based entirely on how children learn. This is precisely why we have emphasized the pedagogy/andragogy distinctions before discussing any training that is directed toward improving patient satisfaction.

Although an in-depth review of adult learning is beyond the scope of this book, a number of practical guidelines were developed by Tracey (1992, p. 409). The following adaptation of these guidelines* can serve to assist you in developing and reviewing your patient satisfaction training:

- *Learner involvement:* Adults learn better and faster by doing—acting, participating, performing, producing. They respond best when they want and perceive a need to learn and when they help design and structure their learning experiences. This is why it is best to involve them in planning and selecting their learning ob-

Table 9–1 Andragogical Versus Pedagogical Assumptions about the Learner

Assumption Type	Pedagogical Assumption	Andragogical Assumption
Concept of the learner	Dependent personality	Increasingly self-directing
Role of the learner's experience	To be built on more than used as a resource	A rich resource for learning by self and others
Readiness to learn	Uniform by age level and curriculum	Develops from life tasks and problems
Orientation to learning	Subject-centered	Task- or problem-centered
Motivation to learn	By external rewards and punishment	By internal incentives and curiosity

*Courtesy of W. Tracey, © 1992, South Weymouth, Massachusetts.

jectives based on their own diagnosed deficiencies and learning needs. Adults are not interested in textbooks full of boring instruction, and hours of lecture turn them off. If they can participate actively in the learning process, the results—true learning—will be much better. Therefore, never simply demonstrate how to do something if an adult learner can actually perform the task, even if coaching is involved and it takes longer that way.

- *Customized activities:* Learning activities should be tailored to the learner's individual needs, skills, abilities, interests, and learning styles. All training strategies and techniques should be learner-centered rather than instructor-centered. Earlier training and past experiences of the learner should be exploited. Therefore, all training activities should start where the learners actually are, instead of where the facilitator thinks they should be. New knowledge should be related to, and integrated with, prior knowledge. In this regard, it is helpful to point out similarities with existing knowledge, but provide a rationale for changing. The key lies with helping the learner see how previous experiences actually lead to new—perceived as better—ways of doing things.

- *Credible problems and situations:* Adults respond best to real-world problems and challenges. If they are learning about their world, learning can take place naturally and effectively. There must be a perceived need for behavioral change coupled with an authentic application for the learning program. Therefore, the strategies, methods, and activities must involve real, job-related tasks, problems, and issues. The idea is to "stick to the point" by limiting information to that which is directly related to the duties and tasks that the learners are (or will be) required to perform on a regular basis.

- *Informal and relaxed climate:* Trying to intimidate adults by inundating them with information will only cause tension that, in turn, inhibits learning. Many adults have unpleasant memories of school days—grading, assigned seats, strict disciplinary rules, and so forth. The instructor should play the role of a partner and helper, not a taskmaster. Exercises and activities must be nonauthoritarian, nonthreatening and, where possible, nonevaluative. The general atmosphere should be pleasant, comfortable (seating and temperature), and satisfying. The facilitator-to-learner, learner-to-facilitator, and learner-to-learner atmosphere should be characterized by mutual respect, acceptance, openness, and trust.

It is best to seat a group of adult learners in such a way that all involved can participate actively, and provide a means for all learners to measure their own progress during the training process. This can take the form of a checklist of items they need to know. You should ask them to check off each item as it is mastered. Furthermore, the use of humor and informal discussion can help eliminate the educational "stigma" associated with traditional (content-push) classrooms.

Adult learning flourishes in a win-win, no-grades environment. Therefore, you should not implement any type of grading system unless the nature of your training absolutely requires it. Instead, offer plenty of guidance when and where it is needed. Checking learning objectives is far more effective than assigning a grade.

- *Variety of methods:* Whenever possible, try to use a variety of training methods and techniques (see a complete description of various techniques later in this chapter). Variety results in a higher level of learning than any single approach. Adults learn faster and better when facts, concepts, principles, and skills are presented in several different ways. Adults today are primarily visually literate and optically centered—they learn best through visual images because that has been their experience.

  Grinder and Bandler emphasized the three ways people process information: auditory, visual, and kinesthetic. Some learners learn best by simply listening, others by listening to and watching a video and then seeing a demonstration. Most learners, however, need hands-on participation or active discussion for learning to "sink in." Variety stimulates and tends to open up all five of the learner's senses. This is why it is important to change the training pace and technique from time to time.

- *Structured tasks:* When adults are asked to participate in learning activities and tasks, the experience needs to be organized and structured. Learning objectives and their associated skill and knowledge foundation must be broken down into manageable units or steps. Within this structured framework, however, there must be enough flexibility to accommodate the unique backgrounds, experiences, abilities, and learning styles of individual trainees. Learners must be provided with guidance, assistance, and suggestions for preventing mistakes during practice. Then, they must be given immediate feedback on their performance.

- *Application of learning:* If you expect the newly learned knowledge, skills, or attitudes to ultimately change on-the-job behaviors, trainees must be given opportunities to apply them in a realistic situation.

Robert Pike, president of Creative Training Techniques, developed "Pike's laws of adult learning" (1992, p. 3). These "laws" are included here as a supplement to the guidelines presented above.*

- *Adults are babies with big bodies.* The kinds of learning activities we did as small children included such things as coloring, drawing, playing games, modeling with clay, finger-painting, and so forth. Then, later in the educational process, these learning activities changed to sitting in rows, being talked *at,* and rarely being permitted to be involved in the learning process. As mentioned above, adults bring a lot of experience with them to the training room. Trainers must acknowledge, honor, and celebrate that experience.
- *People don't argue with their own data.* If a facilitator or instructor says that something is true, learners may or may not accept it as true. However, if you say it, for you, it is true! If trainees draw their own conclusions about which information that you presented will have immediate application back on the job, it reinforces the value of the training and demonstrates that people don't argue with their own data.
- *Learning is directly proportional to the amount of fun you have.* This is not referring to jokes or pointless games or entertainment. Rather, this is talking about the sheer joy of learning that can come from involvement and participation. Few trainers can truly entertain for hours on end. Fortunately, this isn't necessary. They can use the energy, involvement, and participation of the audience to put into their personal learning experiences.

    Humor itself (clean, nonoffensive to anyone), the kind that produces genuine, heartfelt laughter, can enhance the learning that takes place. This can be quite valuable in relaxing adults so they are more open to the learning process. The humor should make a point and not simply provide amusement. Furthermore, it should be used judiciously to enhance the learning process and enable participants to derive greater benefit.
- *Learning has not taken place until behavior has changed.* Plato has been credited with saying that "knowledge is power;" but I would like to suggest that applied knowledge is the real power! In train-

---

Source: Reprinted with permission from R. Pike, *Creative Training Techniques Handbook,* pp. 13–15, © Lakewood Books.

ing, it is not what you know, but what you can do with what you know that counts. That is why skill practice is so important in training sessions. If you want people to do things differently, then it is essential that you provide them with many opportunities to be comfortable accepting new ideas in a nonthreatening environment. Later in this chapter, when we discuss "transfer of training," we will see that there are a number of ways (in addition to practicing during the training session) to facilitate on-the-job application of the newly learned skills, attitudes, and/or knowledge.

- *It doesn't matter what I can do or what I can teach you to do. Ultimately what matters is what I can teach you to teach others to do.* This is one confirmation of the learner's competence—the ability to pass what you know on to someone else. Maslow developed a valuable conceptual framework to understand how we learn *anything*. This involves four sequential stages.

  1. *Unconscious incompetence:* Essentially, we don't know what we don't know. At the age of 5, we are unconsciously incompetent when it comes to driving a car. There has never been an opportunity or need for the 5-year-old to know; thus he or she is oblivious to the incompetence in this skill.

  2. *Conscious incompetence:* We now know what we don't know. When that same 5-year-old reaches the age of 15, he may bribe his 17-year-old brother to let him drive the car, just around the block. In a moment of weakness, big brother tosses the keys to a very surprised 15-year-old, who suddenly panics, realizing, "I don't know what to do. How do I start the car? How do I back the car up?" and so forth. The 15-year-old is now well aware of what he doesn't know.

  3. *Conscious competence:* With careful, conscious attention to the task at hand, it can be performed competently. The 15-year-old completes a driver's training course and is now capable of driving safely provided he pays close attention to the details of what he is doing while driving. Should he load his favorite compact disc, crank up the volume, and add two or three friends to the mix, the distractions may well compromise the safety of his driving.

  4. *Unconscious competence:* We don't have to think about knowing what we know. Continuing the driving analogy, this is the stage most experienced drivers are at. They can carry on a conversation with one or more passengers and drive quite safely at the same time, paying only limited conscious attention to the mechanics of driving.

It is important to realize that the level of competence can change with the situation. For example, after driving in the United States for many years, I was clearly at the unconscious competence level. Then, when attempting to drive a manual transmission automobile in Great Britain—on the left side of the road with the steering wheel on the right side of the ve-hicle—I experienced a quick slide to conscious incompetence. Now (at the time of writing), with several thousand miles under my experience belt, I am clearly sitting on the fence between conscious competence and unconscious competence. We have all experienced this type of transition in various aspects of life; such experiences repeatedly validate this model of learning.

Pike (1992) added a fifth stage to the model, which he termed "conscious unconscious competence" (p. 6).

5. *Conscious unconscious competence:* At this stage, not only are we competent and can run on "auto pilot," but we can also verbal-ize to others the how-tos of how we are able to do what we do.

According to Pike (1992), it is relatively easy to work our way up to unconscious competence, but it is far more difficult to reach conscious unconscious competence. Witness only the common situation where you ask someone who has truly mastered their craft, "How do you do that?" and they unwittingly respond with, "I don't know. I just do it."

Now we have a solid theoretical background for Pike's fifth "law of adult learning."

Identifying Training Needs

The process of systematically identifying training needs is somewhat like the work of a detective. You are aware that there is a problem (detec-tive = a crime to be solved; instructional designer = a performance prob-lem associated with skills, knowledge, or attitude to be solved) and you must search for clues that will help you solve the problem. This all starts with a clear definition of the current situation. Consider what you al-ready know about your situation, based on inputs from patients, patient family members, providers, staff, and outside sources.

In the context of assessing training needs for improving patient sat-isfaction, you already know a great deal based on all of the input previ-ously gathered (as outlined in Chapter 8). Exhibit 9–5 summarizes the information sources you have to identify improvement needs care-fully. Your behavior-based improvement priorities have already been

Exhibit 9–5 Sources of Input for Assessing Patient Satisfaction Improvement Training Needs

Improvement Needs Input Source	Mechanism for Receiving Input
Patients	• Patient satisfaction survey • Patient focus groups; advisory panels • Patient complaints • Patient grievances • Patient "defection" or disenrollment
Patient family members	• Complaint on behalf of patient
Employers	• Indirectly—employee satisfaction survey re: health care coverage • Directly—contract negotiations
Third-party payers (private insurance companies; Medicare)	• Contract negotiations; their own patient satisfaction surveys
Accrediting agencies	• Joint Commission on-site assessment • NCQA HEDIS evaluation
Health care organization employees ("nonmedical") • Receptionists • Appointment secretaries • Switchboard operators	• Employee suggestion program • Performance improvement teams • Direct patient observations/listening
Health care organization employees ("medical") • Health care providers • Nursing staff • Specialty services	• Performance improvement teams • Direct patient observations/listening
Health care organization management • Managers • Directors • Senior management	• Patient satisfaction performance gap analysis • Direct patient observations/listening • Communicating commitment to patient satisfaction • Allocating resources to improve patient satisfaction where needed

established for each of your facilities and/or departments, depending on the design of your patient satisfaction measurement system and the other sources used for input.

All of these sources combine to define your current situation clearly. The next step is to create a vision of where you want to be in the future. In other words, "What would it look like (in each of the respective improvement need areas) in the future if your training efforts were successful?" If the objective is to score higher in applicable areas of your health care organization's next patient satisfaction survey, define how much higher. If you wish to reduce patient complaints, state by how much. Are there any organizational issues that affect the success of your training efforts? These may need to be addressed prior to the onset of training.

By listing your current situations in detail, along with your vision of the "new improved" view of those same situations, you are now ready to perform a *gap analysis*. Table 9–2 shows a sample gap analysis demonstrating the basic format.

The ultimate objective of training interventions will be to develop a means of bridging the behavior-based performance gaps that have been identified. This leads us to the development of specific training objectives.

Table 9–2 Sample Gap Analysis Format

Current State	Gap Indicating Changes Needed To Move from Current to Future States	Ideal Future State
82% of patients rated doctor explanation of medical condition to be "very good or excellent" on recent patient satisfaction survey	Improved ability and willingness of doctor(s) to explain medical condition clearly to patients (training to be provided)	95% of patients rated doctor explanation of medical condition to be "very good or excellent" on next patient satisfaction survey
Five complaints per month regarding receptionist's attitude toward patients	• Coaching for improved performance • Appropriate training re: courtesy to patients	Zero complaints per month regarding receptionist's attitude toward patients

Developing Measurable Training Objectives

Once you have decided that training in the area(s) of skills, knowledge, or attitude is the best way to bridge the performance gap, the next step is to create training objectives. An objective is simply a description of a performance you would like your learners to be able to exhibit before you consider them competent. In other words, you are describing, in specific terms, your intended result of instruction, rather than the process of instruction. Mager (1984), the world-renowned expert on the design, development, and implementation of instruction, emphasized three important reasons for developing objectives (p. 5).

1. Without clearly defined objectives, there is no sound basis for the selection or design of instructional materials, content, or methods. If you don't know where you are going, it is difficult to develop a suitable means for getting there.
2. Objectives establish the "mileposts along the road of learning." In order for instructors to determine whether or not the training has accomplished what they set out to accomplish, whether by testing or otherwise, objectives must be in place.
3. Objectives provide learners with a means to organize their own efforts toward accomplishment of those objectives. With clear objectives in view, students at all levels are better able to decide what activities on their part will help them get to where it is important for them to go.

The main function of objectives, then, is to communicate in measurable terms. When objectives are sent in a clear fashion, instructors can do a better job of instructing and trainees can do a better job of learning. Precisely stated objectives provide an essential ingredient for evaluating the effectiveness of instructors—agreement between the evaluator and the one evaluated about what the instruction should accomplish.

We mentioned earlier that training is capable of modifying behavior in the areas of skills, knowledge, and attitude. Therefore, we will briefly examine the contents of objectives for each of these training types.

- *Knowledge-based objectives* require the learner to recall information to accomplish some task. This may involve recalling rules, facts, names, places, terminology, titles, formulas, definitions, concepts, or principles. For example, the trainee may be asked to list three of your health care organization's personal interaction standards. Knowledge often supports, and may be a prerequisite to, the development of a particular skill or set of skills. It is important to clarify what you mean by indicating to learners that you want them to "know" something. This could mean many different things. Until you have specifically stated this in terms of what the learner ought to be able to do, you have said very little at all! Thus, a performance objective should be communicated clearly and precisely enough that there is little room for misinterpretation. This can be accomplished best by using a format that contains the learning objective characteristics described later in this chapter.

- *Mental skill-based objectives* require the learner to identify, classify, or solve problems that involve cognitive processes. For example, the trainee may be asked to analyze a case study to determine which personal interaction standards were not followed in events leading up to a patient complaint about the receptionist's behavior. Mental skills objectives involve identifying symbols; classifying objects, symbols, and concepts (such as MOTs vs. SPs); using principles and rules; discriminating or detecting differences; using verbal information; decision making; and problem solving.
- *Physical skill-based objectives* require the learner to perform some physical or manipulative activity. These objectives involve the performance of gross motor skills; steering, guiding, and positioning movements; and voice communicating. For example, the trainee may be asked to answer an incoming telephone call appropriately, place the patient on "hold," and then transfer the call.
- *Attitude-based objectives* are usually not observable, but are reflected in the decisions or choices people make. These typically require the learner to make a choice or decision. For example, the trainee may be presented with a typical workplace situation whereby an elderly patient is confused about where to go for his or her laboratory tests (not-so-obvious location). The trainee may be asked to choose between a verbal description combined with "pointing" or escorting the patient personally to the radiology department. The learner who chooses to escort the confused patient can be said to have displayed an attitude of "going the extra mile" to help patients.

According to Mager (1984, p. 21), the optimum format for effectively communicating the intent of an objective answers three important questions.

1. What should the learner be able to do?
2. Under what conditions (if any) do you want the learner to be able to do it?
3. How well must it be done?

In terms of descriptive characteristics, the answers to these questions translate into the following:

- *Performance:* An objective should always state what the learner is expected to do; this often describes the product or result of the doing. If the performance happens to be somewhat covert, add an indicator behavior to the objective by which the main performance can be known. Make the indicator the simplest and most direct one possible. The learned behavior may involve the application of knowledge or the demonstration of a specific skill or constellation of skills.
- *Conditions:* An objective always indicates the important conditions under which the performance is to occur. If it seems useful, add a sample test item. Add as much description as is needed to communicate the intent to others. For example: "Without references, be able to recall (write) the five steps involved in the 'recovery' process used in managing a nonmedical patient complaint."

   In summary then, the conditions of the objective should identify what learners will be given to use in doing the performance (tools, equipment, job aids, references, materials). Also, anything that will be denied during the performance should be listed (tools, equipment, references, etc.). Furthermore, indicate what assistance (if any) learners will have, what supervision will be provided, and the physical environment in which they must perform (climate, space, light, etc.).
- *Criterion:* To the extent possible, an objective should detail the criterion of acceptable performance by describing how well the learner must perform in order for performance to be considered acceptable. You should try to include words that clearly describe your criterion for success. Keep in mind that you are not trying to specify the minimum or "barely tolerable" criterion. Rather, you are looking for ways to express the desired criterion.

   One of the most common criterion descriptors is the speed with which the performance is to take place (i.e., a time limit). This is particularly valuable if speed of performance is important in the actual workplace. For example, "Acknowledge/greet a patient (in the prescribed manner) within 15 seconds of arrival." On the other hand, if speed is unimportant, you should not impose this limitation in the context of training.

   Sometimes, accuracy is more important than speed; other times, both speed and accuracy are important. For instance, "Obtain test results from the clinical laboratory and communicate them to the doctor with no errors and no details omitted." In other cases, quality may be the critical issue, not speed or accuracy. Most specifically, this would communicate the acceptable deviation from perfection. Yet other times, the quantity of work products produced may be important and should be designated.

Elements of Adult Instruction

With a clear understanding of the adult learner in mind, and with clear learning objectives in hand, you are now ready to consider the optimum elements to be included in the instruction. First, the essential ingredients for learning to remain an active process will be presented. Then, a set of practical guidelines to help you with designing your PSI training will be provided.

Meyers and Jones (1993) identified four key elements associated with active learning that we all use to create new mental structures: talking and listening, writing, reading, and reflecting (p. 21). These cognitive activities allow learners to clarify, question, consolidate, and appropriate new knowledge. "The brain engages in different thinking processes, or operations when we talk, listen, read, write, and reflect—an observation supported by research on teaching and learning" (p. 21). A brief look at the functional implications of each of these elements will help underscore the importance of incorporating them in your instructional design.*

- *Talking and listening:* Although learners should learn from the insights of instructors, and verbal presentation can be a valuable prelude to active learning, *the problem is not that instructors talk.... it's that they talk too much!* There comes a time when, after listening to an instructor for a while, everyone needs to speak in order to clarify what they have heard, read, observed, or experienced. In other words, talking clarifies our thinking in a way that merely absorbing the words of others cannot. In fact, we often don't really know what we think about a given topic until we try to put it into words. Speaking forces us to organize and structure our comments so that they make sense to the listener. By providing learners with time and activities to talk and listen to each other, they are actually gaining the self-discipline to be clearer about their thinking.
- *Writing:* Just as speaking clarifies our thinking, so does writing. The specific purpose of having learners write is that it helps them

---

*Source: Reprinted with permission from C. Meyers and T. Jones, *Promoting Active Learning*, p. 21, © 1993, Jossey-Bass Publishers.

to explore their own thinking about concepts and issues. Toby Fulwiler, a nationally respected writing educator, advises that writing "is an essential activity to create order from chaos, sense from nonsense, meaning from confusion: as such it is the heart of creative learning in both the arts and sciences" (1987, p. 44).

A helpful writing format I have used as an instructor in both college and workshop settings for adults involves the learners reflecting on the subject matter recently discussed. More specifically, I ask them to use the "What? So what? and Now what?" approach to this reflection. To clarify how this is to be carried out, the following description of each component is provided:

1. *What?* This question helps the learner briefly describe his or her understanding of the content discussed. This typically leads the learner to review his or her notes or any handout materials in preparation for paraphrasing the material.
2. *So what?* This question helps the learner to reflect on the specific relevance of the content to his or her life or work requirements. In other words, have the learner describe why a specific aspect of the content is particularly relevant to what he or she is doing or attempting to do as part of daily home or work life.
3. *Now what?* This question helps the learner succinctly formulate what he or she will do differently as a result of the new knowledge or information. This makes the content "actionable" for the learner. This can come in one of two forms—looking backward as critical self-reflection of a situation in the past or looking to the future when an appropriate opportunity for knowledge application occurs.
   - *Reading:* This requires learners to think in a slightly different manner because the purpose is to understand what others think, as opposed to primarily clarifying their own thoughts by talking and writing. Additionally, reading uses higher level thinking skills because learners must connect ideas and sources of information, identify faulty logic in argumentation, recognize biases or hidden agendas, and locate unsupported ideas. Using the so-called "selective attention theory," it is best if learners are given a set of questions to keep in mind before they start the reading, or to be prepared to summarize the key points in the reading. This functions to improve their comprehension of the reading. In Adler's classic article "How To Mark a Book" (1940), readers are encouraged to mark up their books—underline, highlight, circle key words, and scribble comments in the

margins. He considered this not to be destructive in any way, but rather that "the physical act of writing, with your hand, brings words and sentences more sharply before your mind and preserves them better in your memory" (p. 11).

- *Reflecting:* This gives the learner the opportunity to foster critical reflection skills. This refers to the ability to identify and critique the preconceptions or seldom-tested assumptions that each of us brings to new learning experiences. In any significant learning experience, we can't help increasing the value of the learning by taking time to reflect on the new information.

Guidelines for Effective PSP Training

As you set about the task of designing your PSI training (behavior-based), the following guidelines regarding their sequence and approach, based on the work of Silber and Stelnicki (1987, p. 266), will help ensure the optimum effectiveness:*

- *Attention/motivation:* It is essential that you get the attention of the learner right from the beginning of the program. If this is done properly, it will serve to motivate learners to pay attention to what follows. The question in the minds of learners in this regard is the same question we all have in mind any time we are asked to invest any of our time or money: "What's in it for me?" Indicate to the learners the importance to them of learning what you will cover. Explain how it may make their life or work more interesting, or how it will help them to be more valuable or productive, which can translate to valued rewards.
- *Influence/credibility:* Often, early in an educational environment (whether training or university work), the question in the mind of the learner is, "Why should I listen to him or her?" This is best answered at the onset of the program. Begin by providing the credentials of the person facilitating the workshop, program, seminar, or whatever. Then, periodic citing of relevant research adds to the credibility because the learners can clearly see that they are not about to be inundated with the preferences and biases of the instructor alone. And finally, providing learners with references sets the stage for them to further research any aspect of what they are learning in the immediate setting. This is comforting because adults by and large

---

Source: Reprinted with permission from R. Craig, *Training and Development Handbook,* p. 266, © 1987, The McGraw-Hill Companies.

engage regularly in self-directed learning, based on the relevance and interest they have in the topic under consideration.

- *Objectives:* The same principles of developing objectives identified above apply to the actual program delivery. Learners must clearly understand the objectives of the learning experience they are about to experience. Objectives must be clearly stated, including a description of any new skills that will be acquired—using the performance, conditions, and criterion format to preclude any misunderstanding.

- *Context/familiarity:* Adults learn best when they can "place" the new information on the specific branch of their existing knowledge tree where similar information already resides. Thus, by helping the learner to recall previous knowledge, then linking the new knowledge to that, the "known" can be perceived as useful building blocks to the "unknown." This is an important strategy for alleviating the anxiety that is often associated with the common adult learning fear based on their dreadful pedagogical experiences.

- *Mental set:* Adult learners feel much more in control when they know the organization, sequence, and format that will be used to present the information that will be covered. Therefore, give them the "big picture," not unlike the "org chart" of a large corporation; this allows them to see how things will be interrelated. It is a sort of map they can use to anticipate where the current topic component is headed.

- *Chunking:* It is much more palatable for the learner—especially if there is a large quantity of information to be learned—to have the information divided in a logical fashion. Each "chunk" should be labeled and presented in the sequence identified at the onset.

- *Illustrations:* The use of visuals supports our understanding of adult emphasis on visual processing of new information. Diagrams or photographs are most helpful if they are captioned and/or explained so there is no room for misinterpretation of the point you are trying to make. The highlights or main points should be emphasized either in the visual itself or in the method of presentation.

- *Intra-organizers:* These let the learner always be aware of how the current discussion fits into the overall instructional "map" described earlier. It may be helpful in this regard to learn from our contemporary shopping malls. They typically provide a large map of every store contained in the mall, along with the much-welcomed "you are here" arrow. Learners feel much more acclimated when they are aware of how the process is progressing according to the original plan. By reusing the same map after each major section, and simply pointing out where the upcoming segment fits, the learner remains fully aware of the current status. This can also be effectively combined with either the facilitator or learner checking off the learning objectives as you accomplish each in progressing through the material.

- *Relevant examples:* The use of examples facilitates the learner in capturing the essential characteristics of the idea being presented. Often, a theoretical explanation of something quite simple sounds somewhat confusing and complex. Then, once a relevant example is provided, the proverbial "light comes on" in the mind of the learner. A useful rule of thumb is to give two good practical examples of each concept being discussed. Once again, this is a valuable move in the direction of clarification for the learner.

- *Frequent relevant practice:* If you allow for questions to be asked either throughout the workshop or, at the very least, at the end of each "chunk" of information, learners are less likely to "tune you out" while you are moving on to other material. If your training is targeted toward a new skill, allow learners two opportunities to practice that skill before continuing. This will reinforce the performance in their minds—increasing the odds that there will later be a "transfer" of the learning to the actual work environment.

- *Feedback:* We learned earlier that the sooner feedback occurs following the behavior, the more effective it can be in influencing that behavior. Therefore, if you wish to encourage the participation that is so necessary to active learning, you should praise and encourage learners who dare to contribute to the discussion. It has been my experience that the best way to get even "introverts" to open up and participate is to demonstrate right before their eyes that speaking up (appropriately) is not only encouraged, but appreciated. Even if learners offer the wrong answer, find something about what they have said to support their contribution. Otherwise, you can bet they will be very hesitant to participate again. On the other hand, when learners offer the correct answer to a question you may pose, let the rest of the group know why that is the correct answer, unless it is intuitively obvious.

- *Review:* As adults, we are accustomed to having things neatly packaged together. This holds true of new information as well. Take the time to tie the essentials together, highlighting the key points. This is even more effective when the information presented is stated in the original way, then restated slightly differently. This way, learners leave the session with a neatly tied together package of information that is placed where it "belongs" on the tree of their existing knowledge, ready for immediate application and retrieval.

Common Instructional Techniques and Methods

When we discussed our guidelines for adult learning, it was recommended that you use a variety of methods to sustain learner interest and motivation. A comprehensive representation of all techniques and methods is well beyond the scope of this chapter. However, a number of training industry books are available that cover each approach with the thoroughness necessary to prepare those who wish to optimize their instruction. For your immediate reference, you may wish to consult one or more of the publications listed at the end of this chapter.

What follows is a brief discussion of several of the more commonly used methods of instruction. Each approach has its own advantages and limitations. It is important that you select the strategies that will best meet your PSI training needs. To assist you in this process, make sure you review your instructional objectives, course content, trainee population, instructor availability, instructional space, facilities, equipment, materials, available time, and costs.

- *Lecture:* This is basically a means of telling trainees information they need to know. Essentially, it is a formal presentation that is used to achieve an instructional objective. Although a lecture should never constitute the entire educational offering, it can be used for specific functions.
  1. Orient trainees to course policies, rules, procedures, purposes, and learning resources.
  2. Introduce a subject, indicate its importance, and present an overview of its scope.
  3. Give directions on procedures for use in subsequent learning activities.
  4. Present basic material that will provide a common background for subsequent activities.
  5. Set the stage for a demonstration, discussion, or performance.
  6. Illustrate the application of rules, principles, or concepts.
  7. Review, clarify, emphasize, or summarize.

The advantage of using a lecture is that it saves time because the instructor can present more material in a given amount of time than by any other method. The presentation can be adjusted to the educational level, training, and experience of the class.

The disadvantage, of course, is that a lecture is essentially a one-way process. The instructor speaks and the learner sits, listens, and takes notes. Most lectures permit little or no interchange of ideas between the instructor and the trainees. Because of this, it is an inappropriate technique for teaching skills such as equipment operation. Although most learning takes place via the visual sense, the lecture (even if supplemented with visual aids) appeals mainly to the auditory sense.

- *Modified lecture:* This is similar to a lecture, except the instructor encourages some group participation. This way, the trainer can rely on the trainee's experiences to generate some form of discussion. It should be made clear right from the beginning that this learning method is intended to be interactive and that audience participation would be appreciated.
- *Question and answer:* This involves one person provoking a response by inquiry, usually from person to person. The advantage of this technique is that it provides for the clarification of information to answer specific needs of the learner. It is also easily combined with other methods. The disadvantage is that it tends to become too formal, threatening, and embarrassing; the group may become bored and lose interest.
- *Conference:* With this method, group discussion techniques are used to reach instructional objectives. These techniques include questions, answers, and comments from the instructor in combination with answers, comments, and questions from the trainees. There are three basic types of conferences.
  1. *Directed discussion:* This type of conference assists trainees with gaining a better understanding and ability to apply known facts, principles, concepts, policies, or procedures. The function of the facilitator is to guide the discussion in such a way that this knowledge is clearly articulated and applied.
  2. *Training conference:* Here the objective is to pool the knowledge and past experience of the trainees to arrive at improved or more clearly stated principles, concepts, policies, or procedures. The primary role of the instructor is to elicit contributions from the group, based on past experiences, that have a bearing on the topic at hand. Balanced participation is the goal.
  3. *Seminar:* This is a meeting of any size conducted for a group of people who have a common need. They are normally led by an expert in the topic area. The purpose of a seminar is to find an answer to a question or a solution to a problem. The seminar leader might present relevant research findings so that the participants can discover the correct solutions based on those find-

ings. The instructor does not necessarily have an answer or a solution. Rather, the primary functions of the instructor are to describe the problem and to encourage free and full participation in a discussion aimed at identifying the real problem, gathering and analyzing data, forming and testing hypotheses, determining and evaluating alternative courses of action, arriving at conclusions, and making recommendations to support or arrive at a solution or decision.

- *Buzz group:* This is when a large group is divided into smaller groups of 5–10 individuals discussing a particular topic and then reporting back to the larger group. The advantage of this format is that it promotes enthusiasm and involvement as it provides opportunity for maximum discussion in limited time. The limitation of this format is that the discussion tends to be somewhat shallow, disorganized, and easily dominated by one or two individuals in the group. This type of group requires a skillful facilitator to handle the process.
- *Workshop:* This is a group of any size with a common interest or background. Workshops are generally conducted so that the participants can improve their ability or understanding by combining study and discussion; they tend to be user-driven, whereby participants may influence the direction of the program from its beginning.
- *Demonstration:* This is where the instructor actually performs a job or task, thereby showing the trainees what to do and how to do it; he or she then explains the process to point out why, where, and when it is to be done. Typically, the trainee is expected to be able to repeat the job or task after the demonstration. The demonstration is often used in combination with another method, such as lecture-demonstration or demonstration-performance combinations.

The basic purpose of a demonstration is to show how something is done. Trainees tend to learn faster and more permanently with demonstration than lecture alone for several reasons.

1. Demonstrations make explanations concrete by giving meaning to the words.
2. Demonstrations provide perspective by showing the complete performance of a procedure. Relationships between steps of the procedure and accomplishment of the objective are clarified.
3. Demonstrations appeal to several senses. Not only do trainees see and hear during a demonstration, but they are often given the opportunity to touch the equipment.

4. Demonstrations provide dramatic appeal. When they are well planned and executed, demonstrations have a dramatic quality that arouses and sustains interest and attention.

- *Performance:* This is a method in which the trainee is required to perform, under controlled conditions, the task, skill, or movement being taught. The various types of performance taught in this setting are: independent practice, where trainees work individually and at their own pace; group performance, where trainees work together in groups at the rate established by the instructor; coach and pupil, where trainees are paired and members of each pair perform alternatively as instructor and trainee; and team performance, where a group of trainees performs a task or function involving teamwork.

- *Role play:* This is a laboratory method of instruction that involves the spontaneous dramatization or acting out of a situation by two or more individuals under the direction of a trainer. The situations that the participants act out are usually related to the workplace and involve situations (such as patient encounters) that the players might be involved in. Then, after the role players have been identified, they act out the parts as they would normally, or perhaps try new behaviors shown to them during training. Once the scenario has been played out, the role players, the rest of the group, and the trainer carry out a critique of the role play, identifying good and bad points and including suggestions for other behaviors and other possibilities.

  Role plays are normally followed by group discussion, and time must be allowed for this very important part of the session. This is an ideal format to use for PSI training because participants can be placed in situations that are directly related to the improvement objectives.

- *Case study:* This method includes a written description of situations that contain enough details so learners can discuss specific recommendations. The advantages of this type of method are that it focuses the discussion and learning experience, it provides a shared understanding of on-the-job problems, and it provides "real-world" applications when it is customized appropriately. The disadvantages of this format are that it may impose time limitations for reading and discussion, it is somewhat difficult to develop and incorporate all the necessary details, and it only builds and demonstrates understanding, not skills.

- *Practice application:* This method involves immediate skill application in a specific patient-contact on-the-job situation the employees are currently facing. The advantages of this format are that learners get practice handling a real-world situation and task using specific skills and behaviors being learned in training, hands-on experience is often more enjoyable for the learner, and there is an opportunity to receive immediate coaching feedback. The limitations are the common resistance of employees to practice in front of peers, the fact that learner focus may be directed toward solving the specific situation rather than practicing the skill being developed and, finally, the realization that some learners prefer to have time to "digest" information first before being put on the spot to apply it right away.

- *Personal action planning:* This involves the identification of specific activities that employees are committed to carry out back on the job. The advantages of this type of format include immediate and focused application of skills, behaviors, and knowledge; facilitation of the documentation and reinforcement of key learnings while still at work; and promotion of personal accountability for learning. The disadvantages of this approach are that some employees may be unwilling to make a commitment to apply training, plans may lack specific follow-up and accountability mechanisms, and reinforcement may come only through punitive consequences rather than rewards.

Learning Materials as an Aid to Training

A variety of learning materials are available for supplementing and potentially increasing the overall effectiveness of training. Before discussing several specific learning tools, we will consider five quality characteristics described by Wade (1995, p. 27).

1. *Visible:* All support materials need to be easily seen by everyone in the audience. This means that you must carefully tailor the size of the print to the size of the audience.
2. *Simple:* Do not present too much material in one visual; the content should be easily "digestible." Limit the amount of information you include. Make use of key words and concepts rather than full sentences and paragraphs. By keeping things simple, learners can easily remember what you want them to.
3. *Accurate:* The information should be up-to-date, factually correct, properly ordered, and complete. If you show something that is perceived as outdated, the credibility of the remainder of the in-

struction may be in jeopardy. If revisions are done between times of presenting the same material, make sure all training materials reflect the changes.

4. *Interesting:* The design, colors, and graphics of all training materials should attract the attention of adult learners. Arrange the information in a creative way to help develop and maintain attention. The illustrations and examples should help promote retention.

5. *Practical:* The program needs to be "easily identified with" from the learner's point of view.

By supporting a presentation with audiovisual aids, you can effectively focus on key concepts, provide clarification of important points, and review selected topics. When your visual training aids are prepared with the characteristics described above, they can serve a number of valuable functions.

- *Simplify complex or obscure material.* A picture, graph, diagram, or model is truly worth a thousand words. It is common for a concept or process to be comprehensible only when it is diagrammed or illustrated. Spatial diagrams can be of tremendous assistance in clarifying complex relationships. As a general rule, if your audiovisual aid simplifies the subject of your discussion, keep it. If it does not, get rid of it and create a different one.

- *Focus attention on the essence of the topic.* Interactive presentations are at high risk for getting sidetracked. A good visual will keep what is important in front of the learners at all times so that everyone remains focused on the topic.

- *Make key points memorable.* Good visual aids can function as "hooks" on which to "hang" your memory of the information. An impressive slide, model, film, diagram, sign, poster, or sound event can be retained far longer than words. Well-prepared visual aids can make a presentation unforgettable.

- *Take the learners where they could not otherwise go.* In this regard, movies and videotapes are best, but slides can also be very effective, especially for fine details. Furthermore, sounds are fantastic for setting atmosphere and mood. These types of techniques enable you to observe providers interacting with patients, tour a particular health care facility, enter into minute spaces, and watch processes that cannot be brought into the room. Always keep in mind, though, that the primary purpose is to aid learning—not just to dazzle and entertain!

- *Create variety.* It is a simple fact that too much of anything becomes boring. By planning a multimedia presentation, you can create a refreshing change of pace or a sense of newness. However, beware that too much variety becomes just as dull as too little, and variety for its own sake wears thin after a while. When combining an overhead projection woven throughout the discussion with a flipchart to capture participant input and periodic videos or video segments to bring things alive, I have found it quite easy to sustain audience interest and attention.
- *Save time.* Having a model to handle or a diagram to refer to not only simplifies the material, but makes explaining the diagrammed or modeled concepts much easier and, therefore, saves time.

The next consideration is to decide which visual aids you wish to supplement your instruction. Table 9–3 lists various audiovisual aids comparing their primary purpose, advantages, and disadvantages.

Purchasing "Off-the-Shelf" Training Programs

An "off-the-shelf" program is one that is mass-produced, like books, and comes as a complete package, ready for trainees. Off-the-shelf programs come in a variety of forms, including the following:

- textbooks covering all required subjects, containing questions at the end of each chapter, or workbooks that accompany the text
- self-study programs that combine explanatory material with study questions and projects
- standard programmed instruction materials
- audiocassette/compact disc learning packages
- audio with slide presentations
- videocassettes on specific topics and general subjects, with or without accompanying facilitator's guide and/or trainee workbooks
- films typically covering key generic concepts (e.g., managing patient complaints)
- computer-based instructional materials
- interactive compact or videodisc instructional programs

There are many commercially available packaged training programs on the market today. A survey of Fortune 500 firms revealed that 85% of them use external suppliers for training programs. Human resources professionals agree that this trend toward more and more available off-

Table 9–3 A Comparative Look at Audiovisual Aids to Training

Visual Type	Primary Purpose	Advantages	Disadvantages
Slides	Take us where we cannot otherwise go (close-ups, enlargements, etc.)	Colorful, varied, easily transportable; give uniform presentation	Require darkened room; no personal contact; possible mechanical problems; overused; passive, not active
Flipcharts and posters	Can develop material interactively with a group; can refer back to earlier material	Flexible, simple, readily available, colorful; show organization of material; enhance interaction in a group; can be referred to several times	Limited sight-lines; limited viewing distance; replacement costs; markers dry out; awkward to transport
Whiteboards and chalkboards	Best when you need to add or remove things in a diagram; excellent for chart development; good scratch pad; useful when reinforcing atmosphere is desirable	Can be colorful; flexible; familiar; universally available	Limited sight-lines; messy, smelly; must be erased; associated with "school"
Overhead projectors	Overlap of transparencies to show layers of complexity in a simple form; good for systems presentation; flowcharting and developmental materials	Universal; readily available; simple to use; flexible, colorful; great with large groups; easy reference to past materials; enhance interaction	Limited sight-lines; distracting if used sloppily; keystoning (top is wider than bottom if projected at an angle upward) of projection
Videotapes	Let you see and evaluate our own performance; action-oriented like film but can be homemade and are easier to update	Dynamic; takes you where you cannot otherwise go; easily updated; easily transported	Incompatible formats (ex. NTSC = USA whereas PAL = UK) can be a problem; fairly high initial cost
Audiotapes	Let you hear yourself as others hear you; let you listen and learn while traveling	Effective for sound-oriented training; portable; create mood	Limited aural attention span; talk at learners, not with them; no interaction; limited sensory input

continues

Table 9–3 continued

Visual Type	Primary Purpose	Advantages	Disadvantages
Computers	Hands-on practice; can be used to give trainees practice on equipment they will actually use; excellent for simulations	Self-paced instruction; interactive; exciting future	Mechanical process with no human contact; high initial expense; time-consuming to program; tied to commercial software; monotonous to use; tendency for information overload
Handouts	Useful for hands-on practice and for giving assignments	Can be referred back to after the course; no sight-line problems	Distracting if distributed while you are speaking
Pointers	Excellent for focusing trainee's attention on one specific detail at a time	Can be used to enhance several other visual aids (slides, boards, posters…)	Distracting if played with; excess movement with no purpose is nauseat-ing!
Models or actual items	Demonstrate how things actually work, look, or will look; show complex relationship of parts in context; show internal movements; allow close inspec-tion and hands-on practice	Real thing; larger than (or as large as) life; help visualization of the abstract; take you where you cannot otherwise go; some easily made	Limited sight-lines; initial cost; unavail-ability; storage and breakage problems; maintenance; distracting if used sloppily; tendency for information overload

the-shelf programs is likely to continue well into the future. So, how do you decide whether to consider this option for your health care organization's PSI training needs? Several factors should be taken into consideration when making this decision.

- *The size of the population to be trained:* When the training popula-tion is relatively small and the per person or per course costs in-curred are less than the costs of developing a new course, purchas-ing makes the most sense. Commonly, when budgets are tight, a program used by many companies will have a much lower breakeven point than a single custom package. When the training population is large and the costs of developing a course are less than the recurring per person or per course costs or a bought course, then in-house development is best.

Even where budget and time allow for custom-developed programs, the variety of available programs may include packages that meet your organization's needs. There is no need to "reinvent the wheel."

- *The nature of the competencies to be trained:* When most of the competencies that your organization needs to focus on are general, functional topics, then purchasing is the best choice. However, when most of the competencies are company- or job-specific, then in-house development makes more sense.
- *The timing of the training:* When training is needed quickly, greater flexibility of training dates is required (assuming a widely available course), or coverage at work is a problem (as employees can only be released in small numbers), program purchase may be better. In-house program development generally needs greater planning and, therefore, longer lead times from conception to delivery.
- *The type of training experiences required:* In some instances, it might be better to have employees from various departments all go through training together in order to gain a wider perspective; this may be more easily facilitated by purchasing an off-the-shelf program. In other instances, however, where there is a need/advantage to have employees trained separately by department/facility—teamwork, communication, and so forth—then developing training in-house that specifically addresses the unique improvement needs of each facility/department is more appropriate.

There are a number of reasons why you may wish to search outside for your PSI training needs. For example, you may not find the proper content specialists, program designers, producers, or production facilities in-house. Even if such resources exist, they may not be available within your time frame. Also, when time, money, or staff limits your options, off-the-shelf programs become a viable choice.

Once you have made the decision to purchase a program from the outside, the next decision involves selecting the best one from those available. A good way to make this decision systematically is to use a comparison ranking. This procedure consists of the following sequential steps:

1. *List the important criteria used to select the program.* This list might include such items as course content, specific to health care in-

dustry, cost(s), instructional method, supplier reputation, ability to customize to your health care organization, media compatibility with what you already have, ease of implementation, and results orientation.

2. *Assign a relative importance weight to each criterion.*
3. *Compare each program under consideration, and rate how it best fits the criteria.* A rating of "3" represents a best fit, a "2" is second best, and "1" is third best (the actual numbers would change if you were, for example, comparing four or five different programs. Then, the ratings would run from "4/5" down to "1").
4. *Multiply the relative importance weight by the rating of each program to yield a criteria-specific program "value" for each program.*
5. *Add the total of program values (i.e., covering all criteria) for each program; this gives a total weighted ranking for each program.*
6. *Select the program with the highest overall weighted ranking because it best meets your criteria.*

Table 9–4 illustrates this procedure when there are three frontline employee PSI training programs under consideration, where Program

---

Table 9–4 Selection Chart for Purchased Patient Satisfaction Training

Selection Criteria	Relative Importance	Program A Rank	Program A Value	Program B Rank	Program B Value	Program C Rank	Program C Value
Course content	30	2	60	3	90	1	30
Health care specific	15	3	45	2	30	1	15
Costs	25	3	75	2	50	3	75
Instructional method	10	2	20	1	10	2	20
Supplier reputation	10	1	10	3	30	2	20
Ability to customize	15	3	45	2	30	1	15
Media compatibility	10	2	20	1	10	3	30
Implementation ease	20	2	40	3	60	1	20
Results orientation	20	1	20	3	60	2	40
Totals:			335		370		265

"B" is the logical choice. This assumes that all three of the "finalist" programs meet your basic program requirements and it implies that others have been eliminated from consideration earlier in the selection process.

DEVELOPING TARGETED PSI TRAINING PROGRAMS

When considering your organization's PSI training needs, it may be best to view off-the-shelf programs as worthwhile supplements to your tailor-made overall approach. For example, the use of the award-winning video entitled "It's a Dog's World" (CRM Films, 1994), functions nicely to introduce the concept of MOTs (and their impact on patient perceptions) to your employees. This is accompanied by an exceptionally well-designed facilitator's guide that assists the trainer in orchestrating organization-specific discussion both before and after video viewing.

The concept of "targeting" your patient satisfaction training refers to two things. First, the information is designed with a particular audience in mind—training for health care providers is commonly different (in some ways) from that intended for nonmedical frontline employees. Second, the training is targeted toward closing a particular performance gap identified during your needs assessment.

Training for Your Health Care Organization's Health Care Providers

Although a variety of PSI efforts may logically be targeted toward health care providers, few deserve the high level of emphasis required for *communication*. Much of the relationship that develops between a health care provider and patient is dependent on positive communication. In a 1995 survey of 1,004 adult consumers and 416 physicians (218 general practitioners and 198 specialists), communication was identified as a major factor in measuring quality of care (Skol Corporation, 1996). This research indicated that consumers who rate communication between themselves and their physicians as excellent were four times more likely to believe that they received excellent medical care than those who did not rate their physicians' communication as excellent (83% vs. 22%).

Few health care providers would argue the importance of communication. Both physicians and patients rate communication-related characteristics as extremely important when evaluating the quality of medical care, but they differ on what constitutes good communication. The Bayer survey revealed that 55% of the patients surveyed, but only 28% of the physicians surveyed, believe that patients share responsibility equally with the physician or even have primary responsibility for establishing good communication (Skol Corporation, 1996). Patients tend to look at communication from a broader perspective than their physicians, rating interactive discussions about their current condition and overall health as most important. Physicians, on the other hand, tend to concentrate on the specific reason for the patient visit, as well as their own ability to explain and discuss treatment options and outcomes with the patient.

The following communication characteristics were rated as "extremely important" by consumers and physicians:

- Physician discusses conditions, options, and outcomes.
  1. Consumers: 80%
  2. Physicians: 78%
- Physician listens to patient's health concerns.
  1. Consumers: 72%
  2. Physicians: 52%
- Physician asks questions about patient's general health.
  1. Consumers: 66%
  2. Physicians: 29%
- Physician discovers and explores patient's beliefs about what is causing the problem and what the physician believes will help the patient.
  1. Consumers: 55%
  2. Physicians: 31%
- Physician encourages patient to state treatment preferences.
  1. Consumers: 53%
  2. Physicians: 31%

According to medical malpractice defense attorneys, communication breakdown is the most important event leading to a patient's decision to litigate (Avery, 1986). The health care provider's ability to communicate effectively has an impact on diagnosis, compliance, patient satisfaction, and health care provider satisfaction. The "Bayer Clinician-Patient Communication To Enhance Health Outcomes," a highly interactive workshop that the author has attended, identifies four communication tasks of the medical encounter (Miles Institute for Health Care Communication, 1992).*

1. *Engage the patient.* During the opening seconds of the encounter, joining takes place. With a new patient, joining takes more time than with a returning patient. Recommended strategies include the following:
   – Communicate warmth and welcome.
   – Be curious about who the patient is as a person rather than the patient's medical problem.
   – Listen to the language of the patient and adapt your language system to meet his or hers.
   – Use open-ended questions.
   – Acknowledge the patient's story.
   – Give the first 2–3 minutes to the patient.
   – Find out all of the patient's complaints.
   – Find out the patient's expectation or goal of the encounter.
2. *Empathize with the patient.* The nonverbal and physical setting of the encounter can facilitate or frustrate an empathetic connection.
   – Greet a new patient while the patient is fully clothed.
   – Do not write and listen at the same time.
   – Sit or stand relative to the patient so that head level is approximately even (not including the actual examination).
   – Do not permit physical barriers to come between you and your patient (i.e., chart and/or desk).
   – Invite the patient to tell you what he or she is feeling or thinking.
   – Acknowledge the patient's feelings and thoughts.
   – Notice the patient's facial expressions.
   – Use self-disclosure when appropriate.
3. *Educate the patient.* Typically, a patient will forget 50% of what the physician says the minute the patient walks out the door. It is important to provide information that fills in gaps and is important to the patient's health care concerns. You can assess the patient's current knowledge by finding out what the patient knows and asking for questions and things he or she wonders

---

*Courtesy of (Bayer Clinic in Patient Communication Workshop Syllabus) Bayer Institute for Health Care Communication, West Haven, Connecticut.

about (i.e., anxieties). The next thing health care providers can do is to provide answers to the patient's "assumed questions," such as

- What has happened to me?
- Why has it happened to me?
- What is going to happen to me—in the short term, in the long term?
- What are you doing to me (examination, tests)?
- Why are you doing this rather than something else (diagnostic or treatment options)?
- Will it hurt me or harm me, for how long, and how much (diagnostic and treatment)?
- When and how will you know what these tests mean?
- When and how will I know what these tests mean?

Remember that education does not truly take place until the patient has learned what he or she was supposed to learn. Therefore, you should ask the patient if he or she has asked all the questions he or she wants to. Then, ask what or how the patient understands (not *if* the patient understands).

4. *Enlist the patient in his or her own health care.* Patients must become partners in their own health care; this, in turn, increases the likelihood of compliance. The Bayer Institute approach to this involves first agreeing on what the diagnosis is. Most patients make a self-diagnosis—this is human nature! If the health care provider's diagnosis differs from the patient's, the patient will follow his or hers. To prevent this, ask the patient what he or she has been thinking the diagnosis is. Then, discuss any discrepancies between your diagnosis and the self-diagnosis. Be careful not to evaluate outside input. You never know the veracity of the patient's report or the patient's relationship to the third party.

   The next important step is to agree on the treatment approach. There are several guidelines for this.

   - Keep the treatment regimen simple.
   - Write out the regimen.
   - Describe both the benefits of the treatment and the timetable for carrying out the treatment and realizing the benefits.
   - Describe the possibility of side effects if appropriate.
   - Have the patient identify barriers to following the regimen successfully. Collaborate on a plan to modify the regimen and/or circumvent the barriers.
   - Ask for feedback from the patient to make sure the patient understands what he or she is going to do.

As you might imagine, there are many resources available for the development of communication training for health care providers. In Chapter 5, we discussed the MOT entitled "provider communication with the patient," wherein a variety of strategies was recommended. In addition to general communication skills, there are a host of other special situations that require consideration, such as

- talking to children
- talking to adolescents
- talking to the elderly
- talking to the dying patient
- talking about pregnancy and reproduction
- talking about sexual function
- aspects of transcultural communication
- breaking bad news to patients
- dealing with angry patients

A list of several resources that may prove helpful to you in addressing these and other special communication issues for health care providers is provided at the end of this chapter.

Based on the findings of your needs assessment (i.e., specifically identifying your health care organization's PSI priorities), other topics may need to be the focus of improvement efforts targeted toward health care providers. Nevertheless, all health care provider training should be laced with relevant aspects of provider-to-patient, provider-to-provider, and provider-to-staff communication skills.

Developing Facility/Department-Specific Training for Staff

During the early stages of planning your organization's approach to measuring and improving patient satisfaction, you carefully identified the elements of patient satisfaction (see Chapter 3) as well as the relative importance of each element component (see Chapter 4). Then, you discovered how patients perceive these factors on the PMRC (see Chapter 5) and communicate their satisfaction/dissatisfaction with each (see Chapters 6 and 8).

With this background in mind, the ultimate organizational preparation for addressing the specific behavior-based improvement priorities of each facility/department would be to prepare for delivering training in all measured patient satisfaction areas. A somewhat more practical approach, however, would be to focus on those areas that your patients have indicated to be most important. This offers several distinct advantages.

- You can begin planning your training efforts at a very early stage of your overall PSI project.
- You will have sufficient lead time to allow for either developing your own in-house training materials or diligently researching off-the-shelf programs that address your needs.
- You will be in a position to respond to facility/department-specific identified "weaknesses"—based on your organization's improvement priority index—shortly after identifying them. This emphasizes to patients, staff, and providers alike that you intend to make the data collected "actionable," and that you are very serious about building a culture of continuously improving patient satisfaction.

Orientation and Reorientation for Providers and Staff

Every service-oriented organization recognizes the importance of formal, structured orientation for new hires. This entails far more than a 30-minute, or even half-day, session, most of which is devoted to filling out employment forms, benefit enrollment forms, and so forth. It must include a carefully planned "indoctrination" of the new employee into your organization's culture, emphasizing the number one organizational message: We exist to provide high-quality service for patients. This segment of orientation should be aligned with (and ideally derived from) those areas that have been identified by patients as especially important. All major areas of patient satisfaction that are measured in your organization's periodic surveys should be touched on at this time. Staff members should leave their basic orientation and training knowing exactly what it takes to get excellent, average, and poor grades on the PMRC. This component of orientation should be introduced by the highest ranking executive available (preferably the chief executive officer) of your organization. This delivers a strong message about your health care organization's commitment to service excellence.

Because change is ongoing in almost any industry, especially one as dynamic as health care, it is essential to update existing employees on a regular basis through the process of reorientation. They must be informed of how any changes impact them in their ability to ensure continued high levels of patient satisfaction. There are always new goals to achieve, new technologies to use, new procedures to follow, and new people to include in the team.

The service-related contents of reorientation should be dynamic so as to reflect improvement needs identified in the patient feedback mechanisms discussed in Chapter 8.

DELIVERING EFFECTIVE PATIENT SATISFACTION TRAINING WITHIN THE FRAMEWORK OF NORMAL OPERATIONS

Nadler and Hibino (1994) referred to the "systems principle [which states] that nothing exists by itself... successful problem solving... hinges on considering the various interrelated elements and dimensions that comprise every solution" (p. 198). Thus, the training "solution" to your organization's behavior-based improvement needs must fit within the "system" that supports normal daily operations. Because the overriding purpose of your health care organization is to serve the needs of patients better than any of your competitors, no PSI strategies should run contrary to that purpose.

In order for training to be effective, it must be properly delivered no matter what training methods or techniques are used. This requires the use of experienced trainers or facilitators using highly developed presentation skills. Furthermore, PSI training can bring value to your organization only if the desired behaviors are exhibited when employees actually interact with patients on the job. This process is referred to as the "transfer of training," which can be either facilitated or prevented by various factors present when the trainee returns to the workplace.

Determining the Logistics for PSI Training

The first question that is likely to arise when the topic of employee training comes up is, "When is the best time to conduct the training?" Is it best to offer full-day, half-day, or 2–3-hour training sessions? Based on the answer to this, you must then determine which days and/ or times of the day will least interfere with an employee's job responsibilities to the patient. The extent to which an organization is willing to adjust normal clinical operations (or employee hours) in order to facilitate the delivery of needed employee training will be directly reflective of the level of executive commitment to PSI.

If such training is viewed as a "luxury," then it will be expected to be "squeezed" in between other "more important" daily responsibilities. On the other hand, if senior management is well aware of the positive correlation between an organization's action-oriented focus on PSI training and patient satisfaction/loyalty, needed training will receive the scheduling priority it deserves.

The next typical question relates to employee compensation for completing training during outside-of-normal hours—alleviating the necessity to infringe on normal patient care hours. On the surface, this is straightforward and can be calculated simply by multiplying the total outside-of-normal hours by the hourly wage levels of each involved employee. This, of course, is required if such training is considered "mandatory" by the organization—in accordance with typical state labor laws. However, the issue becomes somewhat more complex when employees are expected to travel to and/or from the training sessions from either homes or their normal workplace, using their own vehicles. Several guidelines regarding employee compensation for travel may be helpful.

- If employees are driving from home to a training site and back home again afterward during outside-of-normal hours, they are entitled to compensation for all miles traveled (at a predetermined per-mile rate) and payment for travel time at their normal hourly wage.
- If employees are driving from home to a training site and then on to their normal workplace to begin work hours, they are entitled to compensation for mileage and time from the training site to the workplace.
- If employees are driving from the workplace to a training site and back to the workplace during normal work hours, they are entitled to compensation for mileage each way.
- If employees are driving from the workplace to the training site and then home afterward, they are entitled to compensation for mileage from the workplace to the training site alone, not for the trip home from the training site. If this occurs during outside-of-normal work hours, then a claim can be made for wage payment for travel time from the workplace to the training site.

It is best to consult with appropriate legal counsel or your local labor board to determine specific compensation requirements that apply to your health care organization.

Another issue that often comes up is whether or not to supply trainees with food and/or refreshments. Some would argue that, especially during a "lunch hour meeting," it is most appropriate to supply lunch. During other times, you may wish to provide some form of refreshments like coffee, tea, and/or soft drinks. Offering these "extras" can help support a positive atmosphere at the training sessions. There is no single "right way," but the matter deserves your consideration during the planning stages—from both a logistical and a financial standpoint.

GUIDELINES FOR EFFECTIVE TRAINING DELIVERY (PRESENTATION SKILLS)

A comprehensive discussion of presentation skills is beyond the scope of this book. For a detailed overview of the subject, a list of references is included at the end of this chapter. These references have been chosen on the basis of practicality of approach and value in technique advice. The quality of training delivery in your health care organization directly impacts trainee reaction. Therefore, to make training most effective, the following factors should be considered.* These are based, in part, on the "Effective Business Presentations" workshop presented by the Zig Ziglar Corporation (1987) and should be adhered to by anyone responsible for PSI training delivery.

- *Appearance:* This refers to the way you groom yourself, the clothes you wear, and the general way you carry yourself. To be appropriate, your appearance should be at or slightly above the level of your audience. This will help both the trainer and the audience feel comfortable and still portray professionalism. Caution: Limit those items, such as jewelry, that may distract attention away from the message; tugging at rings or cufflinks can be distracting.
- *Posture:* The speaker's stance should begin with a balanced and comfortable posture that communicates confidence. The arms should be at the side and squared to the audience, with feet spread with weight evenly balanced, although slightly up on the balls of the feet. Caution: Avoid hip sway, foot shuffle, and movement without purpose.
- *Eye contact:* Random eye contact with various members of the audience (which is sustained for a period of 3–5 seconds) is most effective. This includes and involves the audience in the message and individualizes your message. It is best to complete a thought or sentence while looking at one person, then move on to another. This is much more natural than "darting" in a shifty-eyed fashion, which tends to erode trust. Focus your eye contact on those who "ask for it" instead of those who are obviously uncomfortable with it. Cautions: Avoid staring or making eye contact for more than 5 seconds. This will assuredly make the listener uncomfortable, feeling as though he or she is being singled out for some

---

**Source:* Adapted with permission from "Effective Business Presentations" seminar. © 1987, The Zig Ziglar Corporation, Carrolton, Texas.

reason. Also avoid a mechanical sequential eye contact because this appears transparent and impersonal.

- *Facial expressions:* It is said that your face is the mirror of your emotions. Therefore, you should smile, frown, and use various facial gestures. Look for opportunities to communicate emotions through your expressions. Your facial expressions set the tone or mood of the presentation. An audience is more comfortable with a speaker who communicates facially. Cautions: These should be "normal" expressions for you. Make sure your facial expressions support the words you are saying. Recall that communication is 55% visual, 38% how we say what we say, and only 7% the actual words used. Therefore, if your body language contradicts the words you are saying, listeners will believe what they see every time.

- *Gestures:* These are arm and hand movements that add clarity by reinforcing key points and increasing overall impact. The movement should be meaningful, painting a visual picture and moving outside the area between shoulders and hips. The presenter should look for natural opportunities to gesture—numbers, directions, comparisons, and action verbs. Caution: Make sure the gestures don't become a distraction, taking away from the message.

- *Voice:* This refers to the clarity and interest of sound. Clarity requires proper pronunciation and annunciation of all words used. The key is to introduce variety with your voice. This can be done by varying your volume, inflection, and pace appropriately with the content of the message. This will add considerable impact to the overall presentation. Caution: A monotone will put any audience to sleep in a relatively short time. No matter how intrinsically interesting the topic, this approach will instill boredom for sure.

- *Padding:* This refers to the use of "nonwords" such as "um, er, uh, ah." This also refers to those words we commonly use as connectors—"and, but, or, so." And finally, those words that don't really work to contribute meaning—"ok, you know, well, now." The "cure" to this problem is to use nothing in their place; instead, use a pause. This adds dramatic impact and allows the audience time to think about what you have just said. A good rule of thumb is to always use complete sentences and become aware of any tendencies you may have to use padding... then consciously eliminate it.

- *Humor:* This can be valuable as long as it is used to help carry your message. Either tell funny things or things funny. Don't rely on a long-winded joke. Some of the best opportunities for humor come from spontaneous interactions with various audience members during the training session. Don't be afraid to laugh at your own expense. Humor also adds impact to your message—the listener will retain the message far longer if it is linked to humor. Cautions: Avoid controversy—no politics, religion, race—and be careful about laughing at someone else's expense. You should also be sure to use language that will not offend even one person in your audience.

FACILITATING THE TRANSFER OF PSI TRAINING TO THE JOB

The transfer of training refers to the trainee's continuous application of the knowledge, skills, and attitudes gained in training to his or her job. Transfer from the training situation to actual on-the-job performance is one of the most important aspects of training design and development: This process is the ultimate goal of nearly any training session. Increased knowledge or skill acquisition means very little if an employee cannot put it into practice once the training sessions have been completed. Clark (1986) coined the term "transfer failure" to describe what happens when trainees return to the workplace and perform tasks using the same procedures that were used before training occurred.

The natural questions at this point are: "Why *doesn't* training transfer to the workplace?" and "What are the barriers that keep trainees from fully applying newly learned behaviors to their jobs?" Kotter (1988) conducted a survey of top executives that revealed four major factors that frequently inhibited the success of training and development efforts to improve the performance of managers (p. 113).

- lack of involvement by top management in the behavior change process—reported by 71% of the respondents
- recognition by respondents that new efforts to improve were too centralized in the top echelons of the organization, resulting in little acceptance by lower level participants—reported by 51% of respondents
- belief by executives that new efforts to improve employee behavior were too staff-centered, with insufficient participation by the direct users—reported by 21% of respondents
- unrealistic expectations from the training programs: too much was expected too soon—reported by 17% of respondents

In another study, Newstrom (1983, p. 36) attempted to identify barriers to the transfer of training by asking trainers what factors inhibited training. Initially, a group of 24 trainers identified the major impediments to the successful transfer of training in their organizations. The responses from this study were then classified into nine distinct categories. Then, a second questionnaire was designed and administered to 31 trainers from a diverse range of organizations. In this case, the respondents were asked to rank order the nine barrier categories according to their perception of the relative influence against training transfer. Exhibit 9–6 presents the results of that study, which identified *lack of reinforcement on the job* as the most significant barrier.

Broad and Newstrom (1992, p. 52) developed a transfer matrix that combined the roles of managers, trainers, and trainees with three distinct times—pretraining, during training, and post-training. By carefully analyzing what each of the people can do in each time frame relative to training, a variety of helpful strategies are presented to facilitate the transfer of training. Much of what can be done before and during training focuses on the use of accurate needs assessments, adult learning principles, and careful performance analysis.

Recommended strategies for facilitating the transfer of learning after the training include the following:

- *Managers'* involvement following training is one of the three most potent role-time combinations for any type of intervention. Specific managerial strategies include the following:
  1. Have managers sit down with trainees immediately on their return from training to debrief them as to what took place during the training, identify mutually foreseen barriers to transfer, and explore possibilities for the use of the training material.

Exhibit 9–6 Trainers' Perceptions of Barriers to Transfer

Rank order	Barrier to transfer of training
1	Lack of reinforcement on the job
2	Interference from immediate (work) environment
3	Nonsupportive organizational culture
4	Trainee's perception of impractical training programs
5	Trainee's perception of irrelevant training content
6	Trainee's discomfort with change and associated effort
7	Separation from inspiration or support of the trainer
8	Trainee's perception of poorly designed/delivered training
9	Pressures from peers to resist changes

Source: From TRANSFER OF TRAINING by MARY L. BROAD and JOHN W. NEWSTROM. Copyright © 1992 by M.L. Broad and J.W. Newstrom. Reprinted by permission of Perseus Books Publishers, a member of Perseus Books, L.L.C.

2. Have managers conduct one-on-one meetings with trainees for the purpose of communicating support for transfer; the manager needs to immediately assure the trainee of continuing mutual interests in transfer and of the necessary support being provided.

3. Have managers remind trainees on their return to the job that it will seldom be as easy to apply new skills as trainers made it sound; that there will inevitably be difficulties, frustrations, and setbacks; and that the path to success will be rocky and circuitous. The basic message is that the manager wants trainees to change to new and preferred behaviors, but they should not expect the process to be easy.

4. Have managers provide trainees with the opportunity to apply new knowledge and skills, and the perception that they have that opportunity.

5. Have trainees participate in transfer-related decisions. Let employees help decide where and how transfer can best take place on the job.

6. Have managers reduce job pressures initially, giving employees a period to experiment and "get up to speed," taking time to solidify new patterns of behavior.

7. Have managers provide positive reinforcement to the trainees. As was mentioned in the beginning of this chapter, this entails the systematic application of a positive consequence to a trainee, contingent on the demonstration of a desired behavior. The principle is simple: Behavior that gets rewarded gets repeated.

8. Have managers make sure that any job aids (checklists, flow charts, diagrams, list cards, etc.) that are available are used on the job. If job aids were not provided during training, they can be prepared by the manager.

9. Have managers publicize employee successes using the new behaviors.

- *Trainers* can take a number of post-training steps to facilitate the transfer of training.

  1. Provide follow-up support. Function as facilitators of behavioral change on the job. Something as simple as calling trainees to ask how things are going in using the skills learned during the training on the job can be helpful.

  2. Provide trainees with refresher/problem-solving sessions. These can help the trainee address some of the inhibiting factors that act as barriers to successful training transfer.

- *Trainees* can have a significant influence on the desired transfer. In order for this to occur, they must have the ability to apply the new skills, the opportunity to use them, the confidence to try, and the perception that there is some value (personal or organizational) for doing so. Specifically, trainees can
    1. Take the responsibility to monitor and manage their own post-training behavior.
    2. Review training content and learned skills. Early and frequent review can help a lack of recall (retention) from preventing a transfer of learning.
    3. Form a mentor relationship with another employee who has mastered the skills and behaviors he or she is attempting to apply on the job. Trainees can use the mentor as a source of feedback, aggressively bouncing new ideas off the mentor and asking for candid advice on the merits of using new approaches.
    4. Maintain contact with training "buddies." For example, fellow trainees might commit to each other that they are going to try the new behaviors on the job, then set periodic time frames to contact one another for a progress check. The entire purpose of the buddy relationship is to increase the likelihood of transfer through the use of interpersonal commitment, mutual support, goal setting, and the availability of an ally who has experienced the same process and can speak the same language.

EVALUATING THE EFFECTIVENESS OF YOUR PSI TRAINING

Kirkpatrick developed the "Kirkpatrick model" for evaluating training programs in 1959 (1994, p. 21). This approach has since become the most widely used approach to evaluating training in the corporate, government, and academic worlds.

Evaluation is an essential component of any organizational project that involves training. This is true for three important reasons.

1. To justify the value of the training by showing how it contributes to your organization's objectives to improve patient satisfaction.
2. To decide whether to continue or discontinue programs.
3. To gain information on how to improve future training programs.

Exhibit 9–7 presents a brief summary of the Kirkpatrick model for evaluating training effectiveness. The four levels (*reaction, learning, behavior,* and *results*) represent a sequence of ways to evaluate programs.

Exhibit 9–7 The Four-Level Kirkpatrick Model of Training Evaluation

Evaluation Level	Description
Level I—Reaction	• This measures how those who participate in the program react to it. • It is important to get a positive reaction because this is a prerequisite to participants being motivated to learn. • Positive reaction may not ensure learning, but negative reaction almost certainly reduces the possibility of learning occurring. • You need to design a form that will quantify reactions; this allows for summarizing participant reactions to each program and documenting it.
Level II—Learning	• The extent to which participants *change* attitudes, *improve* knowledge, and/or *increase* skill as a result of attending the program. • Use a paper and pencil "test" to measure knowledge and attitudes, and use a performance test to measure skills. • It is important to measure learning because no change in behavior can be expected if no learning has taken place.
Level III—Behavior	• The extent to which change in behavior has occurred because the participant attended the training program. This requires four conditions: 1. The person must have a desire to change. 2. The person must know what to do and how to do it. 3. The person must work in the right climate. 4. The person must be rewarded for changing. • Allow time for behavior change to take place before measuring it. • Evaluate behaviors both before and after the training if practical. • Survey and/or interview one or more of the following: trainees, their immediate supervisor, their subordinates, others who often observe their behavior.

continues

Exhibit 9–7 continued

Evaluation Level	Description

Level IV—Results	• Determination of what final results occurred because of attendance and participation in your patient satisfaction improvement training.
	• Use existing results measures that identified your behavior-based improvement priorities in the first place:
	  – Patient satisfaction surveys (comparing before/after training)
	  – Patient focus groups
	  – Patient complaint and grievance data

Source: Reprinted with permission of the publisher. From *Evaluating Training Programs: The Four Levels,* copyright © 1994 by D. Kirkpatrick, Berrett-Koehler Publishers, Inc., San Francisco, CA. All rights reserved. 1-800-929-2929.

According to Kirkpatrick, "Each level is important. As you move from one level to the next, the process becomes more difficult and time-consuming, but it also provides more valuable information. None of the levels should be bypassed simply to get to the level that the trainer considers most important" (1994, p. 21).

Throughout this chapter, we have directed your attention toward various aspects of addressing behavior-based improvement priorities. Training, as an intervention, provides a foundation for changing attitudes, increasing knowledge, and improving skills. When this is carried out in an organizational climate that supports the transfer of training, then the desired behaviors prerequisite to improving patient satisfaction (desired results) can be anticipated. Chapter 10 will focus on systems-based improvement priorities. This will form yet another important component of your health care organization's continuous improvement efforts.

CONCLUSION

Special attention must be given to those employee behaviors associated with the management of each MOT. This is an essential prerequisite to improving patient satisfaction continuously. Behavior is best influenced in terms of its rate or frequency by altering the consequences associated with it. Two behavioral consequences, positive reinforcement and negative reinforcement, increase behavior; punishment and extinction decrease behavior. The greatest practical application of this information is for an organization to carefully design consequences (e.g., with reward and recognition programs) in such a way that behaviors that produce desirable outcomes (i.e., favorably contribute to patient satisfaction) are positively reinforced. Simply put: "Behaviors that get rewarded get repeated."

Another important requirement for addressing behavior-based improvement priorities is that clearly defined behavior expectations in the form of performance standards be in place. These specific, concise, and measurable standards need to be focused on behaviors and actions that are very important to patients, can actually be improved, and are challenging but realistic. Standards should be developed for the important satisfaction elements of each of the six categories of patient satisfaction defined in Chapter 3 (access, convenience, communication, perceived quality of care, personal caring, and health care facilities/equipment). They should be written into job descriptions and performance reviews so as to function as credible and respected management tools that are fairly enforced organizationwide.

Training is a means by which we attempt to close the gap between an individual's present performance levels and his or her desired performance levels. More specifically, it is the process of equipping people with the attitudes, skills, and knowledge needed to carry out their responsibilities. In order to ensure optimum effectiveness of your organization's PSI training, the principles of *andragogy* or adult learning must be adhered to. A variety of training tools and techniques are available to promote active learning; a selection of them has been presented in the text of this chapter for the reader's review. All training should be developed on the basis of a thorough needs assessment and measurable training objectives.

Then, the "make or buy" decision regarding training materials can be based on the availability of materials that can support the achievement of your objectives. All training should be offered within the "system" of your organization—supportive of normal daily operations and facilitated by training professionals.

The effectiveness of training should be evaluated on Kirkpatrick's four levels.

- *Reaction:* Did the trainees enjoy the training experience?
- *Learning:* Did the trainees learn the content presented?
- *Behavior:* Did the trainees' behavior reflect the application of newly learned skills on the job?
- *Results:* Did the level of patient satisfaction related to the training actually increase?

The next consideration for making the training valuable to the organization is "transfer of training." The transfer of newly acquired attitudes, skills, and/or knowledge to the job is, in large part, contingent on the organization fostering a supporting environment for behavioral change. The top two barriers to the transfer of training are "lack of reinforcement on the job" and "interference from immediate (work) environment." In Chapter 10, we will focus on addressing systems-based improvement priorities.

ACTION STEPS

1. List the resources that are currently available in your organization for PSI training. State if and how training content is (or should be) driven by identified PSI needs.
2. Review service standards that are (or should be) in place in your organization to clearly define how each important MOT and SP should be positively managed. Consider whether behaviors that are/are not aligned with these standards are linked to your performance appraisal and reward/recognition systems.
3. Determine whether your organization's current training methodologies are engaging and interactive, reflecting the principles of adult learning or simply one-way "content-push" lectures. Develop a list of training methodologies ideally suited for your PSI training needs.
4. Identify all methods of training effectiveness evaluation your organization currently uses. Divide these into Kirkpatrick's four levels (I = "reaction," II = "learning," III = "behavior," IV = "results"). Determine what mechanisms are in place to ensure that the training effectiveness data are "actionable," resulting in continuously improving training programs.
5. Assess your organization in terms of existing "barriers" to or "reinforcers" for the transfer of training to the job.

REFERENCES

Adler, M. (1940, July 6). How to mark a book. *Saturday Review*, 11.

Avery, J.K. (1986, July/August). Lawyers tell what makes some patients litigious. *Medical Malpractice*.

Broad, M.L., & Newstrom, J.W. (1992). *Transfer of training: Action-packed strategies to ensure high payoff from training investments*. New York: Addison-Wesley.

Clark, R.C. (1986). Nine ways to make training pay off on the job. *Training Magazine*, 23(11), 83–87.

CRM Films, Inc. (1994). *It's a dog's world.* CRM Films [Videocassette].

Daniels, A.C. (1994). *Bringing out the best in people: How to apply the astonishing power of positive reinforcement.* New York: McGraw-Hill.

Friendly Hills HealthCare Network. (1994a). *Network service standards.* La Habra, CA: Author.

Friendly Hills HealthCare Network. (1994b). *Personal interaction standards.* La Habra, CA: Author.

Fulwiler, T. (1987). *Teaching with writing.* Portsmouth, NH: Cooks Publishers.

Geary, Rummler, G., & Brache, A. (1995). *Improving performance.* San Francisco: Jossey-Bass.

Kirkpatrick, D.L. (1994). *Evaluating training programs: The four levels.* San Francisco: Berrett-Koehler.

Knowles, M.S. (1987). Adult learning. In R.L. Craig (Ed.), *Training and development handbook* (168–179). New York: McGraw-Hill.

Kotter, J.P. (1988). *The leadership factor.* New York: Free Press.

LeBoeuf, M. (1985). *The greatest management principle in the world.* New York: Berkley Books.

Mager, R.F. (1984). *Preparing instructional objectives* (2nd ed.). Belmont, CA: Lake.

Martin, W.B. (1989). *Managing quality customer service: A practical guide for establishing a service operation.* Menlo Park, CA: Crisp.

Meyers, C., & Jones, T.B. (1993). *Promoting active learning: Strategies for the college classroom.* San Francisco: Jossey-Bass.

Miles Institute for Health Care Communication. (1992). *Physician-patient communication workshop syllabus.* West Haven, CT: Author.

Nadler, G., & Hibino, S. (1994). *Breakthrough thinking: The seven principles of creative problem-solving* (2nd ed.). Rocklin, CA: Prima.

Newstrom, (1983, August). The management of unlearning: Exploding the "clean state fallacy." *Training and Development Journal*, 36.

Pike, R.W. (1992). *17 ways to get more into and out of your training.* Bloomington, MN: Resources for Organizations.

Scholtes, P. (1988). *The team handbook.* Madison, WI: Joiner & Associates.

Sibler, K.H., & Stelnicki, M. (1987). *"Writing training materials" Training and development handbook* (3rd ed.). New York: McGraw-Hill.

Skol Corporation. (1996). Is good communication synonymous with high patient satisfaction? *The Back Letter, 11*(2), 15.

Thomas, B. (1992). *Total quality training: The quality culture and quality trainer.* London: McGraw-Hill.

Tracey, W.R. (1992). *Designing training and development systems* (3rd ed.). New York: AMACOM.

Wade, P.A. (1995). *Producing high-impact learning tools.* Irvine, CA: Richard Chang Associates.

Ziglar Corporation. (1987). Effective business presentations. *Syllabus for two day workshop.* Carollton, TX: Author.

SUGGESTED READING

Albrecht, K. (1988). *At America's service.* Homewood, IL: Dow Jones-Irwin.

Albrecht, K. (1992). *The only thing that matters.* New York: Harper Business.

Bader, G.E., & Bloom, A.E. (1994). *Make your training results last.* Irvine, CA: Richard Chang Associates.

Bailey, E.P., Jr. (1992). *A practical guide for business speaking.* Oxford, England: Oxford University Press.

Bell, C.R., & Zemke, R. (1992). *Managing knock your socks off service.* New York: AMACOM.

Bonwell, C.C., & Eison, J.A. (1991). *Active learning: Creating excitement in the classroom.* Washington, DC: The George Washington University School of Education and Human Development.

Carr, C. (1990). *Front-line customer service: 15 keys to customer satisfaction.* New York: John Wiley & Sons.

Carr, C. (1992). *Smart training: The manager's guide to training for improved performance.* New York: McGraw-Hill.

Chang, R.Y. (1994). *Creating high-impact training: A practical guide to successful training outcomes.* Irvine, CA: Richard Chang Associates.

Connellan, T.K., & Zemke, R. (1993). *Sustaining knock your socks off service.* New York: AMACOM.

Craig, R.L. (Ed.). (1987). *Training and development handbook* (3rd ed.). New York: McGraw-Hill.

Decker, B. (1988). *The art of communicating: Achieving interpersonal impact in business.* Menlo Park, CA: Crisp.

Denton, D.K. (1989). *Quality service: How America's top companies are competing in the customer-service revolution...and how you can too.* Houston, TX: Gulf.

Disend, J.E. (1991). *How to provide excellent service in any organization: A blueprint for making all the theories work.* Radnor, PA: Chilton Book.

Drummond, M.E. (1993). *Fearless and flawless public speaking with power, polish and pizazz.* San Diego: Pfeiffer and Company.

Dunckel, J., & Taylor, B. (1988). *The business guide to profitable customer relations: Today's techniques for success.* Seattle, WA: Self-Counsel Press.

George, S., & Weimerskirch, A. (1994). *Total quality management: Strategies and techniques proven at today's most successful companies.* New York: John Wiley & Sons.

Glass, L. (1987). *Talk to win: Six steps to a successful vocal image.* New York: Perigee Books.

Goad, T.W. (1982). *Delivering effective training.* San Diego: Pfeiffer & Company.

Harrington-Mackin, D. (1994). *The team building tool kit: Tips, tactics, and rules for effective workplace teams.* New York: AMACOM.

Hayes, J., & Dredge, F. (1998). *Managing customer service.* Hampshire, England: Gower.

Haynes, M.E. (1988). *Effective meeting skills: A practical guide for more productive meetings.* Menlo Park, CA: Crisp.

Hinton, T., & Schaeffer, W. (1994). *Customer-focused quality: What to do on Monday morning.* Englewood Cliffs, NJ: Prentice Hall.

Hoff, R. (1988). *"I can see you naked": A fearless guide to making great presentations.* New York: Andrews and McMeel.

Hoops, A. (1992). *Art of caring.* Bloomington, MN: Service Quality Institute.

Hunsaker, P.L., & Alessandra, A.J. (1980). *The art of managing people: Person-to-person skills, guidelines, and techniques every manager needs to guide, direct, and motivate the team.* New York: Simon & Schuster.

Katz, J.M., & Green, E. (1997). *Managing quality: A guide to system-wide performance management in health care* (2nd ed.). St. Louis, MO: Mosby-Year Book.

Kaufman, R., Rojas, A., & Mayer, H. (1993). *Needs assessment: A user's guide.* Englewood Cliffs, NJ: Educational Technology.

Kaufman, R., Thiagarajan, S., & MacGillis, P. (Eds.). (1997). *The guidebook for performance improvement: Working with individuals and organizations.* San Francisco: Pfeiffer.

Knowles, M.S. (1980). *The modern practice of adult education from pedagogy to andragogy.* Englewood Cliffs, NJ: Prentice Hall.

Kreps, G.L., & Kunimoto, E.N. (1994). *Effective communication in multicultural health care settings.* Thousand Oaks, CA: Sage.

Kroehnert, G. (1995). *Basic training for trainers: A handbook for new trainers* (2nd ed.). New York: McGraw-Hill.

Kupsh, J. (1993). *How to create high impact business presentations.* Chicago: NTC Publishing Group.

Lee, C. (1990). Motivating and managing performance. *Training magazine.* Minneapolis, MN: Lakewood Books.

Leebov, W. (1988). *Service excellence: The customer relations strategy for health care.* Chicago: American Hospital.

Leebov, W., Vergare, M., & Scott, G. (1990). *Patient satisfaction: A guide to practice enhancement.* Oradell, NJ: Medical Economics Books.

Leland, K., & Bailey, K. (1995). *Customer service for dummies.* Chicago: IDG Books Worldwide.

Miller, W.R. (1990). *Instructors and their jobs.* Homewood, IL: American Technical.

Mitchell, G. (1993). *The trainer's handbook: The AMA guide to effective training* (2nd ed.). New York: AMACOM.

Myerscough, P.R., & Ford, M. (1996). *Talking with patients: Keys to good communication* (3rd ed.). Oxford, England: Oxford University Press.

Nelson, A.M., Wood, S., Brown, S., & Bronkesh, S. (1997). *Improving patient satisfaction now: How to earn patient and payer loyalty.* Gaithersburg, MD: Aspen.

Nilson, C. (1991). *Training for non-trainers: A do-it-yourself guide for managers.* New York: AMACOM.

Peoples, D. (1992). *Presentations plus: David Peoples' proven techniques* (2nd ed.). New York: John Wiley & Sons.

Perret, G. (1989). *Using humor for effective business speaking.* New York: Sterling.

Phillips, J.J. (1991). *Handbook of training evaluation and measurement methods* (2nd ed.). Houston, TX: Gulf.

Phillips, J.J. (1997). *Return on investment in training and performance improvement programs: A step-by-step manual for calculating the financial return.* Houston, TX: Gulf.

Pike, R.W. (1994). *Creative training techniques handbook: Tips, tactics, and how-to's for delivering effective training.* Minneapolis, MN: Lakewood Books.

Piskurich, G.M. (Ed.). (1993). *The ASTD handbook of instructional technology.* New York: McGraw-Hill.

Piskurich, G.M. (1993). *Self-directed learning: A practical guide to design, development, and implementation.* San Francisco: Jossey-Bass.

Reichheld, F.F. (1996). *The loyalty effect: The hidden force behind growth, profits, and lasting value.* Boston: Harvard Business School Press.

Robson, G.D. (1991). *Continuous process improvement: Simplifying work flow systems.* New York: The Free Press.

Rummler, G.A., & Brache, A.P. (1995). *Improving performance: How to manage the white space on the organization chart* (2nd ed.). San Francisco: Jossey-Bass.

Sanderson, (March 1994). *Needs assessment: Training design and development.* Workshop presented in Longmont, CO, at the National Institute of Corrections, The United States Department of Justice.

Shelton, P.J. (1997). *Straight-A's program—Training modules I, II and III.* Carlsbad, CA: Friendly Hills HealthCare Network.

Smalley, L.R. (1994). *On-the-job orientation and training: A practical guide to enhanced performance.* Irvine, CA: Richard Chang Associates.

Sparhawk, S. (1994). *Identifying targeted training needs: A practical guide to beginning an effective training strategy.* Irvine, CA: Richard Chang Associates.

Tate, P. (1997). *The doctor's communication handbook* (2nd ed.). Oxon, England: Radcliffe Medical Press.

Walters, L. (1995). *What to say when...you're dying on the platform: A complete resource for speakers, trainers, and executives.* San Francisco: McGraw-Hill.

Wellington, P. (1995). *Kaizen strategies for customer care: How to create a powerful customer care program—and make it work.* London: Pitman.

Whiteley, R.C. (1991). *The customer-driven company: Moving from talk to action.* Menlo Park, CA: Addison-Wesley.

Whiteley, R., & Hessan, D. (1996). *Customer centered growth: Five proven strategies for building competitive advantage.* Menlo Park, CA: Addison-Wesley.

Wilson, J.B. (1994). *Applying successful training techniques.* Irvine, CA: Richard Chang Associates.

Wilson, J.B. (1995). *Mapping a winning training approach: A practical guide to choosing the right training methods.* Irvine, CA: Richard Chang Associates.

Zeithaml, V.A., & Bitner, M.J. (1996). *Services marketing.* London: McGraw-Hill.

Zemke, R., & Schaaf, D. (1989). *The service edge: 101 companies that profit from customer care.* New York: NAL Books.

CHAPTER 10

Addressing Systems- and Process-Based Improvement Priorities

The normal daily operation of any health care organization involves the performance of a large variety of tasks, some of which are closely related and others that are completely separate. Task performance frequently involves some form of interaction among those persons employed by the organization (providers and/or staff) and patients. In order for people to perform the myriad of tasks required optimally, they need to have the necessary skills, knowledge, and attitudes—all of which can be developed/improved with the provision of effective, "transferable" training (as discussed in Chapter 9). However, this can only contribute to improving patient satisfaction continuously to the extent that organizational procedures, processes, and systems are designed to support the delivery of quality service to patients.

All health care and other organizations are made up of a unique combination of systems that should be designed to meet the needs and perceived needs of its external customers. The term "system" as it is used in this chapter refers to a group of related processes. A process is a sequential grouping of tasks (and subtasks) directed at accomplishing a particular outcome.

Goodman (1986) stated that "80% of customers' problems are caused by bad systems, not bad people." This emphasizes the fact that we cannot expect optimum service outcomes for our patients—no matter how well trained and motivated our people are—unless appropriate, effective, and efficient supportive systems are in place. For example, if the system your health care organization has in place for scheduling patient appointments is poorly designed, resulting in routine errors and long delays, no amount of employee skill, knowledge, or positive attitude will prevent patient dissatisfaction.

Deming viewed organizations as systems designed to serve customers. Furthermore, he believed the following (Scholtes, 1988):

- In order to meet or exceed customer expectations consistently, an organization must constantly improve its systems.
- All work is done through step-by-step processes.
- Most improvement potential can be found in the process, not in the human performance factors.
- Eighty-five percent of all customer dissatisfaction is the result of poor process design.
- Fifteen percent of all customer dissatisfaction is the result of people failure.

While attending the "8th Annual Customer Satisfaction and Quality Measurement Conference" of the American Marketing Association, I listened to several organizational presentations wherein customer satisfaction survey data were responded to by providing targeted, well-designed, and effective employee training. However, each presenter discovered, albeit retrospectively, that the resulting incremental improvements in customer satisfaction (as documented by subsequent surveys) plateaued after a period of approximately 2 years. All of the presenters concluded that the reason for this plateau was their failure to address needed system improvements. They also conceded that further improvements in customer satisfaction could take place only if they revamped their organizational systems. This was a significant revelation that motivated me to ask one of the presenters the following question: "Do you see any reason why an organization could not address both behavior-based and systems-based improvement needs simultaneously?" The response reinforced my convictions: "No, and in hindsight, this is the approach we probably should have taken in the first place."

This chapter will provide an overview of the basic principles of systems and process thinking that apply to health care. Then, health care process improvement through continuous process improvement (CPI) and process reengineering will be examined. Next, important tools and techniques for continuous quality improvement (CQI) will be presented within a practical framework. Then, an interdisciplinary team approach to process improvement will address the "people factor" of collaborating to bring about positive change. Finally, the issue of CQI training will be discussed.

BASIC PRINCIPLES OF SYSTEMS AND PROCESS THINKING

Technically, a *process* is a series of value-added activities or tasks that, when linked together, turn an input from a "supplier" into a product or service output for an internal or external "customer" (Figure 10–1). Almost everything we do in life is a process—getting ready for work in the morning, cooking a meal, planning a vacation, and so forth.

The points where a process starts (inputs) and ends (outputs) are referred to as "process boundaries." The "owner" of a process has the critically important dual responsibilities of clearly defining and communicating the requirements (i.e., specifications) for all inputs to any and all process suppliers and determining, in explicit terms, the specific output requirements as defined by the customer of the process.

For a process to proceed smoothly, the supplier must furnish the input(s) according to the requirements of the process owner; then, in turn, the process owner ("producer") provides output according to the requirements defined by the customer(s) of the process. An internal customer is any individual, group/team, or department that works for the same organization as the producer. Although two or more processes may produce outcomes for internal customers, ultimately, something (a product and/or service) is produced for external customers according to their requirements (needs and expectations).

Most organizations operate through hundreds of processes and subprocesses. In order to remain truly customer-driven, it is essential that the communication of requirements between suppliers, process owners, and customers is an ongoing process in itself. Because the satisfaction requirements of our patients (external customers) can and do change from time to time, it must be kept in mind that the needs and

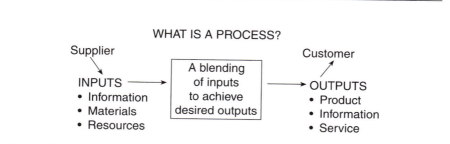

Figure 10–1 Overview of a Process.

expectations of our internal customers will change as well. In order to remain aligned with the essential organizational objective of constantly meeting or exceeding patient expectations, we must be postured for change through CPI.

CPI AND PROCESS REENGINEERING IN HEALTH CARE

It is important to recognize the difference between CPI and process reengineering. CPI is used when an existing process requires an incremental improvement of 10% or less (it is good, but needs to be somewhat better). When a change of 30% or more is desired, process reengineering, or total redesign of the process, is required. Often, radical change mandates designing a new process from scratch. As you might imagine, process improvement is much faster and less disruptive than process reengineering.

If your health care organization needs or is seeking to make significant advances, so-called "breakthroughs," then both CPI and process reengineering may be required. Therefore, a thorough understanding of the fundamental differences between these two methodologies is essential. Then, based on your knowledge of the differences, you will be in a position to appreciate when CPI should be used and when nothing short of process reengineering is required for your organizational improvement.

The scope of CPI tends to be much narrower and to involve frontline employees more than with process reengineering, where the scope is more broad-based and cross-functional. Because changes in organizational structure and job design often result from process reengineering, management commonly needs to be involved on a "hands-on" basis. As a result, process reengineering brings about much more radical organizational change (with breakthrough improvements) than CPI, where more subtle changes (incremental improvements) occur over an extended period of time. Also, in CPI, management takes more of a "hands-off" approach, allowing for greater autonomy among employees directly involved in the process.

When CPI is undertaken, team members are chosen on an "as-needed" part-time basis over a prolonged period of time. Process reengineering, on the other hand, demands the full-time participation of team members operating within much tighter time constraints, with a greater sense of urgency. Additionally, because process reengineering requires a radical new approach to achieving a particular outcome, more "out-of-the-box" creative thinking—without the constraints of how things were previously done—is needed. Table 10–1 summarizes the differences between CPI and process reengineering.

Process reengineering is geared toward bringing about dramatic improvements in the performance of existing processes. This typically entails a fundamental rethinking and redesigning of the tasks that make up the process. The key is to focus on those processes that are critical (of high relative importance—as discussed in Chapter 4) to pa-

---

Table 10–1 Comparison of Continuous Process Improvement (CPI) to Process Reengineering

Comparison Category	Continuous Process Improvement (CPI)	Process Reengineering
Scope of processes changed	• Narrowly defined processes (or subprocesses)	• Broad-based cross-functional processes
Magnitude of change throughout the organization	• Relatively small incremental process improvements • Limited disruption of existing jobs • Limited change in management systems or organizational structure	• Radical process changes • Begets further organizational changes: –job redesign –management systems –training and retraining –organizational structure –information technology
Management participation	• Somewhat limited role, leaving employees at all levels to improve processes on their own	• "Hands-on" role due to high impact on overall organizational function
Improvement team member time commitment	• Part-time on an "as-needed" basis • Minimal intrusion on normal work activities • Over extended time frame	• Full-time, highly intense • Interruption in normal work activities required • Over condensed time frame
Improvement magnitude	• Small, incremental • Many processes at once	• Large, dramatic • Single large process focus
Frequency of use	• Ongoing	• Periodic

Source: Adapted with permission from R. Chang, *Process Reengineering in Action*, p. 16, © 1995, Richard Chang Associates, Inc.

tient satisfaction. By classifying your health care organization's improvement priorities as outlined in Chapter 8, you have a head start on identifying which processes to focus on for improvement or reengineering—systems- and process-based improvement priorities. Later in this chapter, we will discuss a team-based approach to process improvement.

The next consideration is when to use CPI and when to use process reengineering. CPI will be most appropriate when one or more of the following conditions exist:

- All tasks and subtasks involved in the process are performed within one or two physical locations.
- Data exchange is not particularly critical.
- You need (or can get) only a low amount of process supplier and customer involvement.
- There is a limited time (part-time) and/or financial resource commitment from senior management.
- Your organization has limited experience with quality improvement procedures.
- The marketplace for your product/service is relatively stable, with little ongoing change.

Process reengineering will be more appropriate when one or more of the following conditions exist:

- The tasks and subtasks of a process span multiple locations.
- The process requires critical data exchange between stages of the process.
- An existing process is failing and the situation is considered drastic.
- Significant improvement must be accomplished in a short time frame.
- Key process suppliers and customers are available to provide input.

Harrington, the international quality advisor for Ernst & Young, emphasized that "expending much more effort to improve our business processes during the 1990's will be a major factor in being competitive in the 21st century" (1991, p. 16). Harrington went on to list a variety of organizational benefits for focusing on the continuous improvement of business processes.

- Enables the organization to focus on the customer.
- Allows the organization to predict and control change.

- Enhances the organization's ability to compete by improving the use of available resources.
- Provides a means to effect major changes to very complex activities in a rapid manner.
- Helps the organization effectively manage its interrelationships.
- Provides a systematic view of organization activities.
- Keeps the focus on the process.
- Prevents errors from occurring.
- Helps the organization with a measure of its poor-quality costs (waste).
- Provides a view of how errors occur and a method for correcting them.
- Develops a complete measurement system for the various business areas.
- Provides an understanding of how good the organization can be, and defines how to get there.
- Provides a method to prepare the organization to meet its future challenges.

Recall that process reengineering involves much more radical change than that associated with CPI. Chang (1995, p. 5) developed a three-phase model that provides a step-by-step approach to the complex topic of reengineering. This model is summarized in Table 10–2. Notice that the sequential effort is not too dissimilar to the steps in CPI.

The FOCUS-PDCA Model for Continuous Improvement

One of the most comprehensive overall approaches to process improvement was developed by the Hospital Corporation of America's Quality Resource Group (Al-Asaaf & Schmele, 1993). This combines the "F-O-C-U-S" method of placing a particular process under a figurative microscope with the Shewhart "Plan-Do-Check-Act" (PDCA) improvement cycle (Figure 10–2). Although there are a variety of different approaches to process improvements, the FOCUS-PDCA method is particularly useful in health care environments.

The following nine sequential steps are involved with this methodology:

1. *Find a process to improve.* This process should be selected on the basis of being important to meeting patient expectations. The best way to ensure this is to direct your attention toward those processes that have outcomes that are directly related to your

Table 10–2 The Chang Reengineering Model

Reengineering Phase	Major Steps	Subtasks
Phase I— Planning	• Determine "new" process requirements.	• Identify who the customers of this process are. • Identify what your patients want. • Forecast future patient requirements. • Observe how competitors are managing this process. • Recognize your operating requirements.
	• Uncover "breakthrough" opportunities.	• Analyze the "as is" capability of the process. –List major tasks. –Create a flowchart. • Envision the desired state. • Identify process performance "gaps."
Phase II—Design	• Map the "ideal" process.	• Address how to fill performance gaps. • Set new goals and establish measures. –simpler process? –eliminate any data? –add technology? –training needed? –reduce time/cost? • Create a new process flowchart.
	• Redefine process support requirements.	• People –role transitions? • Technology/support tools • Financial support –cost/benefit analysis
	• Develop a change management plan.	• Who will be impacted? • Emotional factors? • How will the plan be monitored? • All involved consulted? • Plan foster involvement?
Phase III— Implementation	• Implement on a "trial run" basis.	• Pilot test the change. • Assess results and make adjustments.
	• Standardize the reengineered process.	• Guidelines published and distributed. • Job descriptions revised. • Encourage participation.
	• Evaluate process performance.	• Regular team meetings. • Ensure guidelines followed. • Identify obstacles. • Celebrate progress.

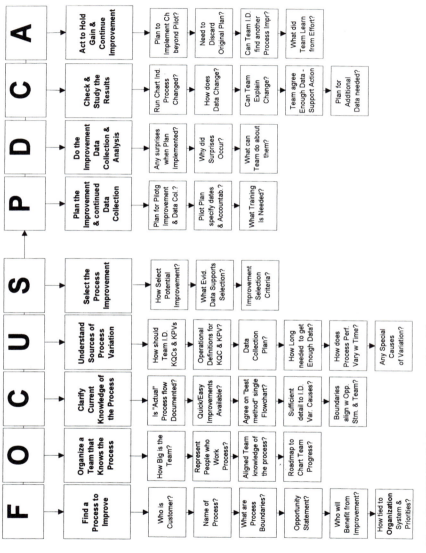

Figure 10–2 FOCUS-PDCA Improvement Model.

organization's carefully identified improvement priorities (as defined in Chapter 8). There may be multiple processes involved in the improvement area you have chosen to work on. In this case, select a process using the following criteria:

- There is current patient dissatisfaction with the process "product" using the mechanisms discussed in Chapter 9 (the dissatisfaction index multiplied by the relative importance index [RII]).
- The product/service that is the output of this process is important to patients (see RII in Chapter 4).
- You have control over improving the process.
- The process can be improved using existing resources (i.e., no significant financial resource requirements).
- There is a clear perceived benefit to the organization for improving the process.
- There is a high likelihood of success (particularly important in the early stages of your patient satisfaction improvement efforts).

   If you have multiple facilities/departments, your improvement priority index may vary from location to location. Therefore, at any given time, different facilities/departments are likely to be focusing on different processes to improve. The remaining stages of step one of the FOCUS model include:

- Identify the supplier(s) and customer(s)—internal and external—for that process. This is essential because you will need to communicate with them to clearly define customer requirements and provide the supplier(s) with input requirements. In the case of patients, your external customers, you have already identified, in general terms, their requirements for the improvement area you have chosen.
- Name the process and determine its starting and completion boundaries.
- Develop an opportunity statement. Remain focused on critical improvement opportunity. Develop a gap analysis chart in order to state specifically what needs to change to get the desired outcome. This will typically relate to timeliness, convenience, communication, personal caring, perceived quality of care, responsiveness, follow-up, accessibility, or knowledgeable employees.
- Demonstrate how improving this process will benefit your organization. One approach is to indicate how it will move opera-

tions to closer alignment with organizational purpose. You need to connect it to the successful accomplishment of the established mission and vision.

2. *Organize a team that knows the process.* This team needs to consist of those people who work directly with the process. Although the team should involve suppliers and customers of the process, it is also important to include those people who carry out the tasks and subtasks that form the building blocks of the process. The assumption that drives this step of the FOCUS model is the notion that the person who performs a task is the most knowledgeable about that process.

3. *Clarify current knowledge of the process.* The first team step is to establish a clear understanding of how the process is currently "working." Good or bad news is unimportant at this stage. Establishing a clear understanding is accomplished by having each individual who works within the process draw a flowchart that includes only the major tasks (see details of flowcharting later in this chapter) representing that person's understanding of the existing process. Recognize that, at this stage, each flowchart may be somewhat different because each person typically understands a process in a different way. The next step is to compare flowcharts and, as a team, develop one final detailed flowchart that everyone agrees accurately represents the process as it is. This allows each team member to develop an understanding of how various people associated with the process carry out their work. Sometimes this procedure alone leads to the discovery of obvious improvements that would be relatively quick and easy to implement.

   A thorough understanding of a particular process requires sufficient detail to allow for measurement to occur. But what do you measure? It could be a result that is delivered directly to the patient (measuring only those aspects that are important to patients), critical points within the process itself—telling you how well the process is performing, or process inputs established separately for each supplier. This is the only way to recognize that variation (the true "enemy" of product/service quality) is or is not occurring with each cycle of the process. The process measures that you identify should be linked to the needs and expectations of patients (so-called "key quality characteristics"). They should also be quantifiable/measurable and easily observable.

4. *Understand sources of process variation.* Deming (1982) communicated the message regarding quality improvement this way: "If I

had to reduce my message to management to just a few words, I'd say it all had to do with variation" (p. 21). Simply defined, variation is the difference in the reproducibility of a particular action. In other words, it is the difference between a particular action and the targeted outcome. Variation is what produces defects (errors of any kind) and less uniform service quality. Reduction and control of variation will lead to the improvement of service.

Once the process is clearly understood by everyone on the team, and there is consensus as to which measures best represent various aspects of the process, the next step is to gather data reflecting the performance of the process over a period of time. The cycle time of the process will help your team decide the length of time needed to gather sufficient data. For example, the process of scheduling patient appointments in person has a relatively short cycle time; therefore, data collection might be planned for a period of several days or weeks. However, the process of grievance management may take a longer time, necessitating the collection of process measurement data over several months.

When your team evaluates the collected data, areas of significant variation (key product variables) should be examined closely. Look for places in the process where different conditions or procedures lead to differences in results. If patient waiting time in the examination room varies from 15 minutes to 90 minutes, something needs to be done to reduce/control the variation. The first step is to look for so-called "special causes" that are not part of the process all of the time, but rather arise because of special circumstances. For example, if a staff member has taken a leave of absence and has not been replaced temporarily, this would be a special cause. Elimination of special causes of variation is a critical first step toward improvement.

So-called "common causes" occur due to a large number of small variations. These causes are much more difficult to detect. One consideration is whether or not there is a way to standardize results to eliminate consistent differences you have identified.

5. *Select the process improvement.* Recognize that most process problems arise, according to Scholtes (1988, pp. 4–6), for one of six reasons.
   a. inadequate knowledge of how a process works
   b. inadequate knowledge of how a process should work
   c. errors and mistakes in executing policies

d. current practices that fail to recognize the need for preventive measures

e. unnecessary steps, wasteful measures that do not add value to the product/service

f. variation in inputs and outputs

If you can identify the root cause of any process problem areas (see fishbone cause-and-effect diagramming later), you can target your improvement efforts accordingly. This ensures that you are dealing with the underlying causes rather than simply quick-fixing the obvious symptoms. Root cause analysis typically entails asking "Why?" on three to five consecutive occasions.

Error-proofing the process can be extremely helpful, particularly if you have identified that a great deal of the variation in output (service/product) is related to errors made while the process is in progress. Thus, you need to consider whether you should

– Change the order of the steps so that a frequently forgotten step is more prominent or more difficult to forget.

– Modify the design of a form so that it is less confusing or more "user-friendly."

– Use a checklist much like airline pilots do in preparation for takeoff.

– Provide graphically illustrated, prominently displayed, and easily understandable instructions placed at key points where process errors commonly occur.

We have all error-proofed a process in our lives at one time or another. Have you ever left the house with the briefcase you wanted to bring sitting on your desk, or office keys sitting in the pocket of a coat you are not wearing? Undoubtedly, you did what I have done—placed the needed item(s) strategically in front of the door you will be exiting from so that you couldn't possibly leave without stumbling over the very things you want to take with you. Admittedly, this is a simplistic example, but nevertheless, it is an effective means of error-proofing a process.

Another consideration lies with whether or not you can streamline the process as it exists now. This occurs when you redesign a process so that you eliminate steps or reduce the activities within the component tasks of the process. If you can identify a step that will add value to the product/service (i.e., better meet customer requirements), then it is worthwhile to consider.

Alternatively, if you identify existing steps that add no value whatsoever for the customer (internal or external), step elimination is probably the better choice.

6. *Plan the improvement and continued data collection.* Carefully plan the process improvement, including such details as what measures will be taken to ensure that the desired result is achieved, what training may be needed in order to implement the change, who will be accountable for what steps in the process, and how a pilot test of the redesigned process should be carried out.

7. *Do the improvement.* Collect and analyze data. Run the pilot test version of the process improvement and see how it goes. If there were any surprises, can the improvement team do anything about them?

8. *Check and study the results.* Examine the data collected subsequent to the implementation of the pilot test of the changed process. Has the desired improvement taken place? If you are not sure, what other measures might be needed to document this?

9. *Act to hold gain and continue improvement.* If the desired outcomes have occurred with the changed process, as demonstrated during the pilot test, plan for implementing the change as a standard. Before finally introducing the changed process to the rest of the organization, have your team take one more critical look to see if it can identify another process change that will improve the outcome (better meet internal customer or patient requirements). If so, plan it and reenter the PDCA cycle.

Figure 10–2 uses a top-down flowchart to illustrate the major functional components of the FOCUS-PDCA improvement model.

The Bay Area Medical Center in Marinette, Wisconsin put the FOCUS-PDCA model into action in early 1996 when management committed to using Press-Ganey survey data as the primary tool to measure customer satisfaction (Press-Ganey, 1997). It further committed that an improvement in customer satisfaction results would be the first priority among all corporate initiatives. Based on the data, several areas of concern were identified and teams were formed to analyze, make recommendations, and develop action plans for improvements.

During analysis, one team identified intravenous (IV) starts and venipunctures as an important issue that could help improve customer satisfaction. Using the FOCUS-PDCA, a venipuncture team developed a "blueprint" for change.

- *Find a process to improve.* The need for better venipuncture procedures was uncovered.
- *Organize a team that knows the process.* The venipuncture team was formed from several departments, including laboratory, nursing, radiology, physical therapy, and ambulance services.
- *Clarify current knowledge of the process.* Four steps helped to clarify the current process: analyzing the patient satisfaction survey scores, reviewing the comments patients had made, reviewing department policies about the procedure, and flowcharting the processes involved in venipunctures.
- *Understand underlying problems.* An analysis of flowcharting and customer data revealed potential problems with staff training, placing orders, equipment, access to the patient, patient education, and selection and care of the venipuncture site.
- *Select the process improvement.* Enhance training for lab and nursing personnel by revising orientation checklists and establishing preceptor programs. Review/revise department policies so they are consistent. Encourage the use of *Emla Cream* as a local anesthetic. Develop a patient education pamphlet that answers patient concerns about the procedure. Improve lighting and access to the light switch at the bedside and limit furniture so as to provide better access to the patient. Educate nursing about different draw priorities and encourage combining tests to reduce the number of blood draws. Standardize equipment. Purchase a new restraining board for pediatric draws. During nursing assessments, discuss the patient's history with venipunctures. Use an identification band that indicates if a particular limb cannot be used.
- *Plan and do (implement) the recommendation.* Recommendations were implemented at the department level.
- *Check.* Customer satisfaction for IV starts was monitored for several months.
- *Act to hold gain.* Recommendations that worked well were made permanent. Scores and patient comments continue to be monitored.

Through the use of the FOCUS-PDCA quality improvement model, all scores relating to the issues of IV starts have improved. And, most importantly, improvements in customer satisfaction is this area have helped to increase the overall hospital score, which has gone from the 75th percentile to the 97th percentile.

USING THE TOOLS AND TECHNIQUES OF CQI IN HEALTH CARE

The Use of Flowcharting in Health Care

In your organization's quest to improve the systems- and process-based components of patient satisfaction, the use of several basic CQI tools may be quite helpful. As we have seen above, flowcharting is an essential part of clarifying a process as we embark on either CPI or process reengineering.

A flowchart is a step-by-step schematic picture that describes a process or system. Figure 10–3 demonstrates the basic standard flowchart symbols. Numerous other standardized symbols are also available for specialized use.

There are several types of flowcharts.

- *Top-down flowcharts* list the major sequential steps across the top of the page and the major substeps needed to arrive at the respective major step underneath. Figures 10–2 and 10–4 show examples of top-down flowcharts. Figure 10–2 depicts the sequential FO-CUS-PDCA process improvement model; Figure 10–4 outlines the approach for establishing policies and procedures for (and implementing them) basic life support training.
- *Detailed flowcharts* describe almost all of the steps in a process, with varying levels of detail. This can be derived by your team by

FLOWCHART SYMBOL	MEANING
⬭	Beginning and ending of a process
▭	Activities in a process
◇	Decision point
⇨	Direction of process flow

Figure 10–3 Basic Standard Flowchart Symbols. *Source:* Adapted with permission from P. Mears, *Quality Improvement Tools & Techniques,* p. 19, © 1995, The McGraw-Hill Companies.

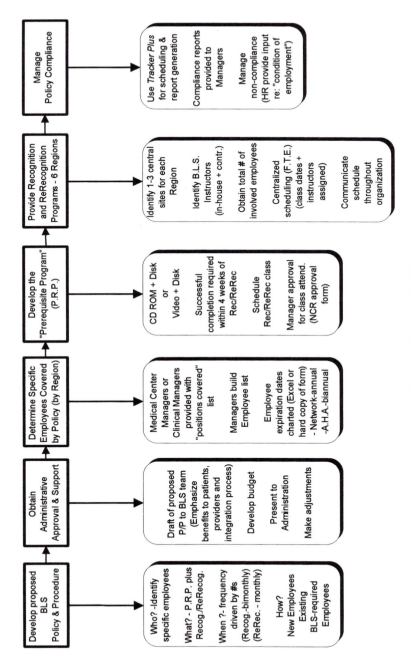

Figure 10–4 Top-down Flowchart of Basic Life Support Training P&P Development.

using an initial top-down flowchart and adding greater detail. Figure 10–5 shows a detailed flowchart of the process of ensuring compliance to a basic life support policy. A detailed flowchart should be looked on as a communication device that helps people develop an objective understanding of the process. This tool was originally developed in order to improve the efficiency of manufacturing processes. It has widespread applications in the health care industry, especially in the development of moment of truth management blueprints.

Once you have organized a team consisting of the individuals involved in performing the tasks of the process (including input suppliers and output customers, where appropriate), you need to work together to brainstorm the sequence of major process tasks. Then, determine if one or more decisions need to be made in conjunction with any of the listed tasks. Generally speaking, decision points are "yes" or "no" answers that steer the process in one direction or another. For example, if an approval is required, whether or not approval has been given will determine the next step in the process.

- *Deployment flowcharts* show both process flow and the people or groups involved in each step. This type of flowchart is constructed by first listing the major steps of a process or project vertically and then listing each of the people working on the process/project across the top, creating columns down from each name. Finally, mark the key action at each step in the appropriate column, indicating which person is primarily responsible for that step.

The Use of Check-Sheets in Health Care

A check-sheet is a structured form that makes it easy to record and analyze data. The best check-sheets are simple to use and visually display the data in a format that can reveal underlying patterns. Table 10–3 demonstrates a check-sheet gathering data pertaining to patient complaints about telephone management.

The first step in developing a check-sheet is to clarify what you are measuring. Be specific with regard to the location being measured. For example, are you only measuring waiting time in the reception room, or will it include waiting time in the treatment room as well? Then, agree on the length of time you will be gathering data for—this is typically determined by the cycle time of the process being evaluated. The longer the cycle time, the longer total duration should be covered by

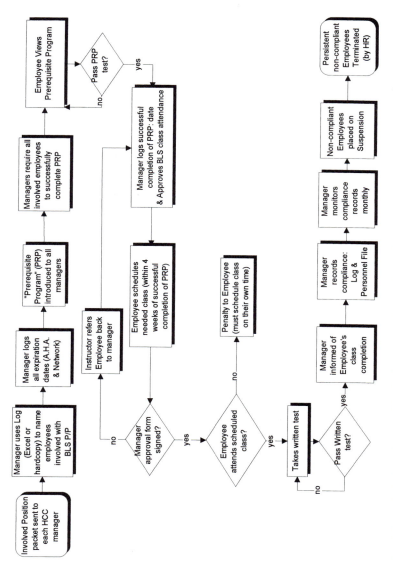

Figure 10–5 Detailed Flowchart of BLS Policy Compliance Procedures.

Table 10–3 Check-Sheet Tallying the Frequency of Patient Complaints re: Telephone Management

Patient Complaint	Mon	Tue	Wed	Thu	Fri	Total
On hold too long	IIIII I	II	IIII	I	IIIII IIIII I	24
Rude operator	II	I	I	I		5
Unhelpful operator	III	II	II	IIIII	I	13
Cut off during call transfer	I	IIIII	I			7
Total	12	10	8	7	12	49

the check-sheet. These comparative data can then be displayed using a bar graph.

The Use of Brainstorming in Health Care

Brainstorming is one of the easiest, quickest, and most enjoyable techniques for generating a list of ideas from your team. Brainstorming affords team members to be as creative as possible without restricting their ideas in any way. It also allows everyone to participate and is a good method for "breaking the ice" because it is free of criticism and judgment. You can maximize the benefits of your brainstorming sessions by creating and distributing a few simple ground rules to your team prior to the start of the session.

- Agree on a single question, issue, or problem that represents the focus of your brainstorming. Write this out clearly at the top of a flipchart page so it is in plain view throughout the session.
- Allow everyone a few minutes of quiet "think time" before beginning the discussion, giving them an opportunity to "mind-storm" their possible contributions to the discussion.
- Go for volume. The greater the number of ideas, the greater the possibility of good ones. Encourage everyone not to hold back ideas, even if they seem "silly" or "off-the-wall." No judgment of ideas is allowed. No one is allowed to criticize or evaluate another's ideas, either verbally or with body language or audible signs of approval or disapproval.
- Encourage participation by beginning with an emphasis on the importance of this session representing the ideas of all team members.
- As ideas are generated, document them on the flipchart by writing each in large easily visible print. Make sure you record the idea in

the same words as those given by the speaker: Do not abbreviate or interpret what the speaker says.
* Encourage people to "hitchhike" or "piggyback"—to build on the ideas already presented.

Brainstorming can be conducted using either a structured or an unstructured format. In *structured brainstorming,* each team member gives an idea in turn. The advantages of this type of brainstorming are that it ensures that everyone will be given the opportunity to contribute, it helps diffuse the effect of a dominant team member, and it appeals to logical, scientific people because it is systematic in approach. The disadvantage, of course, is that it can make more timid, introverted members feel somewhat intimidated or put on the spot. This can be partially offset by allowing all team members to "pass" on their individual turn if nothing comes to mind.

Unstructured brainstorming follows all the same rules as outlined above. However, with this type of brainstorming, team members give their ideas as they come to mind, rather than wait for a turn. There is no need to "pass" because ideas are not solicited in rotation. The advantages are that this creates a free-flowing positive environment and it fosters greater spontaneity in connecting one idea to another. The disadvantage is that it requires careful facilitation to maintain a balance of contributions among team members. When using the unstructured format, consider using the following hint: If you reach a point where it seems that there is too much tension or hesitation to contribute (particularly if a "high-ranking" team member seems to be dominating the discussion), transition over to structured brainstorming partway through the process.

The Use of Affinity Diagramming in Health Care

This procedure functions as a natural follow-up to brainstorming because it provides a mechanism for natural grouping of the brainstormed ideas. With this technique, each idea is recorded on a Post-it note of its own. Then, the team sorts the various ideas into five or six related groupings. Finally, a group title or heading that clearly indicates how the ideas in the group are linked is created. The headings should be short and should describe the main theme/focus of the group each represents. If you discover that two or more groups are very similar, the next step is to combine them into a new group with a different all-inclusive title or heading. This process should be continued until everyone on the team agrees to the groupings.

Figure 10–6 demonstrates the basic format of the completed affinity diagramming exercise.

The Use of Cause-and-Effect Diagrams in Health Care

This type of diagram was invented by Kaoru Ishikawa to identify and organize possible causes of problems or factors needed to ensure success of some effort (Mears, 1995). It consists of a pictorial diagram of a list of factors that are thought to affect a problem or desired outcome. Each diagram consists of a large arrow pointing to the name of the problem. The branches off of the large arrow represent main categories of potential causes or solutions. Typical main categories might include such areas as policies, procedures, environment, equipment, and people. Figure 10–7 is an example of the basic recommended structure. The main categories should be developed to reflect your topic.

This tool allows a team to identify and display all possible causes related to an adverse outcome (i.e., problem) or condition in order to discover its root causes. This type of diagram focuses attention on causes rather than symptoms. Once you uncover a potential cause with a given category, continue to explore the cause underlying that cause by asking "Why?" Next, members should come to an agreement

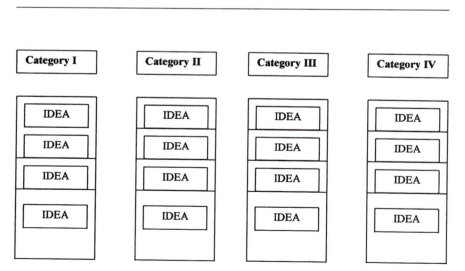

Figure 10–6 Basic Format for Affinity Diagramming.

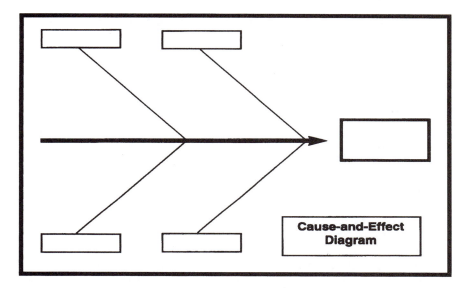

Figure 10–7 Cause-and-Effect Diagram Format.

as to what the most likely causes are. This may require gathering further data to convert "potential/possible" causes to "actual" causes. This sets the stage for long-term improvement/solutions as opposed to quick-fix "Band-Aid" approaches.

I have found it quite helpful to precede the construction of a cause-and-effect diagram with an affinity diagramming exercise as outlined above. In this way, the main categories have already been established and ideas within each category can be combined and listed as subcategories connected to each main branch.

The Use of Force-Field Analysis in Health Care

Force-field analysis is a technique developed by Kurk Lewin for identifying the forces that are present to facilitate or prevent a particular change (Mears, 1995). In this model, change is viewed as the outcome of a struggle between driving forces that are seeking to upset the status quo and restraining forces that are attempting to maintain the status quo. Driving forces are things like actions, skills, equipment, procedures, culture, people, and so forth that help move you toward the change. Restraining forces attempt to prevent the change from taking place. If the driving forces are stronger, the restraining forces will be overcome, and change will occur. When the restraining forces are equal to or stronger than the driving forces, there will be no change. The format for a force-field analysis is demonstrated in Figure 10–8.

Once your team has identified that a change should take place, brainstorming can be used to identify driving forces and restraining forces in the situation. Then, a force-field action plan can develop in terms of either strengthening the driving forces or reducing the restraining forces. This is very helpful when you are at the stage of implementing a change in one of your processes involving a facility or department as a whole. By identifying the restraining forces, your team can determine what needs to be done to eliminate them and then concentrate on reinforcing the driving forces. By anticipating resistance and contingency planning around the restraining forces, I have seen organizations in both the private and the governmental sectors successfully bring about radical change that was previously resisted.

Force-field analysis forces people to identify and think through the specific facets of a desired change. Furthermore, it helps teams identify the relative priority of the specific driving and restraining forces, which, in turn, provides a prioritized action plan.

CQI Must Be Organizationwide

In this section, we have listed only a limited number of tools and techniques that are commonly associated with CQI efforts. These

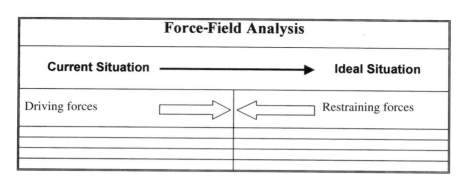

Figure 10–8 Force-Field Analysis Format.

should be introduced to everyone in your organization who will be involved in improving the systems and processes within which they work on a daily basis—virtually every employee or provider needs to know them. As their experience using them increases, so will their confidence level.

A coordinated organizationwide educational effort is needed to make sure the regular use of these tools becomes a part of your organization's culture. Policies and procedures should be established that afford all employees the chance to identify an improvement opportunity, coordinate a team to study the involved process(es), and see the idea through to the stage of successful change implementation. Multiple teams should be working on the various areas identified (as discussed in Chapter 8) as needing improvement. Many, much more sophisticated tools and techniques are available for your continuous patient satisfaction improvement efforts. Although these are beyond the scope of this book, a selected list of references that may prove helpful to you in this regard is provided at the end of this chapter.

GUIDELINES FOR TEAM FUNCTION IN YOUR APPROACH TO PROCESS IMPROVEMENT

We, in America, do not grow up learning how to function in teams. Granted, various athletic endeavors afford the limited opportunity to function in this capacity, but our cultural norms generally encourage otherwise. In school, we never receive a team report card or win team scholarships. Weisbord (1987) summarized this nicely: "Teamwork is the quintessential contradiction of a society grounded in individual achievement" (p. 21). This self-centered mentality runs contrary to the needs of contemporary organizations—to implement new ideas, develop more efficient processes, and apply better technology to compete with.

This section is not intended to provide a comprehensive overview of the complex topic of teamwork—that would be far beyond the scope or intention of this book. However, we will consider several practical issues related to team function. This material is intended to supplement the reader's existing knowledge about how organizational teams work (or don't work).

First, we will discuss basic small group discussion skills—a fundamental step that is often overlooked as teams come together. Next, several common discussion problems encountered by teams (along with possible solutions) will be briefly mentioned. Then, various team roles will be presented, along with a brief summary of the duties associated with each role. Once agreement is established about how discussions will be conducted, how discussion problems will be handled, and who will take responsibility for each role, an important early-stage task is to develop "team rules" that will govern how the team will function. Although this must be established by consensus within the team, several suggested rules will be provided for you to begin with. Then, you will be given a mechanism for evaluating the productivity and effectiveness of your organization's team meetings. Finally, the main elements necessary for overall team success will be discussed briefly.

Basic Small Group Discussion Skills for Teams

As a consultant to the U.S. Department of Justice, I have had the opportunity of facilitating a number of 5-day (Monday through Friday) CQI workshops at the National Institute of Corrections training center in Longmont, Colorado. While facilitating this workshop for my first time, I noticed that the small subgroups seemed to get bogged down with discussion problems whenever a timed exercise was assigned. As a result, their overall productivity and enthusiasm were somewhat dampened.

On the final day of this training, each small group was responsible for presenting a comprehensive application of CQI methods, tools, and techniques in the form of a plan for improvement in their respective agencies or departments. As expected, some groups performed better than others. However, it seemed to me that if they could have worked more synergistically throughout the week, the result could have been a better and more valuable product. After carefully reviewing the workshop curriculum with other consultants, we agreed to move the small group discussion skills segment from Thursday morning to Monday morning, immediately following introductions and the workshop overview. To make a long story short, the consequences of this relatively small modification were nothing short of phenomenal! Each small group remained enthusiastic and excited throughout the week of working together. They moved through various team exercises with much greater ease and with better results. As you might imagine, the quality of presentations made on the final day was superb: All groups were far better than I had observed before. Granted, other variables may have come into play, but I think the lesson learned applies to any team or other group of people hoping to work together toward a common goal.

It is hoped that the following general guidelines* (Scholtes, 1988, pp. 4–36) will help your health care organization's patient satisfaction improvement teams work more harmoniously together:

- *Ask for clarification.* If the topic being discussed or the logic of a group member's discussion is unclear, ask someone to define the purpose, mission, and focus of the discussion. Further clarification might be achieved by asking team members to repeat ideas in a different way or rephrase them. An ideal mechanism for ensuring clarification is to provide examples, pictures, diagrams, and so forth.
- *Act as a gatekeeper.* Everyone at various times throughout a discussion should function as a gatekeeper. That is, they should attempt to encourage equal participation among group members. This involves making openings for less aggressive members by directly asking for their input.
- *Listen.* Keep in mind that we were born with two ears and one mouth, yet seldom are they used in this proportion! In order to facilitate group discussion, it is essential that active listening be used in order to explore one another's ideas, rather than defending or debating each idea that comes up.
- *Summarize.* Periodically, the purpose of clarity is best served by restating to the group what has been said so far in a summary form. Then, make sure everyone agrees that the summary accurately reflects what has been discussed so far.
- *Contain digression.* Many times, when adults are participating in a discussion, they feel compelled to provide extensive examples from their own personal experiences. Often, this may be irrelevant to the material being discussed. By agreeing at the beginning that the group's objective is to remain focused on the agreed-on task or subject, those who digress can be reminded of the primary purpose of the meeting.
- *Manage time.* One or more individuals within the group should function as a time monitor to remind the group of deadlines and time allotments. This is of particular importance when the group has been given a limited amount of time to accomplish the task scheduled for the meeting.
- *End the discussion.* Many people feel compelled to continue discussing an issue even though nothing is to be gained from further

---

Source: This section through next section, "Common Discussion Problems and How To Handle Them," © 1999 Oriel Incorporated. All Rights Reserved. Used here with permission.

discussion. Therefore, teams should agree in advance that once everyone's opinion has been heard and sufficient discussion has taken place, it is acceptable to recommend that the discussion be ended.

- *Test for consensus*. Once the discussion has apparently been brought to an end, it is important to state the decision that seems to have been made. At this point, summarize the group's position on the issue, and check to see if the team agrees with the summary. Remember that any one member of the group has veto power (a primary rule of consensus). It does not mean that there is a unanimous vote or a majority vote, but rather it is a solution or a selection that everyone can support or "live with."

Common Discussion Problems and How To Handle Them

There are several strategies for dealing with group problems that can be helpful if decided on at the beginning of the team meeting. First, anticipate and prevent group problems whenever possible. Most problems can be anticipated or prevented if the team spends time getting to know each other, establishing group rules, discussing norms for group behavior, and agreeing on an objective to constantly improve group process.

When a problem occurs, and one will inevitably occur, it is important not to blame an individual, but to accept the problem as a group problem.

Finally, don't overreact or underreact to the problem. Many behaviors are only fleeting disruptions in the group's progress. Some behaviors are very disruptive and can seriously slow down the team's discussion progress. As a rule of thumb, if the disruption is not a chronic problem and doesn't seem to inhibit the team's progress, it is best ignored. On the other hand, if a particular behavior becomes chronic in nature, it is best that a general reminder be issued to the group about the rules of discussion so as not to point out an individual. If this does not seem to be productive, then it may be appropriate to have a discussion away from the group or team setting.

Common group or team discussion problems include the following:

- *Floundering:* Many times, a group will have problems starting or ending. The group may suffer from false starts or directionless discussions and activities. Problems at the beginning suggest that the group is unclear or overwhelmed by its tasks. Startup problems may also indicate that group members are not yet comfortable enough with each other to engage in real discussion and decision making. On the other hand, floundering at the end of the discussion indicates that the group members have developed a bond and are reluctant to separate. This can best be managed by examining how the project is being run, reviewing the mission and plan, understanding the causes of confusion, and discussing what is needed to move on.

- *Overbearing participants:* These people usually have a position of authority or an area of expertise on which they base their authority (i.e, legitimate or position power and expert power, respectively). These individuals can be detrimental to the group when this discourages or forbids discussion encroaching into their authority or area of expertise (or signals the "untouchability" of an area by using technical jargon or referring to present specification, standards, regulations, or policies as the ultimate determinants of future actions). Furthermore, this person of authority or expertise may regularly discount any proposed activity by declaring that "it won't work," or may cite instances when it was tried unsuccessfully in the past.

  The best way to deal with overbearing participants is to reinforce the agreement that no area is sacred during discussion (Kriegel & Brandt, 1996). It should be agreed that each group member has the right to explore any area that pertains to the objective of the team. Next, it is helpful for everyone to agree that it is important that the process or problem be fully understood by every member of the team in all discussions. That is, if something is unclear to any given individual, it should be accepted as the group's responsibility to clarify that point before moving forward. This requires a spirit of cooperation and patience.

- *Dominating participants:* We have all experienced the occasion where people in a discussion simply like to "hear themselves talk" and rarely give others a chance to contribute. This can be detrimental to the team because it discourages others from participation.

  The best way to minimize the detrimental effect of a dominating participant is to begin the discussion by agreeing as a group what the limits of an individual's participation can be. That is, structure the discussion so that it encourages equal participation by all members of the team. Remember to practice the skills of gatekeeping.

- *Reluctant participants:* Due to shyness or insecurity with a knowledge base relative to the subject matter being discussed, individuals often feel hesitant to contribute to the discussion. Being an introvert is neither wrong nor right. However, problems can develop in a group discussion when there are no built-in activities that encourage introverts to participate and extroverts to listen.

Managing reluctant participants can best be accomplished by having someone function as a gatekeeper and simply ask if anyone has any additional ideas about the matter under discussion. This is most effective when facing the individual who has been a reluctant participant. More directly, it may be advisable to ask the reluctant participant specifically what his or her experience has been or what his or her opinion is. (This, by the way, is one of the most potent questions you can ask anyone!)

- *Unquestioned acceptance of opinions as facts:* When a team member asserts a statement with a great deal of confidence, many times, other group members accept that statement as factual. Members are hesitant to question a self-assured statement from another member. The danger here lies in having the group proceed on the basis of a false assumption (which was perceived as "fact").

  The best approach to managing this situation is to use a traditional axiom of debate that simply indicates that if a speaker presents something as fact without legitimate supporting evidence, the listener does not need to have evidence in order to respond with skepticism. The best way to manage this type of participant is to ask him or her point blank whether or not the statement is an opinion or fact. If they indicate fact, ask, "Do you have data to support this?" It is also beneficial at this point to have the group reconfirm their agreement to proceed with their group process using a scientific approach—information being presented is based on data gathered or factual information that can be referenced to its source.

- *Rush to accomplishment:* Because it is a common tendency to confuse activity with accomplishment, many times, a team member will become impatient because of his or her need to "do something." This type of individual may urge the team to make hasty decisions and discourage any further efforts to analyze or discuss the matter. Under these circumstances, it is best to remind all members of the team that they had agreed in the beginning to pursue the scientific approach. Therefore, they will not compromise this or circumvent any of the steps involved. It may be beneficial to remind group members that exerting too much pressure to rush to accomplishment may lead to a series of random, unsystematic efforts to achieve the team's discussion objectives. This is like hunters shooting blindly at silent birds in a heavy fog: They are satisfied that they are "doing something" and pray that at least one shot will hit the target.

The most valuable means of managing team members who are rushing to accomplishment is to confront them with constructive feedback, reminding them of the detrimental effects of the behavior.

• *Discounts or "plops":* We have all had the experience of having someone else ignore what we said or, worse yet, ridicule something we stated, based on our perspectives or values. Typically, no one acknowledges what you said, and the discussion picks up on a subject that is totally irrelevant to the statement you made. Recall the feeling of emptiness that this produced while you wondered why there was no response to your statement.

If this occurs in your team with frequency, it is worthwhile to remind the team of the importance of active listening, so that they recall that every group member deserves full eye contact and body language indicators of attentiveness during the time he or she is speaking. It is also helpful to offer support to the person who received the "plop" so that you "relegitimize" the value of his or her participation. I have seen this make a tremendous difference among mature adult students in a postgraduate university setting as well.

If one member of the team seems to discount the statements of other team members frequently, it may be more productive to speak to that individual away from the team setting, from a constructive standpoint. This is best accomplished by reminding the individual of how this inhibits the full participation of other team members who have been "plopped" on.

• *Wanderlust, digression, and tangents:* When members of the team have become very close and familiar with one another, or if they are about to discuss an issue that is very sensitive, there is a tendency for discussions to wander off in many directions. This may take the form of "speaking of…" or "that reminds me of…." We have all experienced this and, quite frankly, after several transitions of this nature, the discussion may take a direction that is considerably away from the mission or objective of your discussion.

It is best to be mindful of time constraints and remind the person who has digressed of the agenda the team developed if there are multiple topics being discussed. It may be beneficial to have the specific topics that are the focus of discussion printed on a flipchart adjacent to the team's meeting site. It is extremely important that the conversation be redirected back to the point to be discussed. This is simply accomplished by using the phrase: "We strayed from the topic, which was _____."

- *Feuding team members:* If a disagreement predates the team meeting, the team is liable to become a field of combat for the involved members who are vying with each other. Clearly, the issue is not the subject they are arguing about, but rather, the contest itself. Of course, the best mechanism for dealing with this is to select group members for discussion carefully so that adversaries are never on the same team. If, on the other hand, it is essential that these folks be on the same team (e.g., they each perform vital tasks within the same process to be improved), it may be wise for them to work out some agreement about their participation in the discussions prior to a formal team meeting.

The best way to manage team members that are taking up team discussion time with a feud is to get them to discuss their issues "off-line." That is, offer to facilitate a separate discussion between the two of them away from the normal team discussion so that they might arrive at some agreement or ground rules for managing their differences without disrupting the team's discussion.

Team Roles and the Responsibilities of Each

In order for a process improvement team in your health care organization to function effectively, a variety of roles must be played by the team members. These are summarized in Exhibit 10–1.

Developing Team Rules

One of the first orders of business for a newly assembled team is to establish rules that will guide their future work together. These rules function as minimum obligations that team members are expected to adhere to within the context of their work environment on the team. The following are a list of common team rules that can be used to "jump start" your team in developing its own rules:

- Use honest, direct communication.
- Seek and expect active participation by all members.
- Differences and disagreements during decision development are okay.
- Provide 100% support of decisions once they are made.
- Maintain confidentiality—agree on what, how, and when to communicate team results.

Exhibit 10–1 Summary of Team Roles and Responsibilities

Team Role	Role Responsibilities
Leader	• Prepare and schedule meetings. • Conduct meetings, following agenda. • Focus the team's attention on the task. • Seek group participation, asking for facts, opinions, and suggestions. • Provide CQI expertise, tools, and techniques. • Oversee data collection. • Make task assignments. • Facilitate implementation of action plan items. • Conduct meeting evaluations/critiques. • Act as primary spokesperson and presenter.
Facilitator	• Serve as advisor and consultant to team. • Agree to remain neutral; nonvoting member of team. • Suggest alternative methods and procedures. • Provide analytic direction and problem-solving support. • Act as coach and motivator of team. • Assist in building consensus. • Recognize team and individual achievements.
Recorder/scribe	• Maintain records of the team's work. • Record information on flipchart for team. • Create appropriate charts and diagrams. • Assist with notices and supplies for meetings (flipcharts, markers, etc.). • Distribute minutes to team members.
Timekeeper	• Help the team manage time. • Notify the team of time remaining on each agenda item during a meeting.
Team member	• Participate in making decisions and developing plans for the team. • Identify opportunities for improvement. • Function as "team players". • Gather, prioritize, and analyze data. • Share information/data in meetings. • Have "expertise" of the process being studied. • Help the team recommend actions to management. • Track effectiveness of solutions.

- Actively support one another.
- Deliver as expected, what is promised, when it is promised.
- Limit speaking to one person at a time.
- Deal directly with one another.
- Value each other's time.
- Recognize that it is okay to say "no."
- Commit to team priorities.
- If a team rule is broken, deal with it immediately.
- The team has the responsibility to enforce rules—not the team leader.
- Do not say anything about another person that cannot be said directly to the team, or that has not been said to the person.
- Honor the commitments of subordinates.

Surely, these rules seem very basic and obvious; however, I have seen teams attempt to function in the absence of team-established ground rules in many instances. The result?....a great deal of time is wasted and productivity wanes.

The following logistical team meeting guidelines may be incorporated into your rules as well:

- Start and end meetings on time.
- Provide the team with education regarding the team function (including small group discussion skills) during the first meeting.
- Establish a team mission during the first meeting.
- Recruit a volunteer minute-taker at the beginning of each meeting.
- Share data with team members.
- Make specific assignments to create involvement.
- Maintain and review a "parking lot" of peripheral issues.
- Distribute an agenda and minutes of the last meeting immediately following the meeting (hand-written minutes are acceptable, if legible).
- Keep an attendance record, which is cumulative over time.
- Contact absent members personally to review meeting actions and provide any materials that were circulated at the meeting.
- Follow team rules.

Evaluating the Effectiveness of Team Meetings

A team should self-evaluate the productivity and effectiveness of meetings on a regular basis. This is especially important during the early stages of team evolution. The evaluation should take approximately 3–5 minutes and should be conducted as the last agenda item of the meeting. The following implementation steps and guidelines may be helpful for you in developing your unique rules:

- Draw a line down the center of a flipchart page. Write a plus sign on the upper left side and a delta sign on the upper right side.
- Conduct a structured brainstorm on the question: "What went well with today's meeting?" List responses under the plus sign.
- Conduct a structured brainstorm on the question: "What could be improved about today's meeting?" List responses under the delta sign.

If time and circumstances permit, solicit ideas (structured or unstructured) on how to make improvements. If this is not possible or appropriate, the team leader should work with the facilitator to make sure the problem areas are addressed before the next scheduled meeting.

- Don't overuse or underuse this technique. Use judgment to sense when the team is getting off track or when things seem to be stalling or waning. Avoid making this a routine exercise, especially when the team has been well established and is functioning very smoothly.
- Avoid personal attacks. Make it a ground rule if necessary.
- Always conclude the evaluation on a positive, human note. Show appreciation for team member involvement and persistence.

Characteristics of Successful Teams

Successful teams exhibit the following characteristics:

- Possess a clearly stated mission and goals.
- Emphasize the importance of fostering creativity.
- Remain focused on the results they were assembled to obtain.
- Clarify the roles and responsibilities of all who are on the team.

- Remain well-organized throughout their tenure as a team.
- Build on individual strengths.
- Support leadership and each other.
- Develop a team climate and culture.
- Resolve conflicts constructively.
- Communicate openly.
- Make objective decisions.
- Evaluate their own effectiveness.

Teamwork—Nature's Answer to Optimum Survival

Next fall, when you see geese heading south for the winter flying along in a "V" formation, you might be interested in knowing what science has discovered about why they fly that way. It has been learned that as each bird flaps its wings, it creates an uplift for the bird immediately following. By flying in a "V" formation, the whole flock adds at least 71% greater flying range than if each bird flew on its own. (*People who share a common direction and sense of community can get where they are going quicker and easier because they are traveling on the thrust of one another.*) Whenever a goose falls out of formation, it suddenly feels the drag and resistance of trying to go it alone, and quickly gets back into formation to take advantage of the lifting power of the bird immediately in front of it. When the lead goose gets tired, he rotates back in the wing and another goose flies point. (*It pays to take turns doing hard jobs—with people or with geese flying south.*) These geese honk from behind to encourage those up front to keep up their speed.

Finally, when a goose gets sick or is wounded by gunshot and falls out, two geese fall out of formation and follow him down to help and protect him. They stay with him until he is either able to fly or dead, and then they launch out on their own with another formation to catch up with their group. This form of interdependence should serve as an excellent example of how teams can capitalize on the inherent synergy of working closely together.

PROVIDING CQI TRAINING

In order to address your health care organization's systems- and process-based improvement priorities, every provider, every medical staff member, and every nonmedical staff member must know how to identify opportunities for system and process improvement. This means that an organizational commitment to providing the necessary training must be made. Anyone who performs a subtask of a process that ultimately serves to provide for patient satisfaction must be empowered to initiate a performance improvement team.

The tools and techniques required for teams to bring about improvement in areas that have been identified by patients as needing improvement are not difficult to use. As stated at the beginning of this chapter, no matter how well-trained staff are in skills, knowledge, and attitudes, they cannot deliver optimum levels of patient satisfaction if the systems and processes that define daily operations are not patient-focused.

Appendix C includes the handouts for a presentation introducing the basic concepts of CPI. Although you may wish to modify this for your specific organizational needs, it serves as a "starting point" for your educational efforts in this area.

In Chapter 11, your attention will be directed toward identified (in Chapter 8) administration-based improvement priorities.

CONCLUSION

A well-trained and motivated staff can only contribute to improving patient satisfaction continuously to the extent that organizational procedures, processes, and systems are designed to support the delivery of quality service to patients. A process is a sequential grouping of tasks that turn an input from a "supplier" into a product or service output for an internal or external "customer." A system consists of a group of related processes. Your health care organization is made up of a unique combination of systems that should be designed to meet the needs and perceived needs of patients. Those people who are in charge of each process ("process owners") have the dual responsibility of clearly communicating input specifications to process suppliers and obtaining input from process customers regarding output requirements.

CPI is the term applied when an existing process requires an incremental improvement of 10% or less; a radical redesign of the entire process is referred to as *process reengineering*. The scope of CPI is much narrower and tends to involve frontline employees more than process reengineering, where the scope is more broad-based and cross-functional. Process reengineering requires more creative, "out-of-the-box" thinking—without concern for the constraints of how things were previously done. The key is to focus on those processes that produce favorable outcomes in areas that are important to patients (as established in Chapter 4). The FOCUS-PDCA method (Figure 10–2) is one of the most comprehensive approaches to process improvement. This method combines the FOCUS method of placing a given process under a figurative microscope with the Shewhart Plan-Do-Check-Act improvement cycle. The sequential steps to the FOCUS method are: find a process to improve, organize a team that knows the process, clarify current knowledge of the process, understand sources of process variation, select the process improvement, plan the improvement and continued data collection, do the improvement, check and study the results, and act to hold gain and continue improvement.

The best way to analyze, and ultimately improve or completely redesign, a process, is to begin with a flowchart that the team, by consensus, agrees represents the way the process is currently being done. Then, the team uses brainstorming to determine what data need to be collected to identify sources of process variation (the true enemy to quality). Check-sheets are used to collect the data, then *cause-and-effect* diagrams are developed to isolate root causes of variation so that process improvements will not be focused purely on symptomatic "quick fixes," but rather on underlying causes that, when remedied, produce long-term improvement. The proposed changes associated with process improvement and/or process reengineering should be analyzed by the team. This is best accomplished by using a *force-field analysis*, whereby both the driving forces and the restraining forces impacting the change are itemized and discussed. A coordinated organizationwide educational effort is needed to make sure the regular use of continuous improvement tools and techniques is the norm, not the exception.

In order for a group of people to function effectively as a team, they need to be trained appropriately. Some of the important issues include: small group discussion skills, team roles and responsibilities, and the establishment of their own "team rules" governing how the team will conduct meetings and manage various challenges (including conflict and discussion problems).

ACTION STEPS

1. Select a process that currently produces outcomes that detract from patient satisfaction. Identify the suppliers and direct customers of the process, flowchart the process as it currently is, and use the FOCUS-PDCA model to bring about improved outcomes.
2. Provide an existing or newly formed team with appropriate training to enhance its overall effectiveness. This should include such information as systems thinking, small group discussion skills, and how to resolve common discussion problems.

3. Make sure all existing or newly formed teams develop their own unique set of team rules that will guide their behaviors when performing team functions.
4. Establish a format for providing CQI training organization-wide. Make it practical, allowing attendees to work out real-world improvement challenges. Get the message out that everyone is responsible for carefully assessing and incrementally improving the processes that are involved with day-to-day operations.

REFERENCES

Al-Asaaf, A.F., & Schmele, J.A. (1993). *The textbook of total quality in health care*. Delray Beach, FL: St. Lucie Press.

Chang, R.Y. (1995). *Process reengineering in action: A practical guide to achieving breakthrough results*. Irvine, CA: Richard Chang Associates.

Goodman, J. (1986). Don't fix the product, fix the customer. *The Quality Review, 2*(3), 6–11.

Harrington, H.J. (1991). *Business process improvement: The breakthrough strategy for total quality, productivity, and competitiveness*. New York: McGraw-Hill.

Kriegel, R., & Brandt, D. (1996). *Sacred cows make the best burgers: Paradigm-busting strategies for developing CHANGE-READY people and organizations*. New York: Warner Books.

Mears, P. (1995). Improvement tools and techniques. New York: McGraw-Hill.

Press-Ganey. (1997). *Press-Ganey Success Stories*.

Scholtes, P.R., et al. (1988). *The team handbook*. Madison, WI: Joiner Associates.

Weisbord, M. (1987). *Productive workplace: Organizing and managing for dignity, meaning and community*. San Francisco: Jossey-Bass.

SUGGESTED READING

Albrecht, K. (1992). *The only thing that matters*. New York: Harper Business.

Bader, G.E., Bloom, A., & Chang, R.Y. (1994). *Measuring team performance: A practical guide to measuring team success*. Irvine, CA: Richard Chang Associates.

Barsky, J.D. (1995). *World-class customer satisfaction*. New York: Irwin Professional.

Bell, C.R., & Zemke, R. (1992). *Managing knock your socks off service*. New York: AMACOM.

Bennis, W., & Mische, M. (1995). *The 21st century organization: Reinventing through reengineering*. Oxford, England: Pfeiffer and Company.

Brassard, M., & Ritter, D. (1994). *The memory jogger II: A pocket guide of tools for continuous improvement and effective planning*. Methuen, MA: GOAL/QPC.

Capezio, P., & Morehouse, D. (1992). *Total quality management: The road of continuous improvement.* Shawnee Mission, KS: National Press.

Chang, R.Y. (1994). *Building a dynamic team: A practical guide to maximizing team performance.* Irvine, CA: Richard Chang Associates.

Chang, R.Y. (1994). *Continuous process improvement: A practical guide to improving processes for measurable results.* Irvine, CA: Richard Chang Associates.

Chang, R.Y. (1994). *Mastering change management: A practical guide to turning obstacles into opportunities.* Irvine, CA: Richard Chang Associates.

Chang, R.Y., & Curtin, M.J. (1994). *Succeeding as a self-managed team: A practical guide to operating as a self-managed work team.* Irvine, CA: Richard Chang Associates.

Chang, R.Y., & Kehoe, K.R. (1994). *Meetings that work!: A practical guide to shorter and more productive meetings.* Irvine, CA: Richard Chang Associates.

Chang, R.Y., & Niedzwiecki, M.E. (1993). *Continuous improvement tools volume 1: A practical guide to achieve quality results.* Irvine, CA: Richard Chang Associates.

Chang, R.Y., & Niedzwiecki, M.E. (1993). *Continuous improvement tools volume 2: A practical guide to achieve quality results.* Irvine, CA: Richard Chang Associates.

Connellan, T.K., & Zemke, R. (1993). *Sustaining knock your socks off service.* New York: AMACOM.

George, S., & Weimerskirch, A. (1994). *Total quality management: Strategies and techniques proven at today's most successful companies.* New York: John Wiley & Sons.

GOAL/QPC. (1995). *Coach's guide to the memory jogger.* Methuen, MA: Author.

Hackett, D., & Martin, C.L. (1993). *Facilitation skills for team leaders: Leading organized teams to greater productivity.* Menlo Park, CA: Crisp.

Hammer, M. (1996). *Beyond reengineering: How the process-centered organization is changing our work and our lives.* New York: HarperBusiness.

Harrington-Mackin, D. (1994). *The team building tool kit: Tips, tactics, and rules for effective workplace teams.* New York: AMACOM.

Harvard Business Review. (1994). *Command performance: The art of delivering service quality.* Boston: Harvard Business School.

Haynes, M.E. (1988). *Effective meeting skills: A practical guide for more productive meetings.* Menlo Park, CA: Crisp.

Heskett, J.L., Sasser, W., & Hart, C. (1990). *Service breakthroughs: Changing the rules of the game.* New York: The Free Press.

Hinton, T., & Schaeffer, W. (1994). *Customer-focused quality: What to do on Monday morning.* Englewood Cliffs, NJ: Prentice Hall.

Kayser, T.A. (1990). *Mining group gold: How to cash in on the collaborative brain power of a group.* El Segundo, CA: Serif.

Kelly, P.K. (1994). *Team decision-making techniques: A practical guide to successful team outcomes.* Irvine, CA: Richard Chang Associates.

Kinlaw, D.C. (1992). *Continuous improvement and measurement for total quality: A team-based approach.* Homewood, IL: Pfeiffer & Company and Business One Irwin.

Leland, K., & Bailey, K. (1995). *Customer service for dummies.* Chicago: IDG Books Worldwide.

Maddux, R.B. (1992). *Team building: An exercise in leadership.* Los Altos, CA: Crisp.

Maginn, M.D. (1994). *Effective teamwork.* New York: Business One Irwin/Mirror Press.

Manion, J., Lorrimer, W., & Leander, W. (1996). *Team-based health care organizations blueprint for success.* Gaithersburg, MD: Aspen.

Mears, P. (1995). *Quality improvement tools & techniques.* New York: McGraw-Hill.

Omachonu, V.K., & Ross, J.E. (1994). *Principles of total quality.* Delray Beach, FL: St. Lucie Press.

Robbins, H., & Finley, M. (1995). *Why teams don't work: What went wrong and how to make it right.* Princeton, NJ: Peterson's/Pacesetter Books.

Robson, G.D. (1991). *Continuous process improvement: Simplifying work flow systems.* New York: The Free Press.

Rummler, G.A., & Brache, A.P. (1995). *Improving performance: How to manage the white space on the organization chart* (2nd ed.). San Francisco: Jossey-Bass.

Senge, P., Ross, R., Smith, B., Roberts, C., & Kleiner, A. (1994). *The fifth discipline fieldbook: Strategies and tools for building a learning organization.* New York: Doubleday.

Sewell, C., & Brown, P.B. (1990). *Customers for life: How to turn that one-time buyer into a lifetime customer.* New York: Pocket Books.

Shaw, J.C. (1990). *The service focus: Developing winning game plans for service companies.* Homewood, IL: Dow Jones-Irwin.

Stamatis, D.H. (1996). *Total quality service: Principles, practices, and implementation.* Delray Beach, FL: St. Lucie Press.

Whiteley, R.C. (1991). *The customer-driven company: Moving from talk to action.* Menlo Park, CA: Addison-Wesley.

Williams, R.L. (1994). *Essentials of total quality management.* San Francisco: AMACOM.

Winwood, R.I. (1991). *Creating quality meetings: Latest techniques for mastering group communication.* Salt Lake City, UT: Franklin International Institute.

CHAPTER 11

Addressing Administration-Based Improvement Priorities

The activities involved in bringing about behavior-based and systems/process-based improvements are relatively straightforward and have been discussed in Chapters 9 and 10. However, the steps involved in addressing the so-called administration-based improvement priorities are not as well defined. First of all, we need to clarify what is meant by the term "administration." Among other definitions, Merriam Webster's Collegiate Dictionary (1997) provides the following relevant description: "performance of executive duties: management" (p. 15). Therefore, for purposes of this book, we will use the term interchangeably with such commonly used descriptors as "senior or upper management," "organizational executives," or simply "organizational leaders."

Establishing an organizationwide laser focus on improving patient satisfaction requires effective, credible leadership. Furthermore, leaders must be committed to creating an atmosphere of obsession for exceeding patient expectations on a daily basis. This chapter will present several ingredients that are considered essential for ensuring administration's commitment and support of your organization's patient satisfaction improvement efforts, including:

- leading and the role of leadership—effectiveness and credibility
- a compelling vision: the spark that ignites a patient satisfaction obsession
- change: the foundation of continuous improvement
  1. changing management paradigms
  2. reengineering management
  3. executive's role in managing organizational change

- administration's obligation to "walk the talk"
- communicating patient satisfaction data to administration

LEADING AND THE ROLE OF LEADERSHIP—EFFECTIVENESS AND CREDIBILITY

The process of leading consists of a leader influencing the behavior of one or more followers using some form of power. Several forms of power are typically available for use as a given leader deems appropriate. *Legitimate or position power* is that which is inherent to the leader's position within the organizational chart. This is the "Do what I say because I'm the boss" mentality. *Expert power,* on the other hand, relates to the ability of a leader to influence the behavior of followers because he or she possesses certain expertise that the follower perceives as valuable. This form of power tends to engender follower respect. The expertise of being an effective communicator, for example, is commonly observed in an effective leader. *Connection power*—"who you know"—constitutes the foundation on which the infamous "good-old-boy" network is based. Although the use of this power base is rampant throughout many organizations, it is not typically associated with true follower respect. Similarly, *coercive power,* influence by brute force, seldom plays a significant role in contemporary organizations and, when it does, fosters disrespect at best.

Referent power, on the other hand, represents the power base that classically produces followers who will "go the extra mile" for the leader—followers who will routinely exert their "discretionary" effort without hesitation. Definition of this power base is somewhat illusive—a combination of charisma (the John F. Kennedy factor), deep respect for the leader as a human being, and a strong follower conviction that the leader's cause is noble and worthwhile. To this, we must add the ingredient of follower acceptance that the leader is acting in the follower's best interest as aligned with organizational objectives. In short, the leader who possesses and uses referent power combined with expert power is likely to be highly effective and command uncommon levels of respect—both within and outside the organization.

So far, we have considered only the process of leading as it relates to the use of various power bases. In comparing the different forms of power, we alluded to leadership "effectiveness." However, the concept of effectiveness requires further attention because it is often the primary determinant of a given leader's success. More than a decade ago, Tom Peters (Peters & Waterman, 1982) clarified the distinction between effectiveness and efficiency: "Efficiency is doing things right, while effectiveness is doing the right things." Management guru Peter Drucker and leadership gurus Warren Bennis and Stephen Covey (1989) made a similar distinction: "Management is doing things right; leadership is doing the right things" (p. 161).

Covey (1989) elaborated on this distinction when he said that "management is efficiency in climbing the ladder of success; leadership determines whether the ladder is leaning against the right wall...effectiveness—often even survival—does not depend solely on how much effort we expend, but on whether or not the effort we expend is in the right [area]" (p. 101). Covey went on to say that "efficient management without effective leadership is...like straightening deck chairs on the Titanic. No management success can compensate for failure in leadership" (p. 102).

In 1982, organizational behavior researcher Paul Hershey (1984) developed the situational ("contingency") model of leadership wherein leaders adjust their leadership style according to the readiness (or "maturity") level of the follower in a given situation. Although a comprehensive discussion of the model is beyond the scope of this book, a brief overview may serve well to further clarify the concept of leader *effectiveness*. Essentially, Hershey defined four leadership styles on a grid, with one axis "task behavior" and the other "relationship behavior." Figure 11–1 demonstrates the resulting four quadrants with their associated leadership styles.

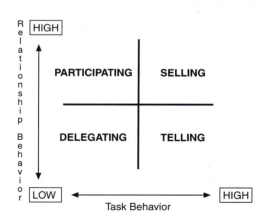

Figure 11–1 Hershey and Blanchard's (1982) Leadership Styles. *Source:* Adapted with permission from P. Hershey and K.H. Blanchard, *Management of Organizational Behavior,* p. 184, © 1993, Prentice Hall.

Note that each leadership style carries a prescribed combination of relationship-based and task-based leader behavior. This is summarized as follows:

- telling = high task and low relationship
- selling = high task and high relationship
- participating = high relationship and low task
- delegating = low relationship and low task

The contingency or situational model of leadership goes on to classify followers in terms of their readiness (a combination of ability and willingness) for performing a particular task in a given situation. Thus, low readiness is designated as an "R-1" readiness level, whereas high readiness is referred to as an "R-4" readiness level. The next step, then, is to align the leadership style of the leader with the properly "diagnosed" readiness level of the follower in each situation. This roughly translates (for each distinct situation) into an R-1 readiness level follower being best led by a "telling" leadership style; an R-2 readiness level follower being best led by a "selling" leadership style; an R-3 readiness level follower being best led by a "participating" leadership style; and finally, an R-4 readiness level follower being best led by a "delegating" style of leadership.

In the context of the situational leadership model, the term *effectiveness* as applied to a leader refers to the leader's practice of consistently adapting his or her leadership style to the identified readiness level of the follower in each situation. Thus, contrary to traditional usage of the term consistent—which would imply the use of the same leadership style all the time—it means consistently adaptable using this model. So far, then, we see that in order for leaders to be truly effective, they must not only carefully use their various power bases, but they must be prepared to adjust how they lead appropriately depending on the follower's readiness and then lead the follower to do the right things. Another essential ingredient for effective organizational leadership is for each leader to be credible—this is the foundation for building follower trust.

Kouzes and Posner (1987, 1993) reported findings based on, among other things, interviews with more than 7,500 followers to determine the most important characteristics needed to make a leader credible. They consistently found that the four most important characteristics were honesty, forward-looking, inspiring, and competent.

One of the most important elements in a health care organization's quest for high patient satisfaction is the belief by the organization's credible and effective leaders that success is directly connected to continuous quality improvement. Without that belief, other efforts to meet or exceed patient expectations can only result in marginal success. Of course, the chief executive officer is a key figure in this regard. He or she must openly and consistently support the service quality movement, not only with words, but also with actions. When resources must be allocated for making needed, patient-identified improvements, the mindset of "investment" rather than "expenditure" must be forthcoming.

Deming believed that the leadership role must include developing a customer-driven mentality (Scholtes, 1988). Thus, senior management must create clear and visible patient satisfaction values and high expectations—the vision and purpose of improvement efforts. Then, reinforcement of the values and expectations requires senior management's substantial personal commitment and involvement. Leaders must take part in the creation of strategies, systems, and methods for achieving service quality excellence.

Organizational systems need to guide all activities and decisions of the health care organization and encourage participation and creativity by all employees. Through their regular personal involvement in visible activities, such as planning, review of company quality performance, and recognizing employees for outstanding patient service quality, senior leaders serve as role models reinforcing the values and encouraging leadership in all levels of management.

Establishing a health care organizational culture that is truly committed to improving patient satisfaction continuously requires leaders who are highly effective. They must be credible in order to maximize their effectiveness, but there is one more essential ingredient—they must also be capable of developing (in cooperation with others throughout the organization), communicating, and implementing a vision.

A COMPELLING VISION: THE SPARK THAT IGNITES A PATIENT SATISFACTION OBSESSION

Recall that Kouzes and Posner (1987, 1993) determined the characteristics of "forward-looking" and "inspiring" to be two of the four most mentioned characteristics that make for a credible leader. Both of these are linked to vision—a vivid picture of an optimistic, ambitious, desirable future state that is connected to patient satisfaction (and loyalty) and is better in some important way than the current state. A vision is value-based and functions as the lighthouse that gives general direction rather than a specific destination. It describes an ideal to strive for without necessarily describing how to accomplish that ideal. A common vision is important for several reasons.

- It provides a source of inspiration—inspiring employees to do their best when it comes to meeting or exceeding patient expectations.
- It gives the organization a philosophical context to operate in—a natural guide for all decision making. Walt Disney reportedly once said: "When your values are clear, decision making is easy" (Capodagli & Jackson, 1999, p. 9). When senior management codevelops a shared patient-focused vision to which they commit themselves, the decisions in favor of allocating resources needed for improving patient satisfaction will be consistently forthcoming.
- It acts as a unifying force, giving everyone in the organization a common goal and direction.
- It provides clarity in uncertain situations. When organizations face a crisis or move in new directions, there are usually few or no precedents and no clear paths to follow. People need guidelines for their day-to-day actions and decisions. They need to know what is expected. A clear, commonly shared vision provides this guidance. The shared vision is like a beacon that guides travelers in the right direction. Even if the people cannot see the path, or if there are obstacles they must steer around, the beacon keeps them heading in essentially the right direction.

Whiteley (1991) stated that the most difficult aspect of making the vision real is imparting it to all the people in the organization so they will share a profound commitment. Thus, it is the effective, credible leader who makes the vision real because he or she

- Communicates the vision constantly.
- Establishes challenging, often seemingly impossible, concrete goals that are driven by the vision.
- Encourages others in the organization to create their own compatible visions for their parts of the business.
- Embodies the vision in day-to-day behavior—"walks the talk" (p. 31).

Leaders must collaborate with one another to establish and "live" a common vision. Some organizational leaders may initially fail to embrace the vision-oriented conceptual framework. If this occurs, it is advisable for his or her fellow leaders to establish a mentor relationship for this purpose. After all, the remainder of the organization cannot be expected to rally around a common vision if leadership doesn't set the example. In Chapter 13, the concept of organizational vision will be explained in greater detail in the context of organizational culture.

When a health care organization clearly declares what it stands for, and its people share this vision, a powerful network is created—people seeking related goals.

CHANGE: THE FOUNDATION OF CONTINUOUS IMPROVEMENT

In an industry as dynamic as health care—particularly in the United States—constant and often radical change have become the norm. The question is not whether change will take place, but how and how fast it will be implemented—and at what expense in terms of financial and human resources. As a result, management needs to change a variety of its operational paradigms. Indeed, management itself (vs. one work process or another) may often need to be completely reengineered. As such, management must be prepared to play an active role in effectively managing organizational change in alignment with the established shared vision.

Changing Management Paradigms

A paradigm functions as a lens through which we view the world around us. It is our framework for perception, understanding, and interpretation. Paradigms tend to dominate the way people think and act. Albrecht (1992, p. 39) maintained that contemporary management must switch from the thing-centered industrial orientation to the new customer-value orientation. This paradigm shift involves 10 key areas of management thinking.*

1. *The business mission:* The industrial business mission of making a good product and then finding someone to buy it must change to a customer-value paradigm where services are designed to win and keep customers—to their exacting specifications. The objective must be to identify the needs and perceived needs of the target audiences and then match the services to meet those needs.
2. *The profit principle:* Old paradigm: Carefully control costs, use capital as efficiently as possible, and deliver outcomes that are

---

Source: Copyright © 1992 by Karl Albrecht. Reprinted by permission of HarperCollins Publishers, Inc.

on a level with those delivered by competitors. New paradigm: Customer value (the quality of the total experience as perceived by the customer—recall the patient's mental report card) drives profit.

3. *View of customers:* Old paradigm: The customer is expendable or replaceable. As long as we keep new customers coming in, it doesn't matter if some of them leave due to dissatisfaction. New paradigm: Customers must be viewed as appreciated assets who not only continue to bring us revenue, but who are in a position to refer other customers as well.

4. *The employees:* Old paradigm: The purpose of employees is to carry out orders given by supervisors. New paradigm: Recognize that customer focus pertains to both internal and external customers. Everyone has customers who must receive process outcomes that meet quality requirements. The outcome may well be an intangible, like a convenient appointment for a patient, or timely results from a laboratory test.

5. *The work:* Old paradigm: Employee attention should be directed toward assigned tasks that must be performed in accordance with standards. New paradigm: The primary objective of the employee is to focus on the quality of the customer's experience at each moment of truth (MOT).

6. *Measurement:* Old paradigm: Frontline employees get measured according to evidence that they have accomplished their tasks. New paradigm: The entire organization is accountable for measuring and monitoring the outcomes of managing each MOT— recognizing that a lot of things need to happen in order to have a MOT managed positively.

7. *Rewards:* Old paradigm: Employees will "malfunction" if you don't give them sufficient money and good working conditions. New paradigm: A sense of pride in quality, ownership of results, and a sense of belonging are valuable payoffs, just as money and material compensation are valuable.

8. *Supervising and managing:* Old paradigm: Middle managers or supervisors are to make sure frontline employees carry out their tasks according to pre-established standards—shaping employee behavior in the direction of task performance. New paradigm: The manager's job is to be resourceful to frontline employees who are in direct contact with and serving customers.

9. *The organization:* Old paradigm: Structure, process, and control are the main apparent components of organizational effectiveness. New paradigm: Organizational structure and systems are

designed to support frontline workers in their efforts to serve customers, not to exert control over them.

10. *Executive roles:* Old paradigm: Senior management's role is to preside over an organization by exerting control using various mechanisms. New paradigm: The primary role of executives is to create and maintain a service culture; all efforts are directed toward putting organizational values aligned with being customer-driven into daily action.

Reengineering Management

In 1990, authors Michael Hammer and James Champy wrote the enormously successful (more than two million copies sold) book, *Reengineering the Corporation,* to improve business performance by showing managers how to revolutionize their operational processes. In Chapter 10, we discussed the role of reengineering in addressing a health care organization's systems/process-based improvement priorities. In 1994, Champy conducted a study in which 621 companies, representing a sample of 6,000 of the largest corporations in North America and Europe, completed an extensive questionnaire. Champy reported that "69% of the 497 American companies responding, and 75% of 124 European companies, were already engaged in one or more reengineering projects, and that half of the remaining companies were thinking about such projects" (Champy, 1996).

Although many companies reported big changes and reaped big rewards, Champy reported that "even substantial reengineering payoffs appear to have fallen well short of their potential" and that "the revolution we started has gone, at best, only halfway" (p. 3). Now, there is an "urgent need to reinvent the processes of management, bend them to the new realities of the marketplace" (p. 9). He goes on to say that "the job for management is two-fold: First, our times require us to reexamine and restate our business purpose; and second, we must use this restatement to fully mobilize our companies for change" (p. 41).

Executive's Role in Managing Organizational Change

Health care organizations everywhere are experiencing massive changes due to downsizing, mergers, response to changing markets, or adjustments to competitive pressure. Change is everywhere and is a fact of life. Unless care is exercised by leadership, a health care organization can get so bogged down responding to immediate conditions that an overall sense of direction is lost. To be sure, the underlying driver of all change in the health care industry ultimately must be to deliver greater value to the customer—whether that customer is an employer, a third-party payer, or, most importantly, the patient.

Change that is poorly managed is confusing at best and counterproductive—producing anxiety and chaos—at worst. Well-managed change, on the other hand, can be a tremendous positive force characterized by success and results. According to McCarthy (1995),

> management's challenge in managing complex or compound transitions is twofold: The first major problem is that [transitions] are simply misread…managers are not schooled in recognizing a transition and determining what to do about it…. Many times, market and competitor changes take place around the unaware company as it continues to operate the same way it always has…. Second, management frequently applies overzealous remedies that are disproportionate to the need. The sum total of change required over a period of years may be immense, but the incremental change required month to month may be almost invisible to the average employee. (p. 25)

Every employee who experiences change in the workplace passes through four transitional phases that move the individual from viewing change as "danger" to viewing it as "opportunity." This process leads from the way things were done in the past toward a new way of doing things in the future. Initially, people focus on the past and deny that any change will take place. Then, they become preoccupied with concerns about where they stand and how they will be affected by the change. This is typically manifested by some degree of resistance to the change. As more information becomes available, people start to look to the future, with exploration for possible personal opportunities—answering the most-asked question whenever one's time or energy is required: "What's in it for me?" Finally, when employees begin working together to facilitate the change, the stage of commitment takes place.

Within a 30-month period, I have personally observed/experienced the radical change shockwaves of three organizational mergers and acquisitions—two as the "acquired" and one as the "acquirer." During the 6 months following Friendly Hills HealthCare Network's acquisition of Cigna Health Care Centers, I facilitated numerous workshops (1,400 employees in all) wherein the "acquired" employees were given the skills and tools needed to help them cope with the change. This was greatly appreciated by the employees and, I believe, contributed to the success of the cultural merging.

During those workshops, the most frequent frustration expressed by participants was the lack of information given to them by top management. Fortunately, our executives responded to this concern. We produced a videotape in which I interviewed each of our senior vice-presidents and they clarified the rationale and wisdom of the merger and what it meant to employees from their perspective. This was shown at our monthly leadership meeting and distributed throughout the organization within a very tight time frame. The response was overwhelmingly positive. Moreover, the value and importance of employees receiving information during change were underscored by its presence on the first instance of being acquired and its absence during the second. For these reasons, I believe that a critical role for executives during organizational change is to communicate to all employees as much information as possible throughout the implementation of change.

Costello (1994, p. 102) recommends the following sequential seven-step communication process:

1. *Describe the change and the reasons for it.* This step increases the employee's general awareness.
2. *Explain the impact the change will have on the employee.* This step adds to the employee's personal awareness regarding the change by providing an opportunity to clarify and express feelings.
3. *Encourage questions and allow for the expression of concerns.* This step adds to the employee's understanding of the change by providing an opportunity to clarify and express feelings.
4. *Respond to any questions and concerns.* This step leads to initial acceptance by the employee.
5. *Restate or reemphasize alternative behaviors and methods.* This step clarifies expectations.
6. *Gain commitment to the change.* This step ensures that the employee has a commitment to adopt and implement the change effectively.
7. *Confirm implementation plans and establish follow-through procedures.* This step further clarifies expectations, progress measurements, and ongoing support necessary for change success.

LEADERSHIP: WORDS INTO ACTION—WALKING THE TALK

Effective leaders help make strategy that is aligned with organizational vision a day-to-day reality. Unless senior management professes the religion of patient service, employees will view the most elegant strategy as just another easily ignored public relations campaign. If service to patients is to be outstanding, leaders must incessantly pronounce their beliefs and back up their words with actions. Management's goal is to nurture a service culture that can shape employee behavior more effectively than rules and regulations. They make service everybody's business and empower employees to act consistently in the patient's best interest.

No health care organization can produce outstanding patient satisfaction (and loyalty) unless its senior managers are visibly, constantly, and sometimes irrationally committed to the idea. Taking exceptional care of patients is so much work that it gets done only if the people at the top lead the charge. When they don't, the organization naturally turns inward and concentrates on internal processes that are less demanding to work on. Everyone succumbs to the pressure of just doing their jobs instead of focusing on getting top grades on the patient's mental report card.

Davidow and Uttal (1989, p. 107) identified three principles that leaders of companies that shine in customer service adhere to. Roughly translated for health care, these are as follows:

1. *Foster a service-oriented culture.* Effective organizational leaders help create and nurture cultures by communicating values. They are personally involved in service activities and back up slogans with dramatic actions. To inculcate values, they stress two-way communication, opening their doors to all employees and using weekly meetings of work groups to inform, inspire, and solve service problems. They put values into action by treating employees exactly as they want employees to treat customers.

2. *Make customer service everybody's business.* Patient satisfaction essentially dies unless every employee assumes responsibility for the patient's experience. Effective leaders encourage each employee to feel and act as if he or she owns the company. They set impossibly high standards and push responsibility for service as far down into the organization as possible, often using upside-down or concentric organization charts to underline the idea that frontline employees are second in importance only to patients.

3. *Declare war on bureaucracy.* Red tape and recalcitrant managers can sabotage patient service. To produce effective, efficient patient service, good leaders keep policies, procedures, and other formal control mechanisms to a minimum, relying instead on

cultural control. They reeducate middle managers and supervisors to focus on serving and supporting frontline employees, measuring their performance by surveying the service they render to internal customers.

COMMUNICATING PATIENT SATISFACTION DATA TO ADMINISTRATION

From the onset of your health care organization's patient satisfaction improvement campaign, senior management needs to be involved in the capacity of reviewing and approving your program proposal. Effective improvement proposals typically align with the purpose defined in the organization's mission statement and with the shared organizational vision already in place. Therefore, by the time patient satisfaction research data are available, executives are typically "hungry" for results presented in a concise and easy-to-interpret format so they can get about the business of influencing improvements through change.

The minimum information that should be included in this communication is the following:

- a brief summary of how the data were collected—your methodology—with a brief explanation of how or why certain aspects may not have gone the way you planned (and what you did about it)
- a summary of those elements of patient satisfaction that your research indicates are most important to your patients—the *relative importance* (as discussed in Chapter 4)
- a graphic representation of overall patient satisfaction for your health care organization as a whole
- a tabular summary of the *dissatisfaction index*—satisfaction elements that received a "fair" or "poor" rating by a significant percentage of respondents on your organization's patient satisfaction survey (as discussed in Chapter 8); if you have multiple facilities/departments, these data should be sorted and presented accordingly
- a brief summary of how the *improvement priority index* is calculated (see Chapter 8)—multiplying the *relative importance index* by the *dissatisfaction index*
- a tabular summary of the top 5 or 10 organizational improvement priorities, divided according to improvement mechanism—behavior-based, systems/process-based, and administration-based; this should be presented in such a fashion that executives can clearly

identify the relative patient satisfaction strengths and weakness of each facility, each department, and the organization as a whole
- a summary of other patient satisfaction/dissatisfaction input—from a variety of other sources (as outlined in Chapter 8) that may influence their improvement prioritization for the allocation of resources

With this information in hand, and with a clear recognition that this represents the "voice of the patient," executives are in a position to allocate resources rationally that support the organizational vision for exceptional patient satisfaction and loyalty. Once the needed funds and human resources are committed to patient satisfaction improvement activities, senior management will be most anxious for indicators of program effectiveness—the proverbial "return on investment." As this information becomes available—in the form of reduced patient complaints, more favorable focus group input, decreased disenrollment, satisfaction survey results, and so forth, it should be communicated to top management with a sense of urgency. This information can function very effectively as the positive reinforcement management needs to continue the investment process.

The next chapter will present methods for measuring and reporting the value—"return on investment"—of your health care organization's patient satisfaction improvement efforts.

CONCLUSION

Effective leadership is essential if a health care organization hopes to create an organizational atmosphere of obsession for continuously improving patient satisfaction. Leading involves influencing the behavior of followers using power. Leaders are effective when they "do the right things" and efficient when they "do things right." Equally as important, leaders need to be credible in the eyes of their followers. Research demonstrates that credibility requires that leaders be honest, forward-looking, inspiring, and competent. In order for organizational leadership to be inspiring and forward-looking, there needs to be a collective vision—a vivid picture of an optimistic, ambitious, desirable future state that is connected to patient satisfaction (and loyalty) and is better in some important way than the current state. Once senior management is provided with the appropriate patient satisfaction research data that represent the "voice of the patient," they are in a position to rationally allocate the human and financial resources that support the organizational vision.

Change is the foundation on which continuous improvement rests, but it must be managed well along the way. Change that is poorly managed is confusing at best and counterproductive—producing anxiety and chaos—at worst. Every employee who experiences change in the workplace passes through four transitional phases that move the individual from viewing change as "danger" to viewing it as "opportunity." This process leads from the way things were done in the past toward a new way of doing things in the future. Initially, people focus on the past and deny that any change will take place. Then, they become preoccupied with concerns about where they stand and how they will be affected by the change. This is typically manifested by some degree of resistance to the change. As more information becomes available, people start to look to the future with exploration for possible personal opportunities—answering the most-asked question whenever one's time or energy is required: "What's in it for me?" Finally, when employees begin working together to facilitate the change, the stage of commitment takes place.

Once senior management makes the commitment to support the changes needed to improve patient satisfaction incrementally, they must communicate this commitment to employees. One way to accomplish this is by following this sequence: Describe the change (and the reasons for it), explain the impact the change will have on the employee, encourage questions and allow for the expression of concerns, respond to any questions and concerns, restate or reemphasize alternative behaviors and methods, gain commitment to change, confirm implementation plans, and establish follow-through procedures. In order to sustain senior management's commitment to changes needed to improve patient satisfaction, there needs to be a constant flow of feedback/data documenting that the desired result is being achieved—patient satisfaction is truly improving.

ACTION STEPS

1. Based on the chapter discussion of situational leadership (coupled with appropriate suggested reading at the end of this chapter), identify your primary leadership style (telling, selling, participating, or delegating). Then, picture yourself using the other three leadership styles in various circumstances.
2. Make a concerted effort to "diagnose" the readiness level of your follower accurately in a given situation within the next

week. Then, adjust your leadership style accordingly so that the interaction will be more effective. Remember that the same individual can, and often is, at different readiness levels in different situations. Therefore, how you lead the individual in each situation may be quite different.

3. List three internal changes that are currently in progress in your organization. Then, for each of these, identify the "driving forces" and "resistors" that impact long-term implementation of the change. Next, work with a group of five colleagues to brainstorm ways to minimize resistance while strengthening the drivers to ensure that the transition from "status quo" to the "new way" progresses smoothly.

4. Take the change "pulse" of your organization by identifying signs of those involved with the changes listed above (or any major organizational change) who are exhibiting resistance, denial, exploration, or commitment.

5. List the steps you feel your organization can, and should, take to facilitate the change process on a day-to-day basis.

REFERENCES

Albrecht, K. (1992). *The only thing that matters*. New York: Harper Business.

Capodagli, B., & Jackson, L. (1999). *The Disney way: Harnessing the management secrets of Disney in your company*. New York: McGraw-Hill.

Champy, J. (1996). *Reengineering management: The mandate for new leadership*. London: HarperCollins.

Costello, S.J. (1994). *Managing change in the workplace*. New York: Irwin Professional.

Covey, S.R. (1989). *The seven habits of highly effective people: Powerful lessons in personal change*. New York: Simon & Schuster.

Davidow, W.H., & Uttal, B. (1989). *Total customer service: The ultimate weapon*. New York: Harper & Row.

Hammer, M., & Champy, J. (1990). *Reengineering the corporation*. New York: HarperCollins.

Hershey, P. (1984). *The situational leader*. Escondido, CA: The Centre for Leadership Studies.

Kouzes, J.M., & Posner, B.Z. (1987). *The leadership challenge*. San Francisco: Jossey-Bass.

Kouzes, J.M., & Posner, B.Z. (1993). *Credibility: How leaders gain and lose it, why people demand it*. San Francisco: Jossey-Bass.

McCarthy, J.A. (1995). *The transition equation: A proven strategy for organizational change*. New York: Lexington Books.

Merriam-Webster's Collegiate Dictionary, Tenth Edition. (1997). Springfield, MA: Merriam-Webster.

Peters, T., & Waterman, R.H. (1982). *In search of excellence*. Glasgow, UK: HarperCollins.

Scholtes, P.R., et al. (1988). *The team handbook*. Madison, WI: Joiner Associates.

Whiteley, R.C. (1991). *The customer-driven company: Moving from talk to action*. Menlo Park, CA: Addison-Wesley.

SUGGESTED READING

Disend, J.E. (1991). *How to provide excellent service in any organization: A blueprint for making all the theories work*. Radnor, PA: Chilton Book.

Gitlow, H.S., & Gitlow, S.J. (1994). *Total quality management in action*. Englewood Cliffs, NJ: Prentice Hall.

Heskett, J.L., Sasser, W., & Hart, C. (1997). *The service profit chain: How leading companies link profit and growth to loyalty, satisfaction, and value*. New York: The Free Press.

Mears, P. (1995). *Quality improvement tools & techniques*. New York: McGraw-Hill.

Phillips, J.J. (1991). Handbook of training evaluation and measurement methods (2nd ed.). Houston, TX: Gulf.

Scheuing, E.E., & Christopher, W.F. (Eds.). (1993). *The service quality handbook*. New York: AMACOM.

Stamatis, D.H. (1996). *Total quality service: Principles, practices, and implementation*. Delray Beach, FL: St. Lucie Press.

Williams, R.L. (1994). *Essentials of total quality management*. San Francisco: AMACOM.

CHAPTER 12

The "Bottom Line": Measuring and Reporting the Value of a Patient Satisfaction Improvement Program

The term "value," from a patient's perspective, refers to a fair return of services/products for the price (in both time and money) paid. In practical terms, consumers generally assign value to purchase situations where they get the highest possible perceived product/service quality for the lowest possible cost. Similarly, organizations typically view value received for allocated human and financial resources in such tangible benefit-related terms as *cost/benefit ratios, returns on investment, increased market share, decreased customer defection,* and so forth.

Health care organizations should also look at a variety of intangible measures—benefits directly linked to improvement efforts that cannot or should not be converted to monetary values. For example, actions leading to improved patient, employee, and provider satisfaction (as evidenced on survey scores) are likely to propel a health care organization toward realizing its strategic direction—aligned with the established organizational vision, mission, values, strategic objectives, and priorities. This is critically important for any enterprise, especially in a competitive industry.

This chapter will provide you with a systematic approach to documenting the overall organizational value of your patient satisfaction improvement (PSI) program using both tangible and intangible measures. Two models will be presented: one for determining overall program value and one for determining PSI program value. The following topics will also be discussed:

- determining program value
- collecting essential documentation data

- isolating the effects of various components of a PSI program
- converting appropriate data to monetary organizational value
- determining and itemizing PSI program costs
- calculating the return on investment (ROI) for a PSI program
- identifying the intangible benefits of the PSI program

DETERMINING PROGRAM VALUE

Determining program value is potentially a complicated and re-source-consuming process. Figure 12–1 illustrates a basic model that attempts to simplify and systematize this process by providing sequential steps. In subsequent sections, we will discuss the actions necessary to complete each step.

COLLECTING ESSENTIAL DOCUMENTATION DATA

There are a variety of data sources available to provide input on the overall value of your PSI program. The more sources you use, the greater will be your capacity to demonstrate organizational value credibly. Common sources and types of data to consider in your health care organization include the following:

- *Organizational performance records:* One of the most useful and credible data sources is composed of the existing records and reports of the organization. These typically include those critical success factors that have business impact; therefore, they should be relatively easy to obtain. This information can be valuable for establishing a "baseline" prior to the onset of your improvement efforts and subsequently after the program has been established to demonstrate favorable change. For example, consider
  1. the number of new patients entering your health care organization per month; ideally, this will already be divided into various groupings representing your organization's targeted patient populations (i.e., senior citizens, employees of local businesses, etc.)
  2. source tracking of all new patients—how many from: marketing efforts (subdivided by specific strategies), patient referral, employer contracts, insurance company contracts
  3. defection or disenrollment figures

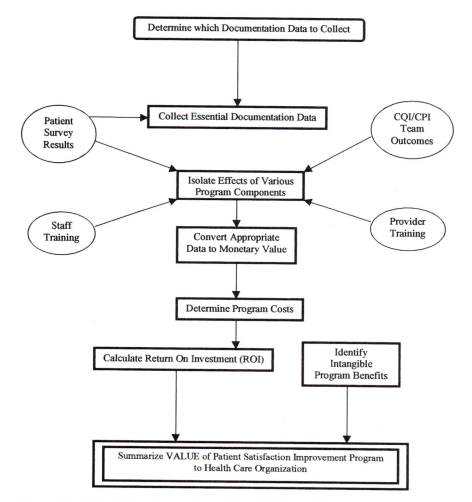

Figure 12–1 Model for Determining Overall Value of Patient Satisfaction Improvement Program. *Source:* Adapted with permission from J.J. Phillips, *Return on Investment in Training and Performance Improvement Programs,* p. 25, © 1997, Gulf Publishing Company.

4. patient (including patient's family members) complaint and grievance data—with particular emphasis on those areas targeted for improvement
5. organizational financial data relating to profitability

6. marketing data pertaining to regional market share
7. number of medical malpractice claims—particularly those triggered by communication breakdown

- *Levels one and two training effectiveness data:* Recall Levels I and II of the Kirkpatrick model for measuring training effectiveness (see Chapter 9). For level I, survey questionnaire response data demonstrate participant reactions to the training; if they respond positively to the training experience, learning is more likely to take place. Level II evaluation—learning—is best documented by the use of comparison pre- and post-training tests that measure training-impacted changes in participant skills, attitudes, and/or knowledge. Application of the new skills, attitudes, or knowledge on the job is highly dependent on whether or not learning actually takes place during the training.

- *Documented key on-the-job behavior changes of PSI program training participants:* For training to be considered successful, it must have practical application. This information is essential if you hope to substantiate the value of your PSI efforts effectively. Although having employees learn new skills, attitudes, and knowledge would seem to be inherently beneficial to the organization, unless it is put into action, it has no real value. Furthermore, program objectives that identify targeted key actions that are to occur following participation in your PSI program should already be in place. Therefore, determine which of these key actions are being taken back on the job as a result of your PSI efforts—reflecting new attitudes, skills, or knowledge. Once this is determined, the next step will be to quantify them:—How frequently and consistently are they being applied? Then you can begin to project the results that will be achieved as a consequence of the new actions.

In order to assess what action is being taken on the job, those individuals who are directly involved with or are affected by the action should provide input. This means that, in most cases, input should be sought from multiple sources.

If an employee has completed a training program aimed at addressing your behavior-based improvement priorities or one directed toward systems-based improvement priorities, you will probably want input from training participants, their supervisors, subordinates, and peers—all four groups are involved in the action. If a single training effort focuses on improving a particular process (say, for example, appointment scheduling), you will want to get input from those people performing the process, those people managing the process, and patients, who are the recipients of the process output.

Supervisors of program participants are another important source of data. They are in a good position to observe participant behaviors that represent an attempt to use the knowledge and skills (or reflect the attitudes) acquired in the program. In this regard, it is important that supervisors maintain objectivity in the assessment process. In some cases, various internal or external groups—program facilitators or external consultants—may provide input on the success of an individual when he or she attempts to apply the skills and knowledge acquired in the program. In comparing these two sources, internal groups may have a vested interest in the outcome of evaluation, thereby biasing results and diminishing credibility; external consultants (who were not involved in providing the training), on the other hand, can make objective observations of on-the-job performance.

Several methods of observation may be considered for identifying and documenting on-the-job behavioral changes. First, a key behavior checklist can be used when recording the presence, absence, frequency, or duration of a participant's behavior as it occurs. The checklist format is particularly helpful because it serves as a guide for an observer to identify which behaviors should and should not occur. The number of behaviors listed in the checklist should be small and the behaviors themselves should be listed in a logical sequence (if they normally occur in sequence). A second approach involves the observer developing a report following the actual observation of behavior. This way, those being observed are not intimidated or distracted by the presence of any forms or other written materials being completed by the observer. Then, in a summary report, the observer reconstructs what has been observed during the observation period. A third, but somewhat more controversial, approach involves the use of either video or audio recordings of interactions between participants and patients. This is an effective way to determine if the desired behaviors are occurring consistently and effectively. In order for this approach to work smoothly, the process must be thoroughly explained to participants in advance of observation.

- *Documented improvement in business results:* Although favorable participant reaction, documented learning, and on-the-job behavioral change are sequentially important, demonstrating results that are aligned with strategic business objectives is critical to establishing overall PSI program value. Inasmuch as the primary business result being sought with your PSI program is improved patient satisfaction, the most important initial success indicator will be multiple follow-up patient satisfaction survey results that document incremental improvement in targeted areas. Then, once the targeted patient satisfaction survey scores are improved, documentation of the anticipated secondary positive organizational impacts should be undertaken. These were discussed in Chapter 1, including such items as greater patient compliance, fewer patient complaints, increased patient referrals, greater patient loyalty (i.e., fewer defections), fewer medical malpractice claims, better meeting payer/employer/accrediting agency demands, improved employee and provider satisfaction, and last, but not least, greater organizational profitability.

Your health care organization may wish to focus on other business result areas that are specific to your improvement needs. Generally speaking, these results can be placed in one of two categories.

1. *Hard results:* These include the easily quantifiable, concrete, objectively observable results. They may be measured in terms of time (e.g., average patient waiting time in reception, average time required for patients to schedule an appointment in person, average time for patient telephone calls to be returned, average time for patients to receive laboratory results, etc.), quality (e.g., number of patient complaints, number of patients seen on time, number of immunizations provided for members, etc.), or output (e.g., number of health maintenance organization patients reenrolling during open enrollment, number of patients referred by other patients, number of third-party payers [insurance carriers or employers] who recontract with your health care organization for insured/employee coverage, etc.)

2. *Soft results:* These are somewhat more difficult to document because these outcomes may be based on employees' behavior and attitudes. These may be measured in terms of work practices (e.g., employee absenteeism or tardiness, number of instances where employees are observed "going the extra mile" for patients, etc.), management skills, or organizational culture.

In addition to having a multitude of *sources* for gathering data documenting PSI program value, there are a variety of *methods* available for gathering those data. Those commonly used for documenting behavioral (Level III) improvements related to PSI program participation include the following:

- *Follow-up surveys* determine the degree to which participants are using various aspects of the training provided.
- *Follow-up questionnaires* uncover specific participant applications of skills, attitude, and/or knowledge obtained during PSI training.
- *Observation on-the-job* is particularly useful for PSI skill application and use. When the observer is either "invisible" or "transparent," the observations will be most valid because awareness of being observed will, in itself, alter behavior. (Recall the "Hawthorne Effect," whereby an attempt was made to document that improving the lighting in a factory would increase productivity of the workers. As it turned out, a number of variables were adjusted, all of which—including a decrease in lighting—produced a transient increase in productivity. The conclusion was that the increase in attention given the workers was responsible for the improved productivity.)
- *Interviews with participants* enable the interviewer to probe the participant to determine the extent to which the learned skills, attitudes, or knowledge have been applied on the job.
- *Follow-up focus groups* are a good format for determining how a group of participants, say, in the same department of your health care organization, have applied your organization's PSI training to department-specific situations.
- *Program assignments* can ensure that the skills or knowledge learned in the program are applied on the job. This is particularly helpful for short-term improvement projects or those involving the development of a new set of habits when dealing directly with patients.
- *Action planning during the program and reviewed later* enables participants to determine whether or not the new skills and attitudes provided for participants during PSI training sessions have been implemented as planned. These plans should be developed by participants. If a review shows that the new skills and attitudes have not been implemented, coaching or counseling should be provided to ensure that they will be implemented.
- *Performance contracting* is a cooperative approach whereby the participant, the PSI training instructor, and the participant's supervisor come to a consensus as to which specific outcomes should result from the PSI training.

- *Program follow-up sessions* provide a setting in which participants can share their special challenges and successes in using new skills, knowledge, or attitudes on the job. These sessions also provide an ideal opportunity to build on the previous learning (and application) by providing the "next tier" of training.

Methods commonly used for documenting business results include

- *Follow-up questionnaires (e.g., patient satisfaction surveys):* These are the "gold standard" for documenting improved patient satisfaction subsequent to the implementation of your PSI program, provided that your organization has conducted patient satisfaction survey research during the process of identifying PSI priorities (see Chapter 8) *and* sufficient time has lapsed since the implementation of your PSI program to allow for behavioral change to take place.
- *Program assignment evaluation:* This evaluation links the outcomes associated with successful assignment completion to various PSI indicators, such as decreased patient complaints.
- *appropriately implemented action plans*
- *performance contracting*
- *program follow-up session(s)*
- *performance monitoring*

ISOLATING THE EFFECTS OF VARIOUS COMPONENTS OF A PSI PROGRAM

The process of establishing a cause-and-effect relationship between a particular program and organizational improvement represents a challenge that, when met, forms the foundation for documenting program value. In this section, a number of steps involved in isolating your PSI program's impact on performance will be presented.

Before proceeding, however, it is important to recognize that there is a chain of impact implied in Kirkpatrick's four levels of evaluation. In other words, if there isn't a positive reaction to the program/training (i.e., Level 1), then learning is less likely to take place. In turn, if learning does not occur, there is little hope of bringing about the desired behavioral changes. Then, in the absence of behavioral changes that reflect learning, there is virtually no hope of giving the PSI program credit for achieving the business result aimed for. Therefore, if the link between business results and your health care organization's PSI program is to be established, data must be collected for documentation on all four levels.

The first step in documenting the impact of your PSI program on organizational performance improvement is to identify all factors that may have contributed to the improvement. Several potential sources for identifying major influencing variables include the following:

- *Program participants,* who may include health care providers, continuous quality improvement (CQI) teams, or frontline staff may be in the best position to estimate accurately how much of the improvement is directly related to the training they have received—and applied on the job—as part of your organization's overall PSI program. Although this is only an estimate, management will likely view this as a credible source because participants are at the center of the change or improvement. It is their actions that have produced the improvement. This impact estimate can be guided by asking each participant a series of questions.
  1. What percentage of the recognized improvement would you attribute to the application of skills/attitude or knowledge gained in the training component of the PSI program?
  2. What is the basis for this estimation?
  3. How confident (expressed as a percentage) are you in the accuracy of this estimate?
  4. Can you identify other factors that have influenced the improvement?
  5. What other individuals or groups would you think could provide an accurate estimate of the impact of training on the overall PSI?

In order to ensure that you are developing conservative training impact estimates, it is advisable to factor the impact percentages by the confidence percentages (i.e., potential error in the estimate). For example, if a participant stated that 60% of the improvement was directly related to training provided, but was 75% confident in the accuracy of this estimate, a *usable training factor* of 45% could be calculated by multiplying the two. This adjusted percentage is then multiplied by the actual amount of the improvement (postprogram minus preprogram value— derived from relevant components of patient satisfaction survey scores).

A word of caution: If a participant makes an extreme, unrealistic, or unsupported claim, it may be included in the intangible benefits, but should be omitted from the analysis.

Because senior management is likely to perceive this approach as an understatement of the success of your PSI program training, the data and process will be considered both credible and accurate.

- *PSI program developers* will typically have thought through the influencing variables when addressing the training transfer issue.
- *Participant's supervisors* may be able to provide insights about performance variables. In many instances, participant's supervisors may be more familiar with other factors influencing performance and therefore may be better equipped to provide estimates of PSI training impact. This may be done using the same questionnaire format suggested above for obtaining participant estimates. The analysis should be carried out in the same manner.

Of course, you may encounter a difference between participant and supervisor estimates (when both have been collected). If there is a compelling reason to believe that one set of estimates is more credible than the other, use that alone. However, it is more likely that each input source should be taken into consideration by averaging the two (i.e., weighting the two sources equally) or assigning a relative weighted percentage to each. On the other hand, the most conservative approach would be to use only the lower of the two values and provide an explanation in your analysis.

This approach is simple and inexpensive and enjoys an acceptable level of credibility. When it is combined with participant estimations, the credibility is enhanced considerably. Then, when factored by the levels of confidence of each source, the value of the analysis increases further.

- *Middle and top management* may be able to contribute based on their knowledge and experience with specific situations. Input from these individuals, although admittedly subjective, may well increase the credibility of the data—a welcome side benefit. Additionally, it is these individuals who often provide or approve funding for the program.
- *Internal or external expert estimations* of the impact of the training component of your PSI program will be helpful if the reputation of the researcher is excellent. Sometimes, management will place more confidence in recognized experts than in their own internal staff, especially if internal staff are in a position of potential gain (bonuses, etc.) for favorable outcomes.

When deciding which strategies to use in estimating your health care organization's PSI program/training impact, several factors should be taken into consideration.

- the feasibility of using the strategy given the infrastructure and operations of your organization

- the degree of accuracy you feel would be afforded by the strategy in question
- the level of credibility inherent in the strategy—taking into consideration that multiple sources will result in greater credibility than one
- the costs involved in designing, implementing, analyzing, and reporting the results of the strategy
- the amount of disruption of normal business operations potentially caused by the strategy
- the amount of time (translated to hourly costs) required for already time-pressured participants, participants' supervisors, consultants, and management.

This approach communicates to all stakeholders that other factors may have influenced the results, emphasizing that the PSI program is not the sole source of improvement. As a result, the credit for improvement is shared with several possible variables and sources. This approach is likely to gain the respect of management—they are accustomed to fielding grandiose and heroic individual claims for results they know full well to be the end product of a team effort.

CONVERTING APPROPRIATE DATA TO MONETARY ORGANIZATIONAL VALUE

Information pertaining to the business results (Level IV) obtained as a consequence of your PSI program needs to be converted to monetary value and compared to program costs in preparation for your ROI calculations (see later in this chapter). Several sources are available for this process. These include, but are not limited to, the following:

- *Participants' (staff or providers) wages and benefits:* These assist with the conversion when the performance improvement results in saving time by decreasing the time needed for key processes or daily activities related to enhanced patient satisfaction. In a team environment (such as an entire department), a program could enable the team to perform tasks in a shorter time frame, or with fewer people. The value of time saved is an important measure of your PSI program's success, and this conversion is a relatively easy process. The average wage with a percentage added for benefits will suffice for most calculations. Of course, the time savings can only truly be converted to a monetary value if the saved time is used for other cost reduction or profit contributions.

- *Incremental third-party payer benefit increases:* Recognizing the importance of high levels of patient satisfaction, third-party payers (employers or insurance companies) often create financial incentives for exemplary patient satisfaction scores. These incentives may be in the form of specific bonuses calculated on a per-covered-patient basis for various components of patient satisfaction targeted for improvement (often based on "industry norms") or, more globally, on tiered levels of "overall satisfaction" reported using your organization's or their own patient satisfaction survey scores. This could amount to significant monetary value. For example, let us say that a particular third-party payer contracts with you to provide health care for 10,000 patients (typically on a capitated basis). Furthermore, they offer a bonus of 5 cents for each covered patient for each satisfaction score percentage above 90% in each of five targeted areas for improvement. If two areas moved from 90% to 95%, and the other three areas moved from 89% to 93%, the following bonuses could be anticipated:
- 90% to 95% = 5 percentage points above 90% in two areas = (2 × 0.05) × 5 × 10,000 = $5,000.00
- 89% to 93% = 3 percentage points above 90% in three areas = (3 × 0.05) × 3 × 10,000 = $4,500.00
- Total bonus earned for the contract year = $9,500.00

These numbers have been provided only for the sake of example. Of course, they will vary based on the nature of any contractual arrangements your health care organization may have.

- *Patient enrollment data—decreased patient disenrollment (increased patient retention) or an increase in the number of new patients:* Most health care organizations maintain data supporting the annual revenue generated per patient, usually subdivided into various demographic attributes such as age, disease states, zip codes, and so forth. By calculating the impact of your health care organization's PSI program on the recorded increase in patient retention (adjusting for other contributing factors as discussed above), you can easily convert the percentage increase into monetary value.

For example, let us say that your total patient population averages 250,000 and you increase your retention by 2%, 50% of which is attributed to your PSI program. This means that 5,000 more patients remain with you than previously. If the average annual revenue received per patient is $1,800, then there is a total revenue increase of

$9,000,000, $4,500,000 of which would be credited to the efforts of your PSI program.

- *Internal or external experts:* Those individuals who have knowledge of the specific area(s) of improvement and the respect of the management group are often the best prospects for expert input. These individuals may be able to provide estimates along with assumptions made in the process of calculating the estimates. For example, if a team-based component of your PSI program results in a decrease in the number of patient grievances filed, the researcher would need to itemize direct costs of handling a grievance, such as employee and management time involved from the time the grievance is filed through the stage of resolution to the patient's satisfaction. Other costs, such as refunded copayments, would also have to be taken into consideration.
- *Estimates from supervisors:* As an offshoot of estimates from participants of the monetary value of PSI program-related improvements, supervisors could review these estimates, providing modifications based on additional information they have at their disposal.

The credibility of monetary value conversions is influenced by a number of factors, including

- *The reputation of the source of data:* How credible is the individual or the groups providing the data? Senior management may place greater credibility on data obtained from those who are closest to the source of the actual improvement or change.
- *The reputation of the source of the study:* Senior management will scrutinize the reputation of the individual, group, or organization presenting the data. Do they have a history of presenting accurate, unbiased reports?
- *Motives of the evaluators:* Do they have a personal interest in creating a favorable or unfavorable result?
- *Methodology of the study:* The target audience for your results (senior management, corporate headquarters, etc.) will want to know specifically how the research was conducted and how calculations were made.
- *Assumptions made during the analysis:* Many calculations or conclusions are made on the basis of certain assumptions. When assumptions are omitted, the target audience will insert their own, often unfavorable, assumptions instead.

- *Realism of the outcome data:* Huge, unrealistic claims often cause considerable suspicion; they may fall on deaf ears, being thrown away before they are reviewed.

DETERMINING AND ITEMIZING PSI PROGRAM COSTS

This step represents the most straightforward component of the overall value determination process. This involves monitoring all of the costs related to your health care organization's PSI program, including each of its components.

A number of cost categories must be taken into consideration when tabulating program costs.

- *Focus group research costs* include those costs associated with determining the relative importance of the various elements of patient satisfaction. Costs here include incentive gifts, staff time, travel time, facilities, materials, preparation time, and result analysis time.
- *Survey research costs* include those costs involved in designing and pilot testing the survey instrument, printing and distributing the survey instrument, administering the survey (particularly if done in person), collecting the completed survey instruments, tabulating the survey responses into a reportable format, and creating an appropriate data display to accurately and clearly communicate the findings.
- *Training material design and development of in-house program and/or acquisition costs* are necessary if portions of your PSI program are purchased from outside vendors.
- *Training delivery costs* include salaries/benefits of facilitators, salaries/benefits of those coordinating and attending the training sessions, program materials and fees, and travel/lodging/meals for participants.
- *Training evaluation costs* include costs incurred in the evaluation of each of Kirkpatrick's four levels (reaction, learning, behavior, and business results).
- *CQI team training and team meeting costs* are especially associated with addressing systems- and process-related PSI priorities (see Chapter 10).
- *General overhead* includes general costs for supplies and equipment.

Because ROI calculations are typically subjected to senior management's rigorous scrutiny, it is best to "fully load" costs, including those costs that company guidelines and philosophy normally don't consider. When you comprehensively report the overall PSI program value to the organization, these "costs" will likely be viewed as "investments" in the organization's future.

CALCULATING THE ROI FOR A PSI PROGRAM

There are two general approaches to calculating the ROI for a PSI program. The first method compares the benefits of the program to the costs in a ratio (benefits/cost ratio [BCR]). In formula form, the ratio is:

$$BCR = \frac{\text{Program Benefits}}{\text{Program Costs}}$$

Essentially, the BCR compares the annual economic benefits of the program to the costs of the program. For example, if the program benefits were estimated/calculated to be $1,224,000, and the costs were tallied at $244,800, the BCR would be 5:1. In other words, for every dollar invested in the program, five dollars in benefits were returned. The main advantage to using this approach is that it avoids traditional financial measures so that there is no confusion when comparing PSI program improvements with other investments in the company.

The second method involves the traditional ROI formula, focusing on net program benefits divided by costs. The ratio is usually expressed as a percentage when the fractional values (ratio) are multiplied by 100. The formula for this method is:

$$ROI\ (\%) = \frac{\text{Net Program Benefits}}{\text{Program Costs}} \times 100$$

The net program benefits are the program benefits minus the program costs.

IDENTIFYING THE INTANGIBLE BENEFITS OF A PSI PROGRAM

In addition to the tangible, monetary benefits of your health care organization's PSI program, there are also intangible, nonmonetary benefits that should be considered when determining overall PSI program value. These would include such items as

- increased job satisfaction for providers and/or staff
- increased organizational commitment of providers and/or staff
- improved teamwork
- improved patient service quality

- reduced patient complaints
- reduced conflicts

Several intangible variables that might be used to include in your overall intangible benefits assessment include

- attitude survey data
- organizational commitment
- climate survey data
- employee complaints
- grievances from employees
- discrimination complaints
- stress reduction
- employee turnover
- employee absenteeism
- employee tardiness
- employee transfers
- teamwork
- cooperation
- conflict
- communication improvement

When summarizing the overall value of your health care organization's PSI program, you should combine your calculated ROI figures with a listing of the reasonable intangible benefits you have identified. By taking this systematic approach, little doubt can remain in the minds of senior management (or any other stakeholders, for that matter) that embarking on a comprehensive PSI campaign has been—and will continue to be—a very worthwhile investment of organizational resources.

PSI must be viewed as an ongoing process rather than a single isolated organizational program, with a finite beginning and end. The next chapter will focus on the processes involved in building and sustaining a service-oriented organizational culture.

CONCLUSION

Organizations typically view value received for allocated human and financial resources in such tangible benefit-related terms as *cost/benefit ratios, returns on investment, increased market share, decreased customer defection,* and so forth. However, health care organizations should also look at a variety of intangible measures, those benefits that are directly linked to improvement efforts that cannot accurately be converted to monetary values. These would include such items as: increased job satisfaction for providers and/or staff, increased organizational commitment of providers and/or staff, improved teamwork, improved patient service quality, reduced patient complaints, and reduced conflicts.

In order to document the organizational value of your PSI program, a systematic approach is essential. The initial stage of documentation consists of gathering data from a variety of sources. These sources include, but are not necessarily limited to, organizational performance records, levels one and two training effectiveness data, PSI program-related on-the-job behavior changes, and documented improvements in business results. The next stage is to isolate the effects of training on performance improvement(s). This can be facilitated by getting feedback from PSI training program developers, participants, participants' supervisors, and middle and top management, as well as internal/external expert estimations. Next, appropriate data need to be converted to monetary organizational value. Sources of these data include participants' wages and benefits (in case PSI results include a saving of employee time), incremental third-party payer benefit increases, patient enrollment data, internal or external experts, and estimates from supervisors.

The most straightforward component of the overall value determination process is that of itemizing PSI program costs. This should include the costs of such activities as: focus group research, survey research, training materials (either internally developed or externally purchased), training delivery, training evaluation, CQI team training and meetings, and general overhead.

There are two general approaches to calculating the ROI for your PSI program. The first method compares the benefits of the program to the costs in a ratio (BCR). In formula form, the ratio is: BCR = Program Benefits ÷ Program Costs. The second method involves the traditional ROI formula, focusing on net program benefits divided by costs. The ratio is usually expressed as a percentage when the fractional values are multiplied by 100. The formula for this method is: ROI (%) = (Net Program Benefits ÷ Program Costs) × 100.

ACTION STEPS

1. List (based on this chapter) the data you currently collect or would like to collect to document the organizational value of your PSI efforts.

2. Next to each item listed above, indicate the specific mechanism by which you collect or intend to collect the data.
3. Develop a plan for isolating the direct/indirect effects of your PSI training on patient satisfaction.
4. Select the sources (from those listed in the chapter) that you wish to use in determining the monetary organizational value of your PSI program efforts.
5. Design a form for organizing and managing the data in calculating the ROI and overall organizational (tangible and intangible) value of your PSI efforts.

SUGGESTED READING

Abrahams, Jeffrey. (1995). *The mission statement book*. San Francisco: Ten Speed Press.

Bell, Chip R., & Zemke, Ron. (1992). *Managing knock your socks off service*. New York: AMACOM, a division of American Management Association.

Brown, Stanley A. (1992). *Total quality service: How organizations use it to create a competitive advantage*. Scarborough, Ontario: Prentice Hall Canida, Inc.

Brown, Stanley A. (1997). *Breakthrough customer service: Best practices of leaders in customer support*. Toronto: John Wiley & Sons Canada Ltd.

Capodagli, Bill, & Jackson, Lynn. (1999). *The Disney way: Harnessing the management secrets of Disney in your company*. New York: McGraw-Hill.

Carr, Clay. (1992). *Smart training: The manager's guide to training for improved performance*. New York: McGraw-Hill, Inc.

Connellan, Thomas K., & Zemke, Ron. (1993). *Sustaining knock your socks off service*. New York: AMACOM, a division of American Management Association.

Craig, Robert L. (Ed.). (1987). *Training and development handbook* (3rd Ed.). New York: McGraw-Hill Book Company.

Deal, Terrence E., & Kennedy, Allan A. (1982). *Corporate cultures: The rites and rituals of corporate life*. Menlo Park, CA: Addison-Wesley Publishing Company.

Disend, Jeffrey E. (1991). *How to provide excellent service in any organization: A blueprint for making all the theories work*. Radnor, PA: Chilton Book Company.

Goad, Tom W. (1982). *Delivering effective training*. San Diego: Pfeiffer & Company.

Kirkpatrick, Donald L. (1994). *Evaluating training programs: The four levels*. San Francisco: Berrett-Koehler Publishers.

Leebov, Wendy, Vergare, Michael, & Scott, Gail. (1990). *Patient satisfaction: A guide to practice enhancement*. Oradell, NJ: Medical Economics Books.

Nadler, Gerald, & Hibino, Shozo. (1994). *Breakthrough thinking: The seven principles of creative problem-solving* (2nd Ed.). Rocklin, CA: Prima Publishing.

Phillips, Jack J. (Ed.). (1994). *Measuring return on investment*. Vol. 1. Alexandria, VA: American Society for Training and Development.

Phillips, Jack J. (1997). *Return on investment in training and performance improvement programs: A step-by-step manual for calculating the financial return.* Houston, TX: Gulf Publishing Company, 25, 89.

Wade, Pamela A. (1995). *Producing high-impact learning tools.* Irvine, CA: Richard Chang Associates Inc.

Wall, Bob, Sobol, Mark R., & Solum, Robert S. (1999). *The mission-driven organization.* Rocklin, CA: Prima Publishing.

CHAPTER 13

Building and Sustaining a Service-Oriented Organizational Culture

The interpersonal contacts between any member of your health care organization and your patients or their family members—the moments of truth (MOTs) on each patient's mental report card—are managed (or mismanaged) based, in large part, on the behaviors of employees. Chapter 9 presented a number of principles and strategies related to influencing employee behavior. These were primarily focused on the improvement of employees' skills, knowledge, and attitudes using appropriately designed and delivered training. However, it is important to look at the "bigger picture" and recognize that employee behaviors are also heavily influenced by the culture, or pervasive norms and values, of the organization within which they function. If improving patient satisfaction and loyalty is to be truly continuous, with all of the associated long-term organizational benefits, then a service culture—one based on a passion for service excellence—must be established and maintained.

This chapter will explore what are considered to be essential ingredients for the development and maintenance of a service-oriented culture within a health care organization. The chapter begins with a discussion of what organizational culture is and what it consists of. Then, the nature and creation of a "compass" that keeps an organization's culture moving toward "true north"—the service vision and mission—are examined. Next, your attention is directed toward the critical role of service employees. This segment addresses the following key cultural issues:

- hiring the right—service-oriented—people
- developing people to deliver quality service, providing them with technical and interactive skills (including conflict management), empowering them, and promoting teamwork

- understanding the relationship between employee and patient satisfaction
- reinforcing service-related behaviors through reward and recognition

THE ANATOMY OF ORGANIZATIONAL CULTURE

Davis defined corporate culture as "the pattern of shared values and behaviors that give the members of an organization meaning, and provide them with the rules for behavior in the organization." Merriam-Webster's New Collegiate Dictionary (1997) defines it as "the integrated pattern of human behavior that includes thought, speech, action and artifacts and depends on man's capacity for learning and transmitting knowledge to succeeding generations" (p. 282).

According to Deal and Kennedy (1982, p. 13), the basic components of culture are as follows:

- *Business environment:* Each company faces a different reality in the marketplace, depending on its products, competitors, customers, technologies, government influences, and so forth. To succeed in the marketplace, each health care organization must carry out certain activities very well. The business environment is the single greatest influence in shaping a corporate culture.
- *Values:* These are the basic concepts and beliefs of an organization. As such, they form the heart of the corporate culture. Values define "success" in concrete terms for employees—"If you do this, you too will be a success"—and establish standards of achievement within the organization. Strong cultural companies typically have a complex system of values that are shared by the employees and management alike. Managers openly discuss these beliefs without any embarrassment and they don't tolerate deviance from the company standards.
- *Heroes:* These individuals personify the culture's values and function as role models for employees to follow. These corporate achievers are known to virtually every employee with more than a few months' tenure in the company. And they show every employee "what you have to do to succeed around here."
- *Rites and rituals:* These include systematic and programmed routines of day-to-day life in the organization. These mundane manifestations show employees the kind of behavior that is expected of them. These rites and rituals may be in the form of ceremonies

that provide visible and potent examples of what the organization stands for.

- *The cultural network:* An informal, but primary, means of communication within the organization, the cultural network is the "carrier" of the corporate values and heroic mythology.

In a somewhat more comprehensive overview of what makes an organization's culture, Wellington (1995, p. 183) stated that there are six basic cultural components.

1. *Symbols* include items such as the company logo/colors/typography, company-specific jargon, and company-identifying products/services.
2. *Power structures* are centers of corporate power that define the company's approach to its market, such as differentiation by price, service quality, patient convenience, innovative methods of service delivery, and so forth.
3. *Organizational structure* can be a traditional hierarchy or contemporarily flatter, bureaucratic or autonomous, centralized or decentralized, inclusive or exclusive of external stakeholders.
4. *Control systems* include items such as the personal performance appraisal system, management information systems, internal perception audits, and corporate policies, mission, and goals.
5. *Routines and rituals* include team meetings, performance/long service/suggestion system awards, consensus or dictatorial decision making, and budget planning.
6. *Myths and stories* include organization origins, accounts of personal successes (or failures), and the genesis of research/product/service breakthroughs.

A patient-focused, service-oriented health care organization will have at its heart a service culture. This is a culture where there is an appreciation for excellent service, where giving good service to internal as well as external customers is considered a natural way of life. Management consultants Bob Wall, Mark Sobol, and Robert Solum (1999) indicated that the values of typical world-class organizations have six cultural elements in common.

1. passionate customer focus
2. urgent obsession with quality
3. continuous improvement

4. high levels of employee participation
5. teamwork
6. ethics and integrity

In their best-selling book, *In Search of Excellence,* Peters and Waterman (1982) identified eight organizational characteristics that tended to be a major feature in the excellent companies. "Hands-on—Value-driven" was the characteristic that most closely reflects the importance given to organizational culture as such. This is broken down into 10 beliefs that reflect that culture.

1. a belief in the importance of enjoying one's own work
2. a belief in being the best
3. a belief that people should be innovators and take risks, without feeling that they will be punished if they fail
4. a belief in the importance of attending to details
5. a belief in the importance of people as individuals
6. a belief in superior quality and service
7. a belief in the importance of informality to improve the flow of communication
8. a belief in the importance of economic growth and profits
9. a belief in the importance of "hands-on management"; managers should be doers, not just planners and administrators
10. a belief in the importance of a recognized organizational philosophy developed and supported by those at the top

Furthermore, in studying the performance of 80 companies, Deal and Kennedy (1982, p. 13) found that the more successful companies were those that had strong cultures. The strong culture was categorized as follows, where the organization:

- Had a widely shared philosophy of management.
- Emphasized the importance of people to the success of the organization.
- Encouraged rituals and ceremonies to celebrate company events.
- Had identified successful people and sung their praises.
- Maintained a network to communicate the culture.
- Had informal rules of behavior.
- Had strong values.

- Set high standards for performance.
- Possessed a definitive corporate character.

In a study conducted by Atkinson (1990), a group of managers brainstormed the factors they thought important in indicating the predominant culture within a company (p. 63). The results are listed in Exhibit 13–1.

Exhibit 13–1 Indicators of Corporate Culture

- Atmosphere: Did it feel good? Was it a nice place to work?
- Ethos: The way things were laid out
- Spirit of teamwork
- Warmth and friendship
- Ideals: Company messages and how they were displayed
- Management style: What people did, not what they said
- How they talk to you: the tone and manner of communication
- Listening to us: Is there evidence?
- Attitudes to employees portrayed through notice-boards
- Involvement: Did people incorporate the ideas of others?
- Ambience: Was it a nice place to be?
- Telephone response: Speed, nice or nasty
- Promises not kept—especially between departments
- Events: Was there evidence of a corporate get-together?
- Criteria for selection/appraisal: Was it a pleasant experience?
- Type of communication
- Negative rumors and the failure to address them
- Reception: Staff entrances and good inwards and outwards
- Stereotypes of departments: What is projected by opinion leaders?
- Answering the phone: Was there a concern for helping?
- Tidiness in all areas
- Participation: Did people participate?
- Belonging: Did they feel at home?
- Motivation: The process—was it carrot or stick?
- Shared corporate values: Were they known by all and displayed?

Courtesy of P.E. Atkinson, © 1996, Edinburgh, Scotland, U.K.

YOUR HEALTH CARE ORGANIZATION'S "TRUE NORTH"

The accuracy, and therefore navigational usefulness, of a compass depends on it being set to "true north." Similarly, the "strategic direction" of any organization must be established on the basis of carefully assessing where it is now, where it ideally envisions being in the future, and how it intends to operate in order to bridge the gap between the two. Throughout contemporary management/business literature, various interpretations of the terms *vision, values, mission,* and *business philosophy* have been promulgated. Chapter 11 presented organizational leadership's responsibility in orchestrating the development of a shared vision, as well as the importance of having such a vision. This was presented in the context of addressing administration-based improvement priorities. In this segment, our objective is to briefly examine each of the key concepts that collectively make up the "true north" on the compass of a health care organization's future.

Organizational Vision

Recall, from Chapter 11, that the vision of an organization is a concise word picture of the organization at some future (preferred) time in a future (preferred) state, which sets the overall direction of the organization. It is the lighthouse that provides general direction rather than the map to a specific destination. It is what the organization strives to be—something to be pursued. More specifically, the vision could be viewed as any of the following:

- picture of a desired future state
- picture of how we would like things to be
- ideal and unique image of the future
- optimistic, preferred future

The characteristics of an ideal organizational vision are summarized in Exhibit 13–2. This provides a context within which to embark on the process of developing a shared vision for your health care organization.

Several questions you might ask to facilitate the clarification of your organization's vision are as follows:

Exhibit 13–2 Characteristics of an Ideal Organizational Vision

---

Organizational Vision

- Specific enough to provide guidance, yet vague enough to encourage initiative
- Future oriented, not constrained by the limitations of today; nonpragmatic
- Idealistic—should at once conjure up thoughts of "apple pie" and produce "goose bumps"
- Uniquely different—not "borrowed" from any other organization
- Radical and compelling—exciting enough to infuse a sense of urgency and excitement

---

- How would you like to change the world with respect to your organization?
- If you could invent the future for your organization, what would it look like?
- What is your dream related to your work within this organization?
- What are the distinctive roles/skills of your organization (compared to competitors)?
- What does your ideal organization look like?

Although the atmosphere for the development of organizational vision should be open, fostering contributions from all levels of the organization—with particular input emphasis placed on frontline employees—two pitfalls should be avoided during the developmental process.

1. Don't be too limited in time. This tends to force reaction to the "urgent" (Covey, 1989, p. 150).
2. Don't base your vision on illusions that ignore proven principles within the health care industry (e.g., the astronomical cost implications of "an MRI for every patient with suspected rheumatoid arthritis" when more cost-effective clinical, radiologic, and laboratory diagnostic modalities will suffice to allow the clinician to

arrive at an accurate diagnosis and formulate a plan for appropriate therapeutic intervention). Furthermore, when a vision is based on illusion, the result may well be the development of "platitudes" that will ultimately result in employees "rolling their eyes" while thinking "here we go with another 'strategic direction' Federal Expressed from the third ring of Saturn—with no connection whatsoever to reality."

The vision statement is a carefully prepared document that captures your company's values (see next section). The organizational vision is the first critical step in making a vision a reality for every member of the organization.

Organizational Values

The values of a health care organization are the collective principles and ideals that guide the thoughts and actions of an individual, or a group of individuals—the maps of the way things should be. They are stable, long-term beliefs that are hard to change. Values define the character of an organization—they describe what an organization stands for. Wall et al. (1999) stated that "the most successful companies worldwide are values-driven. That means a bedrock of common, positive values underlies the thinking and the creativity of everyone in those organizations" (p. 57).

Values function as the building blocks of your organization's culture. They cannot be proven or disproven, but they can be substantiated or refuted by the actions of key people in your health care organization. Values define what is "right" or "wrong," "good" or "bad," and "correct" or "incorrect." They are often hard to articulate in words but still have a great deal of influence on how individuals behave within any organization. Exhibit 13–3 shows values that are commonly listed among health care and related organizations.

Organizational Mission

An organization's mission is summarized in a statement that specifies the organization's purpose or "reason for being." It represents the

Exhibit 13–3 Common Health Care Organizational Values

- Patient-focus: Everything we do must ultimately result in meeting the needs of our patients.
- Outstanding patient service: Patients should consistently perceive that they are receiving better service at our health care organization than they could by patronizing *any* of our competitors.
- Respect: We will treat all individuals with dignity and respect and be honest, open, and ethical in all our dealings with customers, with shareholders, and with each other.
- Responsiveness: We will strive continually to understand and meet the changing requirements of our customers through teamwork, empowerment, and innovation.
- Teamwork: We will work together as a team, or as committed members of various function-specific teams.
- Employee-focus: We will strive to have existing employees refer like-minded, service-oriented friends and family to join our employee team. We will further strive to sustain an atmosphere of working conditions that, when combined, function as an incentive for employees to remain with us in the long term. We wish to recognize and reward employees for helping our organization avoid the patient service complications associated with unscheduled absences.
- Resourceful problem-solving: We wish to foster an environment that encourages all employees to be resourceful in solving various problems encountered by patients (or those serving patients) so that they consistently have their expectations exceeded when it comes to handling "glitches" in the service delivery process.
- Cooperation with major change: We recognize that, in an industry and marketplace as dynamic as health care, we must be postured to embrace needed change on an ongoing basis. Each change can only hope to be successful (i.e., result in the intended improvement) to the extent that our employees help design and cooperate with that change.
- Good place to work: We want our organization to be a safe place to work—no matter what role an employee is playing in the overall function of serving patient needs. Furthermore, we particularly wish to encourage those behaviors that foster goodwill in the workplace.
- Results: We will consistently keep our commitment to provide value to our customers, to shareholders, and to one another.
- Opportunity: Each employee is entitled to the opportunity to maximize his or her potential.

continues

Exhibit 13–3 continued

- Employee self-responsibility: We wish to have each and every employee take personal responsibility for his or her actions; more specifically, to consistently act with integrity (i.e., your behaviors should reflect universal, personal, and organizational values) and to strive to constantly improve your own level of knowledge and skills as they relate to serving patient needs better.
- Communication: We will communicate honestly with the highest standards of ethics, trust, and integrity.

---

primary objective toward which the organization's plans and programs should be aimed. A mission is something to be accomplished, whereas a vision is something to be pursued. Every health care organization should develop its own unique mission statement that answers four key questions.

1. Who are we?
2. What do we do?
3. For whom do we do it?
4. Why do we do it?

There are several important functions of a well-articulated mission statement.

- It establishes the purpose of the organization.
- It coordinates the actions and efforts of the organization. If it is developed and communicated properly, it can be a powerful organizing tool, providing essential direction for all involved. If everyone understands and believes in the mission, they are much more likely to work in harmony like a well-directed orchestra. This prevents people from working at cross purposes.
- It provides broad boundaries within which employees can channel their creativity. This creativity is sparked by the inspirational aspect of the mission statement—catalytic in nature, focusing and uniting action from those who read it (which should include ev-

eryone in the organization). Creativity is especially important to any organization—like health care organizations—that deals with a variety of clients.

Abrahams (1995) recommended the use of a five-step approach to developing a mission statement for an organization. The following adaptation may assist you with the process:

1. *Decide who is going to write the mission statement.* If you are hoping to gain the "buy-in" of all employees, whereby they embrace the content and spirit of the mission statement, consider the wisdom of gathering representative input from employees (and providers) from every department. This way, everyone will have the opportunity to feel as though they had a voice in the statement's creation.
2. *Agree on when the statement is going to be written.* Because this is a process that could potentially drag on over a long period of time, it is best to impose a deadline and stick to it. Decide whether the statement will be formulated on-site, off-site, or a combination of locations. Also, determine whether it will be written during business hours or in evening/weekend sessions, and how much time will be allowed for the developmental process? An evening? A weekend? A month? Three months?
3. *Determine the target audience(s).* It is important to decide who you are talking to before you can figure out what to say. In a health care organization, there are a variety of target audiences: patients, visitors, providers, employees, third-party payers, regulators, accrediting agencies, and so forth.
4. *Decide what kind of language is appropriate.* Begin with a list of key words that apply to your business. You might wish to begin with a brainstorming session with a group of people from your target audience(s). Exhibit 13–4 lists a variety of key words that often appear in organizational mission statements.
5. *Adopt a format.* Will it be printed in a frameable high-quality document or distributed in a brochure or pamphlet? As wallet-sized cards? Printed on coffee mugs? Or T-shirts? Displayed at the front door of each health care facility?

Exhibit 13–4 Key Words Commonly Found in Organizational Mission Statements

Ability	Empower	Leadership	Risk
Accomplished	Enthusiasm	Life	Security
Accountability	Environment	Long-term	Serve
Asset	Ethics	Mission	Service
Best	Excellence	Mutual	Shareholders
Change	Exciting	Passion	Solution
Commitment	Fair	Performance	Strategy
Communicate	Fun	Potential	Strength
Communities	Future	Pride	Success
Conscience	Goal	Principles	Support
Corp. Citizen	Goodwill	Productivity	Team
Customers	Growth	Profit	Teamwork
Dedicated	Harmony	Quality	Tomorrow
Dedication	Individual	Relationships	Trust
Dignity	Initiative	Reliable	Unique
Direct	Innovation	Respect	Value
Diversity	Joy	Responsibility	Values
Employees	Leader	Return on equity	Vision

Source: Reprinted with permission from *The Mission Statement Book.* Copyright © 1995, by Jeffrey Abrahams, Ten Speed Press, PO Box 7123, Berkeley, CA, 94707. Available from your local bookseller or call 800-841-2665. Or visit us at www.tenspeed.com.

The mission statement itself should be "supercharged" with energy and downright exciting! It must be written in such a way that it inspires and invites employee commitment—to make the organization's goals their own. This creates a future for the organization, establishing a foundation for the changes needed to meet the demands of the twenty-first century. It must focus on the needs of patients, now and in the future. During the evolution of a true service-oriented culture, a health care organization begins to unleash authority toward the front lines, and the traditional spans of control begin to disappear. The resulting confusion can render the organization virtually immobile. A well-developed, strong mission statement is the most important tool you can have to ensure that this does not happen.

One hospital's mission statement included the following phrase: "We will care for the physical, spiritual, and emotional needs of our patients." This was enthusiastically embraced by all employees—it meant something to them. Furthermore, it helped to clarify that they were committed 100% to their patients. It was an active statement that became part of the lives of everyone who worked at the hospital.

In order for a health care organization to realize the strategic benefits of having a well-articulated mission, everyone working in the organization (providers and staff members alike) must embrace, know, and be able to recite that mission statement. Victor Kiam, the individual who took over Remington Corporation, recognized that he would have to change the strategic direction of the company if it were to prosper. Among his first actions was to develop a mission statement designed to instill a sense of mission among employees to increase production. After communicating it widely throughout the company, he began a practice of randomly reinforcing the importance of everyone knowing that mission statement. Once each week, he would walk onto the production floor and randomly select an employee, greeting him or her with a $10 bill in hand and saying the phrase, "If you can recite the company's mission statement to me, the company will give you the $10. If not, it goes into the other pocket, which is mine." After several weeks of disappointment, finding that the employees could not perform as hoped, he began to meet with success. Every week thereafter, each employee earned the $10! With great pride, Mr. Kiam stated that "it only costs me $520 a year to make sure everyone in my company knows the company's mission statement." Granted, this does not ensure that employees will act on that knowledge, but you can rest assured that if they don't know it, they will never act on it.

The mission-driven organization provides an excellent "litmus test" you can use for documenting that you have effectively communicated your health care organization's mission statement: "If you ask three or four of your frontline employees (at random) to recite the mission of your company and you do not receive a consistent answer, then in fact you have no mission."

Business Philosophy

The business philosophy establishes a set of "rules of conduct" for operating the organization. This serves to translate the values (as reflected in the vision) and the purpose (as reflected in the mission) into more concrete descriptions of how they will be applied in day-to-day organizational operations. In *The Disney Way: Harnessing the Management Secrets of Disney in Your Company,* authors Capodagli and Jackson (1999) discussed Walt Disney's 10 beliefs that are at the heart of Disney methodology. Your health care organization may well benefit from incorporating Disney's beliefs into an overall business philosophy. Those beliefs are as follows:

1. Give every member of your organization a chance to dream, and tap into the creativity those dreams embody.
2. Stand firm on your beliefs and principles.
3. Treat your customers like guests.
4. Support, empower, and reward employees.
5. Build long-term relationships with key suppliers and partners.
6. Dare to take calculated risks in order to bring innovative ideas to fruition.
7. Train extensively and constantly reinforce the company's culture.
8. Align long-term vision with short-term execution.
9. Use the storyboarding technique to solve planning and communication problems.
10. Pay close attention to detail.

THE CRITICAL ROLE OF SERVICE EMPLOYEES

Even if patient expectations are well understood and you have designed the appropriate management of each MOT and surrogate perception to conform to those expectations, the service that patients experience may fall short of optimum. When such a "service-performance gap" exists—when service is not delivered as specified—the critical role of frontline employees becomes evident.

The familiar adage, "If you're not serving the customer, you ought to be serving someone who is," underscores the fact that frontline employees and those supporting them from behind the scenes are critical to the success of a health care organization. These employees deserve particular attention because, for all practical purposes, they *are* the service and they *are* the health care organization in the patients' eyes.

Failure on the part of employees to deliver services as designed and specified can result from a number of factors. In this segment, we will consider several of them: hiring the right people, developing people to deliver quality service, promoting teamwork among employees, understanding the relationship between employee and patient satisfaction, reinforcing service-related behaviors through reward and recognition, and documenting/celebrating incremental service quality successes.

Hiring the Right—Service-Oriented—People

Schneider and Schechter (1991) recommended that potential service employees be screened for two complementary capacities: service competencies and service inclination. *Service competencies* are the skills and knowledge necessary to do the job. In many instances, these competencies may be validated by achieving particular degrees or certifications. In other cases, service competencies may not be degree related, but may instead relate to relevant experience, basic intelligence, or physical requirements. Because service quality is multidimensional in nature—quality service is reliable, responsive, and empathetic—service employees should be screened for more than their service competencies.

Service employees should also be screened for *service inclination*—their interest in doing service-related work. This inclination or interest is reflected in their attitudes toward service and their orientation toward serving customers (internal and external). Research conducted by Hogan, Hogan, and Busch (1984) indicated that service effectiveness is correlated with having service-oriented personality characteristics such as helpfulness, thoughtfulness, and sociability. This same research defines service orientation as a characteristic complex including elements of good adjustment, likability, social skill, and willingness to follow rules. Ideally, health care organizations should strive to use selection processes that assess both service competencies and service inclination, resulting in new employees who are high on both dimensions.

The Walt Disney organization popularized the idea of "casting" for performers in a role rather than simply hiring employees. All Disney frontline employees are referred to as cast members. Researchers Bell and Zemke studied 400 exemplary service organizations to determine the practices they had in common (1992, p. 4). They reported that in virtually all instances, painstaking thoroughness was built into every step of the selection process. For example:

- When Nordstrom opened its first East Coast store in Tyson's Corner, Virginia, it interviewed 3,000 people to fill 400 frontline jobs.
- For the grand opening of the Grand Hyatt Wailea, one of the crown jewel Hawaiian resorts, 6,000 people were screened to fill 1,200 positions.

Bell and Zemke (1992) identified three key differences between merely filling a job opening and "casting" for the proper person to play each role. Adapted for health care, these are*

- *Great service performers must be able to create a relationship with the audience.* From the perspective of a patient, every performance is "live" and hence unique. It earns the best reviews when it appears genuine, perhaps even spontaneous. It should never be rigidly scripted––certainly not canned.

    Implication: Frontline health care "cast members" must have good person-to-person skills. Their speaking, listening, chatting, and interacting styles should seem natural, friendly, and appropriate to the situation—neither stiff and formal nor overly familiar.
- *Great service performers must be able to handle pressure.* In a health care setting, there are many kinds of pressure—pressure of the clock, pressure from patients, pressure from fellow cast members, and pressure from the desire to do a good job for both customers and the organization, even though the two may be in conflict.

    Implication: Members of your patient service cast must be good at handling their own emotions and calm under fire. They should not be susceptible to "catching the stress virus" from upset patients (or fellow cast members). At the same time, they have to

---

acknowledge and support their patients' upsets and problems and demonstrate a desire to help resolve the situation in the best way possible.

- *Great service performers must be able to learn new scripts.* When dealing with patients, cast members need to be flexible enough to adjust to changes in the cast and conditions surrounding them, make changes in their own performance as conditions warrant, and still seem natural and knowledgeable.

  Implication: Patient service cast members need to be lifelong learners—curious enough to learn from the environment as well as the classroom, comfortable enough to be constantly looking for new ways to enhance their performance, and confident enough to ask "Why is that?" and constantly make observations throughout the organization to learn how things really work. Those who are comfortable with change and handle it well can be the most helpful to patients and need minimal hand holding from their managers.

The following "tips for casting well" are also adapted from Bell and Zemke (1992, p. 6):

- *Treat every vacancy like an open role in a play.* Think in terms of the role the prospective cast member will have to play and how he or she will have to relate to other members of the cast. Give equal weight to technical knowledge and people skills ("service inclination") in the casting/hiring process.
- *Identify the skills needed for the role.* What traits or personality characteristics do you want new cast members to possess? Friendliness? Courtesy? Optimism? Creativity? How will you judge the presence or absence of these traits to your satisfaction?
- *"Screen test" your applicants.* Consider the way applicants treat your secretary or receptionist. That may be a good indication of how they will treat your patients and their fellow cast members if hired. Try role playing difficult patient situations with applicants or posing "What would you do if..." questions based on the kinds of situations likely to occur on the job. Listen for orientation and attitude. Don't be so concerned if they don't use the exact words you prefer—this can be modified with appropriate training.
- *Use multiple selection methods.* Consider multiple interviews, each with different objectives. If teamwork is important in the position being screened for, consider having peer interviews. The viewpoints of potential fellow cast members can be helpful. You can also use job-validated testing and job previewing.

- *Emphasize mutual selection.* Potential cast members need to make as good a selection decision as you do. If the "match" is incorrect, you may end up with a competent, but unhappy cast member who will "jump ship" at the first opportunity for greater job satisfaction.
- *Recruit actively.* Consider where your best people have come from and revisit that source. Reward existing cast members for referring new ones (as mentioned earlier in this chapter) who are capable of filling roles in your patient-focused "production."

In the words of William Shakespeare: "All the world's a stage, and all the men and women merely players."

Developing People To Deliver Quality Service

Once a health care organization has selected the right "cast member" for a given role, the next step is to provide appropriate training to ensure service performance. Chapter 9 presented training in detail. In addition to technical skills training, service employees need training in interactive skills that allow them to provide courteous, caring, responsive, and empathetic service. Process skills such as listening, problem solving, conflict management, communication, and interpersonal relationships are of paramount importance.

In addition to frontline direct patient contact employees, support staff, supervisors, and managers need service training as well. Unless frontline "cast members" experience the same values and behaviors from their supervisors, they are unlikely to deliver high-quality service to patients. Furthermore, training should be ongoing, not just something offered to new cast members—especially in an environment where continuous process improvement (see Chapter 10) is the norm.

The next component of developing people to deliver service involves empowerment. Many service organizations have recognized that to be truly responsive to customer needs, frontline employees need to be empowered to accommodate customer requests and to recover on the spot when things go wrong. Essentially, the term empowerment refers to the process of giving employees the desire, skills, tools, and authority to make decisions on the customer's behalf. Authority alone is not enough. Frontline employees need the knowledge and tools necessary to allow them to make these decisions, and they need incentives that will encourage them to make the right decisions. This must be more than lip service, for very specific reasons.

- If employees are told that they have the authority to do whatever it takes to satisfy the customer, they don't believe it, especially if your organization has functioned hierarchically or bureaucratically in the past.
- Employees don't often know exactly what "do whatever it takes" means if they have not received specific training that includes guidelines and tools for making such decisions.

Although the term *empowerment* was introduced some time ago (by Peter Block), and it continues to be one of the contemporary managerial "buzz words," there are several sound reasons why true empowerment works to the benefit of an organization's customers (our patients).

- Most service workers (health care included) don't want to be robots. They are in the industry, for the most part, because they enjoy serving people. Therefore, they would like to make their own decisions about how to do that best. Thick volumes of rules and procedures typically overwhelm employees and may inhibit employee judgment. If the answer is not in the rule book, they don't know what to do. Thus, one of the hallmarks of the empowering organization is that it has a relatively thin employee rule book.
- Empowerment pushes decision making down into the organization and encourages people to think and use judgment for the benefit of the customer. Frequently, an empowered frontline employee will be making decisions that were limited to his or her supervisor in the past.

Bowen and Lawler III (1992) listed the following benefits of frontline employee empowerment (p. 31):

- *Quicker on-line responses to customer needs during service delivery:* These bypass what is often a long chain of command or, at least, a discussion with an immediate supervisor.
- *Quicker on-line responses to dissatisfied customers during service recovery:* By decreasing the time it takes to make the situation right in the eyes of the customer (patient), there is a greater likelihood that the dissatisfied customer can potentially be turned into a satisfied, even loyal one (who not only remains with the organization, but enthusiastically refers others to it).
- *Employees who feel better about their jobs and themselves:* Empowerment gives frontline employees ownership for customer (patient) satisfaction. Research supports the fact that employees are more satisfied with their jobs when they have a sense of control and of doing meaningful work. The resulting organizational indicators of this are lower turnover and less absenteeism.

- *Employees who interact with customers (patients) with more warmth and enthusiasm:* When employees feel better about themselves and their work, positive feelings "spill over" into their interactions with customers.
- *Empowered employees who are a great source of service ideas:* When frontline employees feel responsible for service outcomes, they will demonstrate creativity when it comes to developing new and better ways to meet and exceed the expectations of customers.
- *Great word-of-mouth advertising from customers:* When employees are truly empowered to function as the customer's (patient's) advocate, they do unique and special things that customers will remember. These "special things anecdotes" get passed along to their friends, family, and associates.

Promoting Teamwork among Employees

Because the positive management of many patient MOTs is contingent on the cooperative behaviors of two or more frontline employees, patient satisfaction is likely to be enhanced when these employees work as a team. Employees who feel supported by a team will, in all probability, feel better able to maintain their enthusiasm and provide quality service. Recall Peter Drucker's description of a contemporary organization: "A continually shifting collaboration of individuals to bring about performance and change." Teamwork, then, can enhance the frontline employee's *ability* to deliver excellent service; his or her *inclination* to be an excellent service provider will increase as a result of the camaraderie and support received from teammates.

As mentioned in Chapter 10, it should be emphasized to all employees that everyone has a customer. That is, even if employees are not in direct contact with patients, they need to know who they do serve directly and how the role they play in the total service picture is essential to the final delivery of quality service. Team goals and rewards also promote teamwork, which promotes team spirit and increases team efforts. When done appropriately, with the proper training provided, teamwork affords tremendous benefits for both customers and employees alike.

The Relationship between Employee and Patient Satisfaction

There is a great deal of evidence that satisfied employees make for satisfied customers (and satisfied customers can in turn reinforce employees' sense of satisfaction in their jobs). Patient perceptions of service quality are highly correlated with both a *climate for service* and a *climate for employee well-being*. In a study conducted by Sears Roebuck (Bowen & Lawler, 1992), customer satisfaction was found to be strongly correlated to employee turnover. In their stores with the highest customer satisfaction, employee turnover was 54%, whereas in stores with the lowest customer satisfaction, turnover was 83%!

Exhibit 13–5 displays the "employee satisfaction = customer satisfaction" experience of Baptist Hospital of Pensacola, Florida.

In a survey of 200 nurses and 700 patients at a tertiary care hospital in the Midwest, researchers Atkins, Marshall, and Javalgi (1996) revealed that health care employee satisfaction has much to do with patient loyalty. Customer loyalty, referrals, and repeat purchase behavior at a hospital can all be encouraged through the image of employee satisfaction. Findings showed that nurses who are unhappy with their jobs have a hard time concealing their feelings from their patients. This research concluded that strong and positive relationships were found between the nursing staff's overall job satisfaction and a patient's recommending the hospital.

The underlying logic of relationships between customer satisfaction and employee satisfaction is best summarized by a diagram created by Zeithaml and Bitner (1996, p. 306). This is represented in Figure 13–1.

REINFORCING SERVICE-RELATED BEHAVIORS THROUGH REWARD AND RECOGNITION

Most employees, when given a choice of all affordable methods of reward and recognition (including merit pay, pats on the back, merchandise awards, prizes, certificates, and more), chose "a pat on the back from my supervisor" as the single, most powerful, meaningful way they believe they can be recognized on the job. In other words, employees at every level in health care want to be noticed and recognized when they reach out to patients and perform well. Leebov, Vergare, and Scott (1990) recommended the following format for giving employees positive feedback for their behaviors toward patients:

- *Describe the positive behavior.* "I noticed that you expressed true concern for Mrs. Johnson when she told you about her husband's heart surgery this afternoon."
- *Articulate the consequences.* "I'm sure the patient felt much better after speaking with you. This is the kind of behavior that makes our organization stand out as having very caring people."

Exhibit 13–5 Baptist Hospital's Employee Satisfaction = Customer Satisfaction Correlation

Driving Change with Reward and Recognition

Employee Satisfaction = Customer Satisfaction

"With our scores [on Press-Ganey Patient Satisfaction Surveys] spiraling downward, we came to grasp the idea that if we didn't make a concerted effort to improve service levels for our patients, we were headed for destitution."

Located in one of the most competitive regions within the country, Baptist Hospital shares its market with two major health systems. All three are fighting for a market that barely has volume for two. With both competitors claiming that they provide excellent service, Baptist had to set and meet "best in the nation" goals for customer satisfaction, quality, and efficiency. In such a competitive market, they decided to use their best advantage, their people.

In February 1996, the hospital began employee satisfaction surveys, and in their own words, "what an eye opener!" What they found was that employee morale was lower than it had been in years. With their scores spiraling downward, they came to the realization that a group effort to improve customer service would be essential to their ability to both flourish and survive.

By June, the hospital had developed "employee roll out sessions" to be conducted by department managers. With each presentation, the managers were finding more opportunities to improve employee satisfaction and morale. Employees, decision makers, front line leaders, and care givers were all given the opportunity to tell the hospital what needed to be done to improve performance. As a result, the hospital developed four key components to its success:

- **Communication**—"If you are only talking, you will only learn what you already know...by listening to employees, we were able to communicate in a way that made them feel part of the team.

- **Reward and recognition**—"Rewarding and recognizing the employees for a job well done has been the cornerstone of our success...of all the tactics used in making an organization successful, this is the most important one.

- **Employee satisfaction**—"If your employees are not happy, you will not be #1 in customer satisfaction. Quite simply, if you want to place in the 99th percentile in customer satisfaction, you must listen to your

continues

Exhibit 13–5 continued

> employees or you'll find yourself in last place both with your customers and your employees."
>
> - **Leadership development**—"We have all heard a chain is only as strong as its weakest link. In comparison, an organization is only as strong as those who are responsible for the leadership."
>
> Through continuous quality improvement, Baptist Hospital received the VHA Leadership Award for its commitment to customer satisfaction and for being a pace setter in its customer satisfaction efforts. **Its Press-Ganey scores also reflect its improvements, as Baptist Hospital has soared from the 17th percentile in 1995 to the 98th percentile in the first quarter of 1997!**
>
> *Source:* Press, Ganey Associates, Inc., *Client Success Stories,* 1998.

- *Express a touch of empathy.* "I realize that you were very busy this afternoon, and taking time to empathize with Mrs. Johnson put extra pressure on you."
- *Express appreciation.* "I want you to know I really appreciate what you did. Thank you."

Deeprose (1994) offered the following 10 guidelines for recognizing and rewarding employees:

1. Determine your goals and get employee input.
2. Specify reward criteria.
3. Reward everyone who meets the criteria.

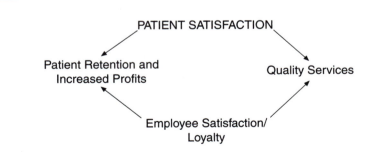

Figure 13–1 Logic of Relationships between Customer Satisfaction and Employee Satisfaction. *Source:* Adapted with permission from V. Zeithaml and M.J. Bitner, *Services Marketing,* p. 306, © 1996, The McGraw-Hill Companies.

4. Recognize behaviors as well as outcomes.
5. Use the "platinum rule" rather than the "golden rule": Do unto others as they would have you do onto them.
6. Say "thank you" frequently.
7. Nurture self-esteem and belonging.
8. Foster intrinsic rewards.
9. Reward the whole team.
10. Be careful. You get what you reward.

Generally speaking, reward systems need to be linked to the organization's vision and to outcomes that are truly important—those that contribute to patient satisfaction. In the context of teamwork, special organizational and team celebrations for achieving improved patient satisfaction or for attaining patient retention goals should be devised and publicized throughout your health care organization. In most health care organizations, it is not only the major accomplishments that count, but the daily perseverance and attention to detail that incrementally improve patient satisfaction. Therefore, recognition of the "small wins" is also very important.

Chapter 14 will focus on the logistical aspects of putting a health care organization's patient satisfaction improvement program together—from concept to implementation and evaluation.

CONCLUSION

Employee behaviors are heavily influenced by the culture, or pervasive norms and values, of the organization within which they function. The basic components of organizational culture include: business environment, values, symbols, routines and rituals, power structures, organizational structure, and control systems. World-class organizations have six cultural elements in common: passionate customer focus, urgent obsession with quality, continuous improvement, high levels of employee participation, teamwork, and ethics/integrity. If improving patient satisfaction and loyalty is to be truly continuous, with all of the associated long-term organizational benefits, then a service culture—one based on a passion for service excellence—must be established and maintained.

The vision, values, and mission of any organization serve to unify the efforts of all levels of management and employees. The vision of an organization is a concise word picture of the organization at some future (preferred) time in a future (preferred) state, which sets the overall direction of the organization. It is the lighthouse that provides general direction rather than the map to a specific destination. The values of your health care organization are the collective principles and ideals that guide the thoughts and actions of an individual, or a group of individuals—the maps of the way things should be. They are stable, long-term beliefs that are hard to change. Values function as the building blocks of your organization's culture. They cannot be proven or disproven, but they can be substantiated or refuted by the actions of key people in your health care organization. Your health care organization's mission should be summarized in a statement that specifies its purpose or "reason for being." It represents the primary objective toward which the organization's plans and programs should be aimed. A mission is something to be accomplished, whereas a vision is something to be pursued.

Frontline employees play a critical role in your efforts to meet or exceed patient expectations. Even if patient expectations are well understood and you have designed the appropriate management of each MOT and surrogate perception to conform to those expectations, the service that patients experience may fall short of optimum. When such a "service-performance gap" exists—when service is not delivered as specified—the critical role of frontline employees becomes evident. Therefore, it is recommended that potential service employees be screened for two complementary capacities: service competencies and service inclination. *Service competencies* are the skills and knowledge necessary to do the job. *Service inclination* refers to the employees' interest in doing service-related work. This is reflected in their attitudes toward service and their orientation toward serving customers (internal and external).

Once your health care organization has selected the right "cast member" for a given role, the next step is to provide appropriate training to ensure service performance. In addition to technical skills training, service employees need training in interactive skills that allow them to provide courteous, caring, responsive, and empathetic service. Process skills such as listening, problem solving, conflict management, communication, and interpersonal relationships are of paramount importance.

Many service organizations have recognized that to be truly responsive to customer needs, frontline employees need to be empowered to accommodate customer requests and to recover on the spot when things go wrong. Essentially, the term empowerment refers to the process of giving employees the desire, skills, tools, and authority to make decisions on the customer's behalf. Additionally, employees must be equipped to function as a team. Because the positive management of many patient MOTs is contingent on the cooperative behaviors of two or more frontline employees, patient satisfaction is likely to be enhanced when these employees work as a team. Employees who feel supported by a team will, in all probability, feel better able to maintain their enthusiasm and provide quality service. Appropriate training, empowerment, and teamwork all combine to contribute to employee satisfaction. Furthermore, there is a great deal of evidence that satisfied employees make for satisfied customers (and satisfied customers can in turn reinforce employees' sense of satisfaction in their jobs). Patient perceptions of service quality are highly correlated with both a *climate for service* and a *climate for employee well-being*.

Finally, service-related behaviors need to be reinforced through reward and recognition. This recognition can range anywhere from a simple "pat on the back from my supervisor" to a sophisticated, customized reward and recognition system whereby employees earn "points" redeemable in a catalog of desirable items. Generally speaking, reward systems need to be linked to the organization's vision and to outcomes that are truly important—those that contribute to patient satisfaction. The sequence for providing employees with positive feedback is: Describe the behavior, articulate the consequences of the behavior, express a touch of empathy, and finally, express appreciation.

ACTION STEPS

1. Form a grid using the six cultural elements of world-class organizations (passionate customer focus, urgent obsession with quality, continuous improvement, high levels of employee participation, teamwork, and ethics and integrity) as the horizontal rows. Then, form three vertical columns to the right of the listed elements. Place the following headings at the top of each column in left-to-right order: "current situation," "gap or opportunity for improvement," and "ideal, but realistic future state."
2. Assess your organization using the above grid.
3. List the values that are currently "alive" (i.e., aligned with common behaviors) in your organization. List the values that are currently "dormant" (i.e., your organization proclaims or aspires to possess these values but they are not evident in common behaviors of individuals within the organization).

4. Design a mechanism for determining whether employees at all levels of your organization know your mission. If you discover that it is not well-known, create a means of changing that. (This, of course, assumes that you have a carefully articulated mission. If not, you know the next step!)

5. Review your "casting" or selection procedures in terms of service competencies and service inclination.

6. List the common patient satisfaction enhancing behaviors (organizationwide or limited to one department or facility) that could be observed in your organization on a typical day. Then, identify what is being done, if anything, to reward/reinforce the repetition of these behaviors. Now list those behaviors that are occasionally observed that detract from patient satisfaction. Finally, identify what is being done to curtail or extinguish these behaviors.

REFERENCES

Abrahams, J. (1995). *The mission statement book*. San Francisco: Ten Speed Press.

Atkins, M., Marshal, Javalgi. (1996, Winter). Happy employees lead to loyal patients. *Journal of Healthcare Marketing*.

Atkinson, P.E. (1990). *Creating culture change: The key to successful total quality management*. London: Pfeiffer and Company.

Bell, C.R., & Zemke, R. (1992). *Managing knock your socks off service*. New York: AMACOM.

Bowen, D., & Lawler, E. (1992, Spring). The empowerment of service workers: What, why, how and when. *The Sloan Management Review*, 31–39.

Capodagli, B., & Jackson, L. (1999). *The Disney way: Harnessing the management secrets of Disney in your company*. New York: McGraw-Hill.

Covey, S.R. (1989). *The seven habits of highly effective people: Powerful lessons in personal change*. New York: Simon & Schuster.

Davis, S.M. *Managing corporate culture*.

Deal, T.E., & Kennedy, A.A. (1982). *Corporate cultures: The rites and rituals of corporate life*. Menlo Park, CA: Addison-Wesley.

Deeprose, D. (1994). *How to recognize & reward employees*. New York: AMACOM.

Hogan, J., Hogan, R., & Busch, C.M. (1984). How to measure service orientation. *Journal of Applied Psychology*, *69*(1), 167–173.

Leebov, W., Vergare, M., & Scott, G. (1990). *Patient satisfaction: A guide to practice enhancement*. Oradell, NJ: Medical Economics Books.

Merriam-Webster's Collegiate Dictionary, Tenth Edition. (1997). Springfield, MA: Merriam-Webster.

Peters, T., & Waterman, R.N. (1982). *In search of excellence*. Glasgow, UK: HarperCollins.

Schneider, B., & Schechter, D. (1991). Development of personnel selection system for service jobs. In S.W. Brown, E. Gummenson, B. Edvardsson, & B. Gustavsson (Eds.), *Service quality: Multidisciplinary and multinational perspectives*. Lexington, MA: Lexington Books.

Wall, B., Sobol, M., & Solum, R. (1999). *The mission-driven organization*. Rocklin, CA: Prima.

Wellington, P. (1995). *Kaizen strategies for customer care: How to create a powerful customer care program—and make it work*. London: Pitman.

Zeithaml, V.A., & Bitner, M.J. (1996). *Services marketing*. London: The McGraw-Hill Companies.

SUGGESTED READING

Albrecht, K. (1988). *At America's service*. Homewood, IL: Dow Jones-Irwin.

Albrecht, K. (1992). *The only thing that matters*. New York: Harper Business.

Albrecht, K. (1994). *The northbound train: Finding the purpose, setting the direction, shaping the destiny of your organization*. New York: AMACOM.

Albrecht, K., & Zemke, R. (1985). *Service America! Doing business in the new economy*. Homewood, IL: Dow Jones-Irwin.

Bader, G.E., & Bloom, A.E. (1994). *Make your training results last*. Irvine, CA: Richard Chang Associates.

Brown, S.A. (1997). *Breakthrough customer service: Best practices of leaders in customer support*. Toronto, Canada: John Wiley & Sons Canada.

Cannie, J.K. (1994). *Turning lost customers into gold:...and the art of achieving zero defections*. New York: AMACOM.

Capezio, P., & Morehouse, D. (1992). *Total quality management: The road of continuous improvement*. Shawnee Mission, KS: National Press.

Chang, R.Y., & Kelly, P.K. (1994). *Satisfy internal customers first!: A practical guide to improving internal and external customer satisfaction*. Irvine, CA: Richard Chang Associates.

Connellan, T.K., & Zemke, R. (1993). *Sustaining knock your socks off service*. New York: AMACOM.

Conomikes, G.S. (Ed.). (1988). *Successful practice management techniques: 329 ideas from Conomikes Reports*. Los Angeles: Conomikes Reports.

Costello, S.J. (1994). *Managing change in the workplace*. New York: Irwin Professional.

Daniels, A.C. (1994). *Bringing out the best in people: How to apply the astonishing power of positive reinforcement*. New York: McGraw-Hill.

Disend, J.E. (1991). *How to provide excellent service in any organization: A blueprint for making all the theories work*. Radnor, PA: Chilton Book.

George, S., & Weimerskirch, A. (1994). *Total quality management: Strategies and techniques proven at today's most successful companies*. New York: John Wiley & Sons.

Harrington, H.J. (1991). *Business process improvement: The breakthrough strategy for total quality, productivity, and competitiveness*. New York: McGraw-Hill.

Heskett, J.L., Sasser, W., & Hart, C. (1997). *The service profit chain: How leading companies link profit and growth to loyalty, satisfaction, and value.* New York: The Free Press.

Hradesky, J.L. (1995). *Total quality management handbook.* New York: McGraw-Hill.

Jerome, P.J. (1994). *Coaching through effective feedback: A practical guide to successful communication.* Irvine, CA: Richard Chang Associates.

Kaufman, R.S., Thiagarajan, S., & MacGillis, P. (Eds.). (1997). *The guidebook for performance management in health care* (2nd ed.). St. Louis, MO: Mosby-Year Book.

Kreps, G.L., & Kunimoto, E.N. (1994). *Effective communication in multicultural health care settings.* Thousand Oaks, CA: Sage.

Leebov, W. (1988). *Service excellence: The customer relations strategy for health care.* Chicago: American Hospital.

Leland, K., & Bailey, K. (1995). *Customer service for dummies.* Chicago: IDG Books Worldwide.

McCarthy, J.A. (1995). *The transition equation: A proven strategy for organizational change.* New York: Lexington Books.

Nadler, G., & Hibino, S. (1994). *Breakthrough thinking: The seven principles of creative problem-solving* (2nd ed.). Rocklin, CA: Prima.

Nelson, A.M., Wood, S., Brown, S., & Bronkesh. S. (1997). *Improving patient satisfaction now: How to earn patient and payer loyalty.* Gaithersburg, MD: Aspen.

Press-Ganey. (1997). *Press-Ganey Success Stories.*

Reichheld, F.F. (1996). *The loyalty effect: The hidden force behind growth, profits, and lasting value.* Boston: Harvard Business School Press.

Scheuing, E.E., & Christopher, W.F. (Eds.). (1993). *The service quality handbook.* New York: AMACOM.

Scott, C.D., & Jaffe, D.T. (1989). *Managing organizational change: A practical guide for managers.* Menlo Park, CA: Crisp.

Scott, C.D., & Jaffe, D.T. (1995). *Managing change at work: Leading people through organizational transitions.* Menlo Park, CA: Crisp.

Shaw, J.C. (1990). *The service focus: Developing winning game plans for service companies.* Homewood, IL: Dow Jones-Irwin.

Stamatis, D.H. (1996). *Total quality service: Principles, practices, and implementation.* Delray Beach, FL: St. Lucie Press.

Thomas, B. (1992). *Total quality training: The quality culture and quality trainer.* London: McGraw-Hill Book.

Whiteley, R., & Hessan, D. (1996). *Customer centered growth: Five proven strategies for building competitive advantage.* Menlo Park, CA: Addison-Wesley.

Williams, R.L. (1994). *Essentials of total quality management.* San Francisco: AMACOM.

Zeithaml, V.A., Parasuraman, A., & Berry, L.L. (1990). *Delivering quality service: Balancing customer perceptions and expectations.* New York: The Free Press.

Zemke, R., & Schaaf, D. (1989). *The service edge: 101 companies that profit from customer care.* New York: NAL Books.

CHAPTER 14

Putting It All Together: Your Health Care Organization's Patient Satisfaction Improvement Program Plan

The great Socrates has been credited with the phrase "knowledge is power." In contemporary organizational reality, however, it would appear that knowledge only provides potential power. Knowledge that is converted to action—applied knowledge—is where the real power lies. Nadler and Hibino (1994) support this belief and emphasize the importance of effectively bridging the gap from *here* (knowledge and needs) to *there* (solutions and results).

Each of the previous chapters has provided you with information to supplement your current knowledge related to the rationale and methodologies for measuring and improving patient satisfaction. In this final chapter, you will be given an approach for putting this information into action in your health care organization. Keep in mind that each health care organization is somewhat different—serving different numbers and types of patient populations, functioning in different marketplaces, offering slightly different services, and operating in differing internal cultures. Therefore, it is important to recognize that you will need to adapt this approach to meet your organization's specific needs. Your patient satisfaction improvement (PSI) program must be in clear alignment with your organization's vision, values, mission, and business philosophy.

A CONCEPTUAL MODEL FOR PLANNING YOUR PSI PROGRAM

Figure 14–1 summarizes the sequential steps involved in planning your PSI program.

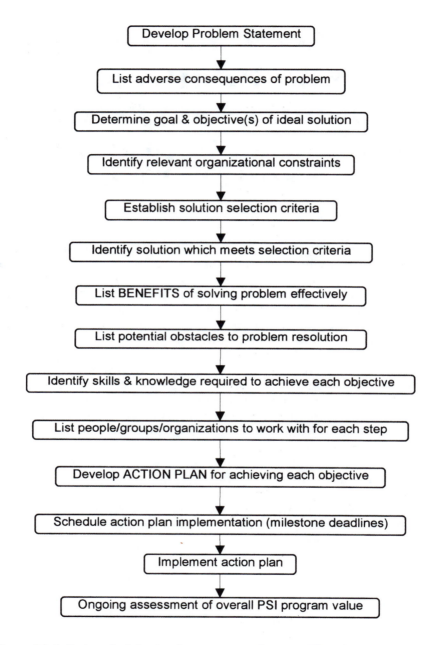

Figure 14–1 Patient Satisfaction Improvement Program Planning.

This can be used as a conceptual framework for several important activities, including the following:

- Develop a program proposal for senior management approval/support.
- Create an integrated organizationwide approach to PSI.
- Establish a unified direction for multidisciplinary PSI teams.
- Introduce a new/renewed PSI program throughout your health care organization.

This sequential approach will also serve as a framework for the chapter. Each step will be discussed in turn—first, in "generic" terms and then, where appropriate, one or more specific examples will be provided for clarification. Finally, references to various relevant chapters throughout this book (for review purposes) will be provided.

Upon completion of this chapter (and, indeed, the entire book), you should be able to:

- Have a global overview of what it takes to systematically measure and improve patient satisfaction.
- Develop and implement a PSI program that specifically meets the needs of your health care organization while enjoying "buy-in" and support at all organizational levels.
- Identify and effectively bridge your organization's patient satisfaction gaps, resulting in valued improvement of business results—aligning day-to-day processes and behaviors with the service vision, values, and mission of your health care organization.

THE PROBLEM OR "OPPORTUNITY FOR IMPROVEMENT" STATEMENT

A "problem" is a condition or set of circumstances that an individual, a group, or an entire organization thinks should be changed. A given situation may be referred to as a *problem* when dissatisfaction with the status quo and/or aspiration for a better state exists. In an organizational setting, problems are typically identified when there is a need to respond to change, adapt to a modified environment, or seek improvement. You may wish to establish a somewhat more positive (albeit euphemistic) tone to this term by phrasing it as "opportunity for improvement." I have seen this seemingly minor semantic adjustment make a major difference in senior management's overall receptivity to recommendations for change.

The critical first step in solving any problem involves the development of an accurate problem/opportunity for improvement definition. We have all heard the old adage that "a problem well-defined is a problem half-solved." When there is a lack of problem definition, those charged with finding a solution may have different perceptions as to exactly what it is they are working on. Consequently, each person's recommendation(s) for solving the problem is likely to be quite different or, worse yet, working at cross purposes with other recommendations. On the other hand, once the problem or opportunity is clearly defined, all involved can focus their energy in the same direction.

When developing your problem statement or, alternatively, opportunity for improvement statement, several guidelines may be helpful in focusing your efforts. The problem statement should be

- *Stated objectively:* The problem/opportunity should be nothing more than a simple statement of fact as it currently exists. There should be no room for misinterpretation or for a biased view of the situation to develop.
- *Focused:* The scope of the problem/opportunity should be limited to that which the involved individual, group(s), or team(s) could be realistically expected to tackle and solve.
- *Written in simple terms:* Avoid marketing or technical jargon whenever possible in order to ensure mutuality of meaning among those reading the statement.
- *Concise:* Limit the statement to 25 words or less.

Exhibit 14–1 shows several examples of problem/opportunity for improvement statements.

Chapter Reference for Review

- Chapter 8: Identifying and Prioritizing Service Quality Improvement Needs

ADVERSE CONSEQUENCES OF THE PROBLEM

Before any individual, group, team, committee, or organization is willing to allocate the necessary resources for solving a problem, they must be convinced that the problem is truly worth solving. The best way to accomplish this is to think through carefully and list the adverse consequences—impacting both external and internal organiza-

Exhibit 14–1 Sample Problem/Opportunity for Improvement Statements

"Currently, there is no standardized, network-wide mechanism at XYZ health care organization for measuring the nonmedical dimension of service quality among ambulatory patients."

"XYZ health care organization does not have a coordinated, systematic approach to improving our currently declining patient satisfaction survey scores."

" Patient satisfaction scores for waiting times in the reception room ('excellent' or 'very good' ratings) have declined from 89% to 81% in the last 12 months."

"The number of monthly patient complaints related to appointment scheduling has increased by 17% over the past 12 months."

tional customers—of the existence of the problem. This serves to "preanswer" the potential question "So what?" in the mind of anyone who reads your problem/opportunity statement.

Because your problem/opportunity statement will probably relate to suboptimum levels of patient satisfaction in one or more service quality areas (as documented by patient satisfaction survey scores and/or other indicators of patient discontent), the adverse consequences might include such items as

- competitive disadvantage, particularly if you can obtain data that document that one or more of your direct competitors (i.e., serving the same patient population, in the same geographic region offering the same or similar services) is achieving higher, similarly derived, patient satisfaction scores
- decrease in market share of patients within your service area
- declining number of new patients per month (particularly from patient referrals) or new enrollees during the "open enrollment" time period in an integrated health network
- increased number of "defectors," patients leaving your health care organization or "disenrolling," especially those who switch to a competitor
- increased number of patient complaints
- increased number of medical malpractice litigation cases wherein the inciting factor can be traced, in part, to an uncaring provider

attitude or poor communication between provider and patient or between provider and staff
- decreased payment levels from contracted third-party payers who offer financial incentives for establishing and maintaining high levels of patient satisfaction

When all of these are combined, the ultimate adverse consequence is decreased revenue and, therefore, diminished profits for the health care organization.

Furthermore, the overall satisfaction level and morale of internal customers—employees and providers—is likely to decline when patients are unhappy with their service experience. As a result of this decline, the organization may suffer the economic and productivity strains associated with increased absenteeism and tardiness among employees. This, in turn, detracts from the establishment or maintenance of a service-oriented organizational culture. In this circumstance, as discussed in Chapter 13, employees/providers are less likely to "go the extra mile" for patients.

Chapter References for Review

- Chapter 1: The Importance of Patient Satisfaction (and Loyalty)
- Chapter 13: Building and Sustaining a Service-Oriented Organizational Culture

THE GOAL AND OBJECTIVES OF AN IDEAL PROBLEM SOLUTION

Recall from Chapter 9 that a patient satisfaction gap analysis compares the way things are now with an improved, much more desirable state—the way things ought to be. Table 14–1 is a reprint of Table 9–2 as a reminder of the recommended format.

Your ideal solution's goal and the supporting objectives should be based on a gap analysis related to the specific problem/opportunity outlined in your problem statement or opportunity for improvement statement. More specifically, the goal should be to bridge the identified gap. For example, if your identified opportunity for improvement pertains to the establishment of a systematic means of regularly measuring the levels of patient satisfaction, Exhibit 14–2 lists a possible goal and supporting objectives for accomplishing this.

Table 14–1 Sample Gap Analysis Format (a Reprint of Table 9–2)

Current State	Gap Indicating Changes Needed To Move from Current to Future States	Ideal Future State
82% of patients rated doctor explanation of medical condition to be "very good or excellent" on recent patient satisfaction survey	Improved ability and willingness of doctor(s) to explain medical condition clearly to patients (training to be provided)	95% of patients rated doctor explanation of medical condition to be "very good or excellent" on next patient satisfaction survey
Five complaints per month regarding receptionist's attitude toward patients	• Coaching for improved performance • Appropriate training re: courtesy to patients	Zero complaints per month regarding receptionist's attitude toward patients

If, however, your health care organization already has a valid and reliable mechanism in place for measuring patient satisfaction (either in-house or externally contracted), your opportunity for improvement will most certainly be focused on continuously improving those measured satisfaction levels. Exhibit 14–3 lists a possible goal and supporting objectives for accomplishing this.

It is important that any proposal for organizational change reflect an intention to support the established vision and mission of the organization. Chapter 13 presented the components and importance of having an organizational vision and mission. Albrecht (1994) stated that "you must have a vision for your success and a direction for getting there. You have to know what train you're going to ride." Albrecht's "northbound train" is a metaphor for achieving a focused vision of the direction your organization must take to succeed and then moving inexorably toward that goal.

Chapter References for Review

- Chapter 9: Addressing Behavior-Based Improvement Priorities
- Chapter 13: Building and Sustaining a Service-Oriented Organizational Culture

Exhibit 14–2 Sample Goal and Objectives for Measuring Patient Satisfaction

Program Goal:	To develop a mechanism for measuring the levels of patient satisfaction with the services each health care provider and each employee category of each department provide:
Objectives:	1. Identify the elements that determine external customer (patient/member) satisfaction. 2. Determine the relative importance ("relative weight") of the various elements within each satisfaction category. 3. Develop and administer a means of measuring current patient/member satisfaction that is organizationwide, as well as region-, health care center-, department-, health care provider-, and employee category-specific. 4. Identify current patient/member perceived service quality (satisfaction element) "strengths and weaknesses" throughout our health care organization.

Exhibit 14–3 Sample Goal and Objectives for Systematically Improving Patient Satisfaction

Program Goal:	To continuously improve the levels of patient satisfaction with services provided by XYZ health care organization.
Objectives:	1. Design an approach for bringing about prioritized improvement in service quality areas perceived as "weaknesses" while sustaining currently perceived service quality areas of "strengths." 2. Deliver education and training designed to improve behavior-based components of patient/member perceived service quality (i.e., satisfaction) "weaknesses." 3. Develop mechanisms for capturing local health care center and departmental suggestions for improving systems and process components of patient/member perceived "weaknesses" in service quality. 4. Continuously evaluate the effectiveness of all patient satisfaction improvement efforts.

ORGANIZATIONAL CONSTRAINTS

Any proposed solution to an identified problem, if it is to be well received and supported, needs to "fit" the operational reality of your organization. Nadler and Hibino (1994) refer to this, in part, as the *systems principle,* which stipulates that every problem is a part of a larger system. By understanding the elements and dimensions of your organization's system framework, you can determine in advance the complexities you must incorporate in implementing your solution. Furthermore, the *people design principle,* another component of breakthrough thinking, emphasizes the importance of having the people who will carry out and use a solution contribute to the development of that solution.

Suppose, for example, you are attempting to address various identified behavior-based improvement priorities (as discussed in Chapter 9) in your organization. Recommending that all frontline employees complete a 3-day training workshop over the next 6 months may not be operationally feasible in light of current understaffing. This would be ignoring the *systems principle.* It would make more sense to break up the training into modules so that there is far less operational interruption involved.

Similarly, the *people design principle* would come into play if you were trying to respond to a systems- and process-based improvement priority. If you were assembling a team charged with the responsibility of improving the efficiency of a particular process (as discussed in Chapter 10), it would be foolish to exclude someone from the team who regularly performs component tasks of that process. This would not only fail to capture the valuable input and creativity of an involved individual, but it would virtually ensure resistance to the implementation of any proposed solution.

Take the time to think through any of your existing organizational constraints. These must be taken into consideration when forming any problem solution or attempting to act on an identified opportunity for improvement. Common categories of constraint include

- *Time:* There may be a sense of urgency among senior management or shareholders for coming up with a solution to the problem. This is likely to be linked with the severity of adverse consequences identified and the degree to which solving the problem is necessary to proceed in accordance with the organization's vision and mission. Furthermore, the individuals or groups needed to implement a solution may be very limited in the amount of time they can devote to the matter.

- *Human resources:* The health care industry is inherently made up of a series of high people-contact processes. Any given patient is likely to interact with a variety of people, each of whom contributes to that patient's overall impression of your organization. This, in turn, drives the grades the patient assigns your organization on his or her mental report card. If you are about to undertake a patient satisfaction survey research project, limitations in available human resources must be taken into consideration. This does not rule out the solution, but a contingency such as using temporary employees should be built into the proposed solution.
- *Financial resources:* Any organization, regardless of size, particularly those operating in a competitive industry and in a competitive marketplace, must be particularly vigilant about the allocation of financial resources. However, when appropriately viewed as an *investment* rather than an *expense*, fund allocation in support of efforts to measure and/or improve patient satisfaction should be given priority.

Chapter References for Review

- Chapter 9: Addressing Behavior-Based Improvement Priorities
- Chapter 10: Addressing Systems- and Process-Based Improvement Priorities

ESTABLISH SOLUTION SELECTION CRITERIA

Prior to proposing a particular approach to solving the identified problem or acting on the identified opportunity for improvement, several (three to six) objective criteria should be developed to assist with the selection process. If you are working as part of a team, it is important that all members participate in brainstorming during criteria development and that they all clearly understand each criterion. Then, in order to prevent each team member from placing greater emphasis on a different criterion, the team needs to decide the relative importance of each one compared to the others. This can then be quantified by assigning a percentage value/weight to each criterion, such that all the criteria values/weights add up to a total of 100% (see Table 14–2).

Although your team needs to develop solution selection criteria of its own, several common ones are

- speed of implementation
- ease of implementation

- minimal in-house human resources required
- probability of success in your organization
- economical and cost-sensitive
- low resistance to implementation

Table 14–2 gives you a format for developing and quantifying your solution selection criteria.

IDENTIFY A SOLUTION THAT MEETS THE SELECTION CRITERIA

Using the process of structured brainstorming (as discussed in Chapter 10), your team should develop several feasible solutions to the problem you are focused on. Make sure consideration is given to new, nonconventional, creative approaches to the problem as well as more traditional approaches. Keep in mind that each of the proposed solutions should be capable of achieving the goal and objectives previously established for the "ideal" solution.

Table 14–2 Format for Defining and Quantifying Your Solution-Selection Criteria

Solution Selection Criteria	Definition of These Criteria	Weight
Speed of implementation	How long will it take to complete all steps required to reach the implementation stage?	25%
Minimal in-house human resources required	How many full-time and part-time employees will be needed to implement this solution?	20%
Low resistance to implementation	How much resistance can we reasonably expect when implementing this solution?	20%
Economical—cost-sensitive	How cost-sensitive (minimizing costs) will this solution be?	15%
Ease of implementation	How easy will it be to implement this solution, given the nature of our operations?	5%
Probability of success in our organization	How likely is it that this solution can actually achieve our PSI objectives?	15%
	Total weighting:	100%

The next step is to rate each of the possible solutions against the criteria your team has established. This is done by first assigning an arbitrary score (1–10) to each solution that meets the first criterion. In other words, your team is rating how well ("1" meaning "just barely" and "10" meaning "perfectly") each proposed solution meets that. Continue on with each of the remaining criteria applied to every proposed solution. Once you have determined how well each of your proposed solutions meets each selection criterion, you are ready to apply the predetermined weights of each criterion—by multiplying the weight by the score in each instance. Finally, the solution with the largest total weighted score should be selected. Table 14–3 provides a format for this process.

THE BENEFITS OF SOLVING THE PROBLEM OR ACHIEVING THE DESIRED IMPROVEMENT

Every individual, team, or organization that is pondering the expenditure of any of its resources (particularly time and/or money) tunes in to the most popular FM radio station in the world—WIIFM. That's right! "What's In It For Me." Therefore, if you are proposing that your solution or improvement should be implemented with the proviso that resources need to be allocated (which they definitely will), then an emphasis must be placed on the likely benefits to be received.

By reviewing Chapter 1, which presented the importance of patient satisfaction, we can develop a number of benefits associated with improving satisfaction levels. These might include, but are not limited to, the following:

- competitive advantage, particularly if you can obtain data that document that you are outscoring one of your competitors in an area important to patients
- increased market share of patients within your service area
- increased number of new patients per month (particularly from patient referrals) or new enrollees during the "open enrollment" time period in an integrated health network
- increased patient loyalty = decreased number of "defectors"—patients leaving your health care organization or "disenrolling"
- ability to better meet third-party payer demands, with potential monetary incentive earnings
- ability to better meet employer and accreditation agency demands
- increased employee and provider satisfaction, fostering a service culture

Table 14–3 Format for Selecting Best Solution Alternative

Selection Criteria	Weight	Solution A	Solution B	Solution C	Solution D
Speed of Implementation	25%	7 × 0.25 = 1.75	6 × 0.25 = 1.5	5 × 0.25 = 1.25	8 × 0.25 = 2.0
Minimal in-house human resources	20%	8 × 0.20 = 1.6	7 × 0.20 = 1.4	7 × 0.20 = 1.4	10 × 0.20 = 2.0
Low resistance to implementation	20%	7 × 0.20 = 1.4	7 × 0.20 = 1.4	5 × 0.20 = 1.0	3 × 0.20 = 0.6
Economical—cost-sensitive	15%	8 × 0.15 = 1.2	7 × 0.15 = 1.05	6 × 0.15 = 0.9	8 × 0.15 = 1.2
Probability of success	15%	9 × 0.15 = 1.35	7 × 0.15 = 1.05	8 × 0.15 = 1.2	7 × 0.15 = 1.05
Ease of implementation	5%	5 × .05 = 0.25	6 × .05 = 0.3	7 × .05 = 0.35	8 × .05 = 0.4
Total points:	100%	7.55	6.70	6.10	7.25

Source: Adapted with permission from P.K. Kelly, *Team Decision-Making Techniques*, p. 94, © 1994, Richard Chang Associates, Inc.

- increased organizational revenue
- improved patient compliance
- fewer patient complaints
- lower medical malpractice claim likelihood

If you are not currently measuring patient satisfaction levels, then the benefits of seizing this opportunity for improvement may be derived, in part, by reviewing the introduction to Chapter 6.

> Seeking and responding to patient feedback regarding their perceptions of service quality is one of the most essential nonclinical endeavors a health care organization can undertake as we approach the new millennium and beyond. Osborne and Gaebler (1994) identified three important principles that underscore the importance of measuring organizational performance:
>
> 1. If you don't measure results, you can't tell success from failure
> 2. If you can't see success, you can't reward it—and if you can't reward success, you are probably rewarding failure and
> 3. If you can't recognize failure, you can't correct it.
>
> By measuring patients' degree of satisfaction with the way all MOTs and SPs are currently being managed, you can determine your organization's current grades on those patients' mental report cards. This then forms the foundation for you to identify specific action(s) needed to increase their satisfaction and loyalty.

Chapter References for Review

- Chapter 1: The Importance of Patient Satisfaction (and Loyalty)
- Chapter 6: Measuring Patient Satisfaction: Determining An Organization's Grades on the Patient's Mental Report Card

POTENTIAL OBSTACLES TO SOLUTION OR IMPROVEMENT IMPLEMENTATION

Having listed the tremendous benefits to be gained from accurately measuring and effectively improving patient satisfaction in your health care organization, enthusiasm for tackling the project is typically quite high. At this stage, it is wise to acknowledge potential obstacles that may be encountered along the way. This allows for effective contingency planning: What would you do to overcome each obstacle? Then, if one or more of the obstacles actually surfaces, the response has already been discussed. In this way, your team can minimize the impact of encountering the obstacle on overall momentum in implementing the desired change(s).

Service quality guru Ron Zemke developed the service management practices inventory database, which includes more than 60,000 surveys from 200 service organizations. Using these data, Connellan and Zemke (1993) identified eight major barriers to high-quality customer service. Adapted for our purposes, they include*

1. *Inadequate communications between departments:* There is a tendency for people to focus on their own departments rather than to see the big picture. Failure to understand what takes place in the radiology department or clinical laboratory may well lead to unrealistic expectations on the part of patients—either in terms of what to expect when they visit these departments, or in terms of how quickly they might expect results.
2. *Employees not rewarded for quality service or quality effort:* Recall from LeBouef (1985) the phrase, "Behavior that gets rewarded gets repeated." In Chapter 9, we discussed in detail the impact of behavioral consequences on employee actions as related to service delivery. If the desired behaviors are not rewarded, or if undesirable behaviors are being reinforced, the net result is diminished service quality and, ultimately, diminished patient satisfaction.
3. *Understaffing:* In health care, service is typically provided on a one-on-one basis. Therefore, when there aren't enough staff to meet patient requirements in a timely fashion, patient waiting time increases, which often diminishes overall satisfaction with the health care organization. Generally speaking, understaffing suggests that either the organization is attempting to cut back on costs (a poor place to cut back), or they don't truly understand patient requirements. If they understand the requirements, perhaps there are no service standards in place (recall Chapter 9 discussion) to ensure that patient requirements are consistently met.

Source: Reprinted from SUSTAINING KNOCK YOUR SOCKS OFF SERVICE by Ronald E. Zemke, et al. Copyright © 1993 Performance Research Associates, Inc. Reprinted by permission of AMACOM, a division of American Management Association International, New York, NY. All rights reserved. http://www.amanet.org.

4. *Inadequate computer systems:* If the system, no matter how technically sophisticated it is, is not adequate to deliver the desired result from the patient's perspective, then it is inadequate for use in a patient-focused culture. When a staff member needs to go through multiple gyrations just to schedule a follow-up appointment for a patient—resulting in more waiting and delays—then, no matter how useful the resulting database of patient visit information, the system needs to be changed, or the way the staff is trained to use the system needs to be adjusted.

5. *Lack of support from other departments:* As was discussed in Chapter 13, a service-oriented organizational culture can only be built when there is ongoing cooperation and support between departments throughout the organization.

6. *Inadequate training in people skills:* Patients obtain two results when they experience health care. The first is an outcome result: Did the patient get what he or she wanted in the first place? For example, a physical examination. The second is a process result: What was the patient's total experience in getting what he or she was after? Throughout this book, particularly in Chapter 5, we emphasized the myriad of patient interactions and observations that all combine to form your organization's grades on their mental report cards. The consistently appropriate management of each moment of truth and surrogate perception can only be expected if sufficient training—coupled with assurances for transfer of skills to the workplace—is provided.

7. *Low morale; no team spirit:* A great deal of research clearly indicates that there is a positive correlation between employee satisfaction and patient/customer satisfaction. Your health care organization cannot hope to satisfy patients consistently if it can't satisfy internal customers first. Employees tend to treat patients the way they are treated by their employer.

8. *Bad organizational policies and procedures:* The purpose of policies and procedures is to make your organization easy for patients to do business with. Bad policies and procedures prevent you from meeting the specific needs and expectations of patients. Recall from our discussion of the dimensions of service quality in Chapter 2 (Figure 2–2) that too much emphasis on procedural matters with little regard for the personal dimension of service results in a "by-the-book" attitude, resulting in such dreaded phrases as, "I've got to follow these rules" or, worse yet, "That's not our policy." When policies and procedures are viewed as laws or holy

writs, the flexibility required to meet a patient's individual needs is lost. Furthermore, employees can't begin to feel empowered to act in a patient's best interest when they are constrained by inflexible policies and procedures.

You may wish to use these guidelines as a framework for identifying potential obstacles to implementing your PSI program. One helpful approach is to use a force-field analysis, wherein "drivers" and "resistors" to implementing change are identified during a brainstorming session. This technique was explained in Chapter 10. Figure 10–8 may be used as a form with which to guide this discussion. Remember that the purpose of this step is to focus your attention on developing predetermined methods for overcoming any and all obstacles to your progress.

SKILLS, KNOWLEDGE, AND PEOPLE REQUIRED FOR ACHIEVING EACH OBJECTIVE

Each step involved in implementing your solution or proposed improvement will require certain skills and knowledge. By carefully identifying these requirements for each objective, you will develop an understanding of who will need to be involved in the project. This, in turn, will help you decide whether or not the use of one or more outside consultants will be necessary. Armed with this information, you will be in a good position to develop projections for the financial, human resource, and time requirements of part or all of your PSI program. Exhibit 14–4 shows a simple format for identifying the skills needed for the implementation of each objective to achieve the overall goal of your PSI program.

Chapter References for Review

- Chapter 3: The Elements of Patient Satisfaction: What Patients Value in Health Care
- Chapter 4: The Relative Importance Index: Determining the Relative Importance of Each Patient Satisfaction Element
- Chapter 6: Measuring Patient Satisfaction: Determining an Organization's Grades on The Patient's Mental Report Card
- Chapter 8: Identifying and Prioritizing Service Quality Improvement Needs
- Chapter 9: Addressing Behavior-Based Improvement Priorities

Exhibit 14–4 Identifying Skills Needed to Achieve Each of Your PSI Objectives

Solution/Improvement Objective	Skills and Knowledge Required
Identify the elements that determine external customer (patient/member) satisfaction.	• Literature review skills—library and on-line • Critical reviewing of survey instruments • Facilitation skills—conduct brainstorming sessions
Determine the relative importance ("relative weight") of the various elements within each satisfaction category.	• Focus group methodology • Basic research statistics • Research report preparation
Develop and administer a means of measuring current patient/member satisfaction that is organizationwide, as well as region-, health care center-, department-, health care provider- and employee category-specific.	• Survey research methodology—objectives, design, testing, validation • Computer design/layout software—*Quark Express* • Commercial printing • Understand scan technology
Identify current patient/member perceived service quality (satisfaction element) "strengths and weaknesses" throughout our health care organization.	• Data analysis, display, and reporting • Designate data tally formats for scan vendor
Design an approach for bringing about prioritized improvement in service quality areas perceived as "weaknesses" while sustaining currently perceived service quality areas of "strengths."	• Quantitative research methodology • Data analysis—determine strengths/weaknesses • Data communication skills • Distinguish behavior-based, systems/process-based, and administration-based improvement priorities (basis of improvement mechanisms)

continues

Exhibit 14–4 continued

Solution/Improvement Objective	Skills and Knowledge Required
Deliver education and training designed to improve behavior-based components of patient/member perceived service quality (i.e., satisfaction) "weaknesses."	• Principles of adult learning • Instructional design • Presentation and group facilitation skills • Kirkpatrick's 4-level effectiveness evaluation model • Transfer of training enhancement techniques
Develop mechanisms for capturing local health care center and departmental suggestions for improving systems and process components of patient/member perceived "weaknesses" in service quality.	• Facilitation skills—small group discussion • Systems thinking • Basic CQI tool and technique application
Continuously evaluate the effectiveness of all patient satisfaction improvement efforts.	• Data analysis, display, and reporting • Kirkpatrick's 4-level effectiveness evaluation model • Trend analysis

ACTION PLAN FOR THE ACHIEVEMENT OF EACH OBJECTIVE

In order to meet the challenge of converting knowledge to action that leads to desired results, there needs to be a detailed plan in place. You may already have an action planning format that you are comfortable with. There are a variety of project planning software programs commercially available. Some are quite simple, whereas others require a rather large "learning curve" investment of time. By all means, use what you have been successful with in the past. At the very least, make sure it contains sufficient detail to both satisfy the most scrutinizing stakeholder—convincing him or her that you have carefully thought the entire project through—and guide you and your team through the patient satisfaction measurement and improvement process.

Exhibits 14–5 through 14–10 contain action steps associated with six different objectives of a patient satisfaction measurement and improvement program.

Most certainly you will want to adapt these to the specific needs of your health care organization. If you enlist the services of an outside market research firm, you will not need various components of this plan—namely, those associated with measuring patient satisfaction.

Exhibit 14–5 Sample Action Plan for Determining Patient Satisfaction Elements

Objective: Identify the elements that determine patient satisfaction.	Starting Date	Ending Date	Completed (X)
1. Read *Measuring and Improving Patient Satisfaction*			
2. Conduct a literature review—on-line re: service quality in health care.			
3. Review existing external customer satisfaction survey instruments. a. Nonhealth care service industry surveys b. Health care patient satisfaction surveys (both managed care and FFS) – any existing within our organization – other health care organizations – other firms consulting to health care organizations			
4. Obtain employee input during established meeting times. a. Facilitate discussions during departmental staff meetings b. Managers conduct brainstorming sessions—using supplied packets – identify local department contributions to the patient's mental report card: *moments of truth* and *surrogate perceptions*			
5. Review accrediting agency patient satisfaction measurement elements.			

continues

Exhibit 14–5 continued

	Starting Date	Ending Date	Completed (X)
6. Attend relevant conference(s) conducted by credible market research firms or American Marketing Association or health care consultants.			
7. Develop your organization's implications of the element categories: access, convenience, communication, quality of care, personal caring, and facilities.			
8. Identify "service quality indicators"—behaviors required to arrive at each satisfaction element in the patient's MRC.			

Exhibit 14–6 Sample Action Plan for Determining Satisfaction Element Relative Importance

Objective: Determine the relative importance of the various elements of patient satisfaction.	Starting Date	Ending Date	Completed (X)
1. Develop a plan for conducting focus group research (decide whether to incorporate electronic keypad response technology to quantify responses).			
2. Establish focus group participant selection criteria. a. By age groups b. By most recent visit to your health care facility			
3. Determine participation incentives—gift certificates?. . . cash?			
4. Randomly select focus group participants from targeted population.			

continues

Exhibit 14–6 continued

	Starting Date	Ending Date	Completed (X)
a. Assign numbers to letters of the alphabet. b. Select a random sequence of alphabet letters (table of random #s). c. Randomly select participants in respective groups.			

5. Design participant contact/ communication sequences.
  a. Telephone call
  b. Confirmation letter
  c. Thank you letters as follow-up			

6. Develop *Focus Group Facilitator's Guide.*			
7. Conduct focus groups.			

8. Report focus group data—producing *relative importance index (RII).*
  a. Comparative tables (by designated groups and quantified totals)
  b. Comparative bar charts to contrast grouping differences			

9. Calculate *relative importance index* for each of your facilities.
  a. Obtain MIS listing of quantity (number and percentage) of each of the focus group descriptors (i.e., age group, etc.) for each facility
  b. Calculate the weighted mean *relative importance index* for each satisfaction element in each satisfaction category.
    – Multiply the percentage of each group by the respective RII.
    – Add all weighted RIIs for each element with each category.
    – Divide sum of weighted RIIs by the # of focus groups conducted.			

Exhibit 14–7 Sample Action Plan for Developing and Administering Patient Satisfaction Survey

Objective: Develop and administer a means of measuring current patient satisfaction that is organizationwide, region-specific, health care center-specific, department specific, employee category-specific, and provider-specific.	Starting Date	Ending Date	Completed (X)

1. Review the file of existing patient satisfaction survey instruments (or contract with an outside survey research firm).
  a. Format
  b. Design and layout
  c. Rating scales
  d. Demographic measurements			

2. Develop survey research objectives.
  a. Measure current patient satisfaction levels—as outlined in objective.
  b. Include all elements identified in Exhibit 14–6 above.
  c. Obtain a response rate in excess of 25%? 30%? 50%?			

3. Create incentive for completing relatively long survey instrument.
  a. 20 $50 awards (green index raffle for "on-site"; yellow for "mail-in" response)
    – 90% of awards (18) for on-site respondents
    – 10% of awards (2) for mail-in respondents
  b. Opportunity to "be heard" re: satisfaction perceptions
  c. Opportunity to contribute to improvement efforts			

4. Design satisfaction survey instrument.
  a. Create sequence of "drafts," each modified to reflect feedback pertaining to layout, visual appeal, ease of understanding instructions, clarity of language for each survey item, logic of category, and element sequencing from:
    – Patients			

continues

Exhibit 14–7 continued

	Starting Date	Ending Date	Completed (X)

– Internal customers—employees of your health care organization
– Marketing consultants, students, experts
b. Final layout and design completed (English version)
c. Spanish (or other needed language) translation
  – literal translation
  – colloquial translation			

5. Satisfaction survey instrument evaluated by marketing research firm contracted to provide *intelligent character recognition (ICR)* scanning of completed surveys.			
6. Arrange for survey instrument printing. a. Determine number (English + Other language) needed b. Price comparison via print broker, etc.			

7. Monitor survey response rates
a. Survey administrators report number of surveys administered daily
  – # completed on-site and returned to survey administrator
  – Given to patient with postage-paid envelope for mail-in
b. Contact each facility to determine total number of patients seen at that facility during the survey day.
c. Market research firm reports number of mail-in surveys (with yellow index-card raffle cards).
d. Market research firm reports number of on-site survey responses received from each facility.			

8. Report of actual response rates. a. Total number of patients seen at each facility on survey date b. Actual number of surveys scanned by market research firm for each facility – Number accompanied by yellow index raffle cards = mail-in			

continues

Exhibit 14–7 continued

	Starting Date	Ending Date	Completed (X)

– Remaining completed surveys = on-site responses
c. Report of response rates for each facility
    – Response rate—on-site survey completion = total # on-site surveys ÷ total # of patients seen at each facility each day
    – Response rate for mail-in survey completion = total # mail-in surveys ÷ total # of mail-in surveys distributed to patients at each facility			

Exhibit 14–8 Sample Action Plan for Identifying Service Quality "Strengths" and "Weaknesses"

Objective: Identify current patient member perceived service quality (satisfaction element) "strengths" and "weaknesses" throughout our health care organization.	Starting Date	Ending Date	Completed (X)

1. Define "strengths" and "weaknesses" in terms of perceived patient satisfaction.
  a. "Strengths" = "satisfied" ("good" + "very good" + "excellent" ratings) with a frequency of 80% or better
  b. "Weaknesses" = "dissatisfied" ("fair" + "poor" ratings) with a frequency of 20% or greater			

2. Design a method of reporting the "satisfaction" data, allowing for easy identification of "strengths."
  a. Data tables showing absolute and relative frequency of "top 3 boxes"
  b. Comparative analysis data provided
    – First visit (yes/no)
    – Age grouping			

continues

Exhibit 14–8 continued

	Starting Date	Ending Date	Completed (X)
– Comparison of each facility to organization composite – Comparison of each facility to region composite c. Data display of "dissatisfaction" deferred* (*Dissatisfaction data will be combined with the appropriate *relative importance index (RII)* to yield the more actionable *improvement priority index (IPI)*)			

3. Develop plan for data distribution.
   a. Determine which data to be provided to whom
   b. Timing of data distribution and special report generation
   c. Format(s) for data distribution to different stakeholder groups			

Exhibit 14–9 Sample Action Plan for Bringing about Prioritized Improvements

Objective: Design an approach for bringing about prioritized improvement in service quality areas perceived as "weaknesses" while sustaining currently perceived service quality areas of "strengths."	Starting Date	Ending Date	Completed (X)

1. Devise a mechanism for prioritizing improvements to be targeted generally, by facility specifically.
   a. *Improvement priority index (IPI) = RII × dissatisfaction index (DI)*
   b. Make sure the RII component of the IPI reflects the differences (age and other demographic descriptors used for your focus groups) in relative importance based on the unique demographic composition of each facility in your health care organiza-			

continues

Exhibit 14–9 continued

	Starting Date	Ending Date	Completed (X)
tion. That is, a weighted figure for the RII will reflect the facility's percentage of each demographic group studied in the focus groups			
2. Identify the top 10–15 improvement priorities for your entire health care organization (i.e., composite of all facilities). a. Mathematically top 10–15 IPI items per facility b. Data display to consist of Pareto Charts for each facility, region, and health care organization composite			
3. Separate improvement priorities into three main categories, based on the mechanism for improvement: a. Behavior-based—requiring training re: "service indicators" (targeted toward both staff and health care providers) – Skills – Knowledge – Attitudes b. Systems and process-based—requiring training, followed by facilitation of teams formed to either improve existing processes or completely reengineer them c. Administration-based—requiring a careful revisiting of the organization's vision, values, and mission; also requiring the development of a service-oriented organizational culture; involves the allocation of financial and human resources for needed changes, particularly those negative "surrogate perceptions" related to the appearance, maintenance, and functionality of facilities and equipment			

continues

Exhibit 14–9 continued

	Starting Date	Ending Date	Completed (X)

4. Identify those patient satisfaction elements that have yielded a grade of "satisfied."
  a. Note those behaviors, processes, procedures (i.e., "best practices")
  b. Standardize the identified "best practices" into organizationwide policies and procedures and performance standards			

Exhibit 14–10 Sample Action Plan for Addressing Behavior-Based Improvement Priorities

Objective: Deliver assessment-driven education and training designed to improve behavior-based components of patient/member perceived service quality (satisfaction) "weaknesses."	Starting Date	Ending Date	Completed (X)

1. Identify "baseline" patient satisfaction skill requirements (including an overview of your organization's PSI program) and deliver to all employees and health care providers in appropriate settings:
  a. New employee orientation
  b. Existing employee reorientation
  c. Ongoing staff development workshops
  d. Provider communication workshops			

2. Identify the top 5–10 improvement priorities for each health care facility.
  a. Determine which improvement priorities are:
    – Behavior-based
    – Systems and process-based
    – Administration-, facilities/equipment-based
  b. Create a prioritized list of behavior-based improvement priorities.			

continues

Exhibit 14–10 continued

	Starting Date	Ending Date	Completed (X)
3. List the "service indicators" (behaviors) that lead to satisfaction in each of the elements listed as a behavior-based improvement priority.			
4. Provide workshops that are modular in design so as to be able to easily be "customized" to meet the identified improvement priorities of each facility. a. Conduct an appropriate needs assessment to clarify specific learning and environmental challenges of each facility. b. Instructional design utilizing adult learning principles, keeping all workshops highly interactive, interesting, and enjoyable.			
5. Follow principles of training effectiveness using Kirkpatrick's *4-level evaluation model* as outlined in Chapter 9.			

However, if you wish to convert the data obtained from the outside firm to actionable change that delivers the business results (improved patient satisfaction and loyalty) you desire, you will need to develop a plan with a similar level of detail, or a level of detail that is greater than what is presented here.

Chapter References for Review

- Chapter 2: The Definition and Dimensions of Service Quality
- Chapter 5: The Patient's Mental Report Card: A Model of How Patients Judge Their Health Care Experiences
- Chapter 9: Addressing Behavior-Based Improvement Priorities
- Chapter 13: Building and Sustaining a Service-Oriented Organizational Culture

ONGOING ASSESSMENT OF OVERALL PSI PROGRAM VALUE

A careful review of the assessment methods discussed in Chapter 12 will serve well to guide you in your planning of the ongoing assessment of your patient satisfaction program.

It is my sincere hope that, with the application of the principles and methodologies presented throughout this book, the patients who patronize your health care organization will acknowledge and appreciate your commitment to making their health care experiences better and better over time. As a direct consequence of this, your organization, assuming other variables to be well managed, can expect to reap the myriad of benefits associated with the establishment of a continuously improving service-oriented health care organization culture.

CONCLUSION

The primary objective of this chapter is to provide a framework for the reader to convert the information presented throughout the book into positive organizational action that will improve patient satisfaction. The PSI planning model (Figure 14–1) is designed to be used generally as an overall approach to your PSI program and individually for each of your behavior-based and systems-based improvement efforts.

Recall that the sequential steps of the model are: develop a problem statement, list adverse consequences of the problem, determine the goal and objectives of the ideal solution, identify relevant organizational constraints, establish solution selection criteria, list the benefits of solving the problem effectively, list the potential obstacles to problem resolution, identify the skills and knowledge required to achieve each objective, list the people/groups/organizations to work with for each step, develop an action plan for achieving each objective, schedule the action plan implementation, implement the action plan, and finally, provide ongoing assessment of success.

The problem (or "opportunity for improvement") is a condition or set of circumstances that an individual, group, or entire organization thinks should be changed. The problem statement should be objectively stated, focused, written in simple terms, and concise—25 words or less. Then, in order to obtain the necessary resources for solving the problem, those individuals responsible for allocating those resources need to be convinced that the problem is worth solving. This is best accomplished by listing the adverse consequences—on both internal and external customers—of the existence of the problem. In the context of patient satisfaction, this includes such items as competitive disadvantage, increased number of patient complaints, increased number of patients leaving, and so forth.

The goal of solving your stated problem should be to bridge the identified patient satisfaction "gap." Also, series of objectives need to be developed to support the achievement of the goal. Next, list any organizational constraints that may limit your ability to achieve the goal. These commonly fall within the categories of time, human resources, or financial resources. Then, with the relevant constraints in mind, develop a list of "weighted" (i.e., assigning a relative importance weight to each) criteria that need to be met by the "ideal solution." This leads directly to applying the criteria to a brainstormed list of possible solutions. The result is appropriate solution selection.

It is extremely important to list the benefits of solving the problem or achieving the desired improvement. This provides sufficient incentive (along with the adverse consequences of the existence of the problem) to get the "powers that be" to allocate the necessary resources for problem resolution. By reviewing Chapter 1, you can develop a general list of benefits. Then, a careful look at the specific improvement desired will reveal more problem-specific benefits for the list. The next step is to think carefully about, and list, the potential obstacles that might be encountered in your attempt to implement the proposed solution. As part of this process, think in terms of how each obstacle might be overcome. Generally speaking, it is more effective to identify and minimize/eliminate "resisters" to change than to attempt to strengthen the "drivers" of change.

The next step involves a clear identification of the skills, knowledge, and people needed to achieve each of the objectives that supports the improvement goal. This will serve as a basis for determining financial, human, and time requirements. Now, develop a detailed (i.e., step-by-step) action plan for the achievement of each objective of the improvement goal. Then commit this action plan to a schedule that lists "starting date" and "ending date" for each item along with a "completed" check-box. Once you have implemented the improvement, periodically evaluate the effectiveness of the change with the intention of further improvement.

ACTION STEPS

1. Select one opportunity for improvement based on your prioritized list of needed improvements. Work through the PSI

planning model presented in Figure 14–1 in planning the needed change(s). Implement the change(s) and make any needed adjustments.

2. Use the PSI planning model along with selected information presented throughout this book to orchestrate a renewed organizational commitment to improving patient satisfaction continuously.

3. Constantly monitor and celebrate the benefits of this renewed commitment.

REFERENCES

Albrecht, K. (1994). *The northbound train: Finding the purpose, setting the direction, shaping the destiny of your organization.* New York: AMACOM.

Connellan, T.K., & Zemke, R. (1993). *Sustaining knock your socks off service.* New York: AMACOM, 13.

LeBoeuf, M. (1985). *The greatest management principle in the world.* New York: Berkley Books.

Nadler, G., & Hibino, S. (1994). *Breakthrough thinking: The seven principles of creative problem-solving* (2nd ed.). Rocklin, CA: Prima.

Osborne, D., & Gaebler, T. (1994). *Reinventing government.* London: Penguin.

SUGGESTED READING

Albrecht, K. (1992). *The only thing that matters.* New York: Harper Business.

Albrecht, K., & Bradford, L.J. (1990). *The service advantage: How to identify and fulfill customer needs.* Homewood, IL: Dow Jones-Irwin.

Davidow, W.H., & Uttal, B. (1989). *Total customer service: The ultimate weapon.* New York: Harper & Row.

Heskett, J.L., Sasser, W., & Hart, C. (1997). *The service profit chain: How leading companies link profit and growth to loyalty, satisfaction, and value.* New York: The Free Press.

Kelly, P.K. (1994). *Team decision-making techniques: A practical guide to successful team outcomes.* Irvine, CA: Richard Chang Associates.

Leland, K., & Bailey, K. (1995). *Customer service for dummies.* Chicago: IDG Books Worldwide.

Wellington, P. (1995). *Kaizen strategies for customer care: How to create a powerful customer care program—and make it work.* London: Pitman.

Whiteley, R., & Hessan, D. (1996). *Customer centered growth: Five proven strategies for building competitive advantage.* Menlo Park, CA: Addison-Wesley.

Zeithaml, V.A., Parasuraman, A., & Berry, L.L. (1990). Delivering quality service: Balancing customer perceptions and expectations. New York: The Free Press.

Appendix A

Focus Group Moderator's Guide

I. **Welcome to Focus Group Meeting**
   A. Greeting to meeting room—provide a name tag (pre-printed)
   B. Provide participants with food and beverages
   C. Interact with participants—small talk

II. **Introduction**
   A. Introduce moderators
   B. Introduce any additional personnel present
   C. Briefly explain the purpose(s) of the session:
      1. "To better understand what is important to you in determining your satisfaction with services provided"
      2. "To help improve services for members"
   D. Clarify that this is *not* designed to measure their current level of satisfaction (this will be measured using other techniques later—surveys etc.)
   E. Alert participants to the audio and/or video recorders that are recording the session (emphasize that these are only for ensuring accuracy of our research)
   F. Inform participants that they will be using keypads during the session, and that they will receive instructions for using them.
   G. Assure confidentiality
      1. Participant names are *not* shared with any providers
      2. The combined information is for research purposes (and may be published at a later date).

Courtesy of Friendly Hills HealthCare Network.

461

    H. Participants introduce themselves
        1. First name only
        2. How long they have been a member

III. Warm-up
    A. "When you think of excellent health care, what comes to mind?"
        1. Have a scribe record these on a flipchart
        2. Use our *service categories* to get the discussion going

IV. Research details provided to participants
    A. Show the 6 service categories (i.e., all at once) that we will be working with one at a time.
    B. Explain that there are various elements of service within each category
        1. For example, under "Access to Care," several elements would include:
           a. Ease of scheduling appointments by phone
           b. Ease of scheduling appointments in person
           c. Length of time you waited between preferred appointment day and day of your visit
    C. Explain that, in order for members to be satisfied with each element of services at your health care organization, our providers or employees need to do a variety of things
        1. For example, under "Ease of scheduling appointments by phone":
           a. Telephone needs to be answered promptly
           b. You prefer speaking to a person (vs. a "machine")
           c. No long periods of time on "hold" etc.
        2. These things are called *service indicators* for purposes of this research
    D. Explain how the research will be conducted:
        1. We will concentrate on one *service category* at a time (Access to Care, Convenience, Communication, etc.)
        2. Within each *service category,* we will ask you, as a group to do **two things:**
           a. Rank the relative importance to you of the various *service elements* (in determining your satisfaction with FHHN)
             1) First you'll view the list of service elements
             2) Discuss which elements are most important to you
             3) Use your keypad to individually rank the elements

     b. Rank the relative importance of the various *service indicators* within each element
       1) First view the list of service indicators
       2) Add any additional *service indicators* they can think of
       3) Discuss which elements are must important to you
       4) Use key pad to rank *service indicators*
   3. After each ranking, you will see the results on the screen
   4. Detailed explanation of key pad use for ranking

V. Key Contents of Research
   A. Proceed through the outline of *service categories, service elements,* and *service indicators* in the order presented
   B. Rank only *elements* of "FHHN Facility" category (i.e., not *service indicators,* since this category consists of surrogate perceptions only)

VI. Conclusion
   A. Thank participants for their hard work and feedback
   B. Distribute incentive items to participants
     1. Gift certificates
     2. Information items re: FHHN services and educational programs

FOCUS GROUP PRE-MEETING CHECKLIST

❑   Determine selection criteria for participation
❑   Obtain list of potential participants
❑   Randomly select desired participants
❑   Randomly select "backup" participants
❑   Determine available dates & times for moderator
❑   Determine availability of needed equipment
❑   Select meeting dates and times
❑   Schedule meeting facilities
❑   Determine participation incentives
❑   Develop dialogue for contacting selected participants
❑   Contact each participant
❑   Create master list of participants for each session
❑   Send confirmation letters to all participants
❑   Arrange for food and beverages to be served
❑   Purchase incentive gifts
❑   Assemble information packets
❑   Orient moderator(s) to format, flow, and content of research
❑   Confirmation telephone calls 24 hours before each session
❑   Prepare name tag for participants and moderator(s)
❑   Arrange for room setup—seating in a "U" shape
❑   Arrange for equipment setup
❑   Review logistics of facilitation
❑   Rehearse welcome and introduction

Patient Satisfaction Survey Instrument

Courtesy of Friendly Hills HealthCare Network.

FRIENDLY HILLS
MEDICAL GROUP
Patient Satisfaction Survey

| Health Care Center | 1 3 |
| Provider | |

Directions

Dear Patient: As part of our continuing effort to improve quality and services, we ask that you assist us by participating in this survey about your recent visit to one of our health care providers.

Below are a number of questions about your **most recent visit**. Please answer each question by checking the box that best describes your opinion. If the patient is a minor child or cannot complete the survey, please make sure that it is completed by a family member. If you have visited a Friendly Hills Health Care Center in the past, please answer only about your **most recent visit** to a health care provider.

As our way of thanking you for your help, your name will be entered into a drawing for a **Cash Award of $50.00**. A total of 20 cash awards will be given out based on a random drawing. Please express your opinions openly and honestly. Your responses will be kept <u>completely confidential</u>, so you are assured that your identity and responses will not be shared with your health care providers at Friendly Hills Health Care Center.

When making your selection, please fill in the box representing your rating: ❑ ➝ ■

Thank you for participating in this survey. Your input is very important in helping us improve our services.

Access: Arranging For & Getting Health Care

How would you grade the:

	Poor	Fair	Good	Very Good	Excellent	Does not apply
1. Ease of scheduling appointments by phone --------	❑	❑	❑	❑	❑	❑
2. Ease of scheduling appointments in person --------	❑	❑	❑	❑	❑	❑
3. Length of time you waited before you could see your health care provider----------------------------------	❑	❑	❑	❑	❑	❑
4. Amount of time waiting in reception room------------	❑	❑	❑	❑	❑	❑
5. Amount of time waiting in exam room before seeing your health care provider-----------------------	❑	❑	❑	❑	❑	❑
6. Access to medical care in an emergency -----------	❑	❑	❑	❑	❑	❑
7. Ease of seeing health care provider of your choice	❑	❑	❑	❑	❑	❑
8. Ease of getting medical information using the Telephone Advice System ------------------------------	❑	❑	❑	❑	❑	❑

Convenience

How would you grade the convenience of:

	Poor	Fair	Good	Very Good	Excellent	Does not apply
1. Location of the Health Care Center you visited-----	❑	❑	❑	❑	❑	❑
2. Hours of the Health Care Center you visited -------	❑	❑	❑	❑	❑	❑
3. Parking at the Health Care Center---------------------	❑	❑	❑	❑	❑	❑
4. Services for getting prescriptions filled --------------	❑	❑	❑	❑	❑	❑
5. Getting prescriptions refilled ---------------------------	❑	❑	❑	❑	❑	❑
6. Getting laboratory work done when ordered by your provider ---	❑	❑	❑	❑	❑	❑
7. Getting X-rays which your provider ordered---------	❑	❑	❑	❑	❑	❑

Communication

How would you grade the:	Poor	Fair	Good	Very Good	Excellent	Does not apply
1. Health care provider's explanation of your medical problem	❑	❑	❑	❑	❑	❑
2. Health care provider's explanation of required medical procedures and/or lab tests	❑	❑	❑	❑	❑	❑
3. Explanation of prescribed medicine(s)	❑	❑	❑	❑	❑	❑
4. Communication between provider and staff	❑	❑	❑	❑	❑	❑
5. Willingness of the health care provider to listen	❑	❑	❑	❑	❑	❑
6. Explanation of any required consents	❑	❑	❑	❑	❑	❑
7. Education about ways to manage your current health problem	❑	❑	❑	❑	❑	❑
8. Education about ways to avoid illness	❑	❑	❑	❑	❑	❑
9. Availability of educational programs which teach healthier living	❑	❑	❑	❑	❑	❑
10. Reminders to use preventive services (PAP smear, Prostate screen etc.)	❑	❑	❑	❑	❑	❑

Quality of Health Care You Received

How would you grade the:	Poor	Fair	Good	Very Good	Excellent	Does not apply
1. Thoroughness of the health care provider's exam	❑	❑	❑	❑	❑	❑
2. Amount of time health care provider spent with you	❑	❑	❑	❑	❑	❑
3. Thoroughness of medical treatment received	❑	❑	❑	❑	❑	❑
4. How well health care provider and nursing staff work as a team to serve your health needs	❑	❑	❑	❑	❑	❑
5. Overall quality of care from health care provider	❑	❑	❑	❑	❑	❑
6. Overall quality of care from nursing staff	❑	❑	❑	❑	❑	❑

Personal Caring

How would you grade the:	Poor	Fair	Good	Very Good	Excellent	Does not apply
1. Friendliness and courtesy shown by health care provider	❑	❑	❑	❑	❑	❑
2. Friendliness and courtesy shown by nursing staff	❑	❑	❑	❑	❑	❑
3. Friendliness and courtesy shown by receptionist	❑	❑	❑	❑	❑	❑
4. Respect shown to you by health care provider	❑	❑	❑	❑	❑	❑
5. Respect shown to you by nursing staff	❑	❑	❑	❑	❑	❑
6. Respect shown to you by the receptionist	❑	❑	❑	❑	❑	❑
7. Personal concern shown by health care provider	❑	❑	❑	❑	❑	❑
8. Personal concern shown by the nursing staff	❑	❑	❑	❑	❑	❑
9. Personal concern shown by receptionist	❑	❑	❑	❑	❑	❑
10. Telephone courtesy when calling Health Center	❑	❑	❑	❑	❑	❑

Friendly Hills Health Care Center Facility

How would you grade the:	Poor	Fair	Good	Very Good	Excellent	Does not apply
1. Overall outside appearance of the Health Center--	❏	❏	❏	❏	❏	❏
2. Appearance of signs on outside of building ----------	❏	❏	❏	❏	❏	❏
3. Cleanliness of the reception area ----------------------	❏	❏	❏	❏	❏	❏
4. Cleanliness of the treatment area ---------------------	❏	❏	❏	❏	❏	❏
5. Comfort of the indoor temperature --------------------	❏	❏	❏	❏	❏	❏
6. Neatness of the reception room -----------------------	❏	❏	❏	❏	❏	❏
7. Neatness of the receptionist's work area ------------	❏	❏	❏	❏	❏	❏
8. Neatness of the treatment area ------------------------	❏	❏	❏	❏	❏	❏
9. Noise level (quietness) in the office --------------------	❏	❏	❏	❏	❏	❏
10. Air quality (freshness) in the Health Care Center---	❏	❏	❏	❏	❏	❏

General Information

1. Was this your first visit to a Friendly Hills Health Care Center?   ❏ Yes   ❏ No

2. How often have you (the patient) seen a health care provider (here or elsewhere) in the past year?
   ❏ Once   ❏ Twice   ❏ Three or more times

3. Are you (the patient):   ❏ Male   ❏ Female

4. What is your (the patient's) age?:
   ❏ under 6 yrs   ❏ 16-25 yrs   ❏ 36-45 yrs   ❏ 56-65 yrs   ❏ over 75 yrs
   ❏ 6-15 yrs   ❏ 26-35 yrs   ❏ 46-55 yrs   ❏ 66-75 yrs

5. How long have you been a member of Friendly Hills HealthCare Network?
   ❏ Less than 1 yr   ❏ 1-2 yrs   ❏ 3-5 yrs   ❏ 6-10 yrs   ❏ 11 years or more

6. Do you intend to remain a member of Friendly Hills HealthCare Network?   ❏ Yes   ❏ No

7. All things considered, how satisfied are you with Friendly Hills HealthCare Network?
   ❏ Completely satisfied, couldn't be better   ❏ Somewhat dissatisfied
   ❏ Very satisfied   ❏ Very dissatisfied
   ❏ Somewhat satisfied   ❏ Completely dissatisfied, couldn't be worse
                     ❏ Neither satisfied or dissatisfied

8. Would you recommend this Friendly Hills Health Care Center to your family and/or friends?
   ❏ Yes   ❏ No

Please place your survey in the SURVEY COLLECTION BOX

THANK YOU FOR YOUR COOPERATION!

COMMENTS

_____

_____

_____

_____

_____

_____

_____

_____

_____

_____

_____

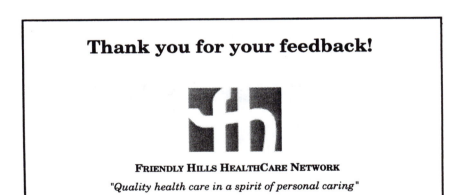

Thank you for your feedback!

FRIENDLY HILLS HEALTHCARE NETWORK

"Quality health care in a spirit of personal caring"

FRIENDLY HILLS MEDICAL GROUP
QUESTIONARIO DE SATISFACION DEL CLIENTO

| Health Care Center | ☐ ☐ |
| Provider | ☐ ☐ |

Instruciónes

Querido Paciente: Como parte de nuestro deseo de mejorar la calídad y los servicos que ofresemos, le pedimos que nos ayúden y participen en esta incuesta sobre la ultima visita que tuvo con su doctor.

Las preguntas que siguen sobre su última visita. Por favor responda cada pregunta marcando el cuadro que mejor indíca su opinión. Si el paciente es un menor de edad no puede completar el questionario, favor de asegurarse que un miembro de la familia lo complete. Si usted a visitado Friendly Hills Health Care Center antes, favor de contestar las preguntas acerca de su última cita.

En agradecimiento por su ayuda, su nombre va hacer puesto en una rifa para recibir $50. Un total de 20 personas van a ganar los $50. Por favor exprese su opinión honestamente. Su repuestas se mantendran completamente confidencial, asi que puede estar segúro que su identidad y sus respuestas no seran compartidas con su doctor de Friendly Hills Health Care Center.

Cuando haga su selection por favor llene el cuadro reprentando su calificacion ☐ ➡ ■
Gracias por participar en este questenario. Su opinion es muy importante ya que nos ayudara a mejorar los servicios le que ofrecemos.

Acceso Obteniendo Cuídado de Salúd

Como classifica usted lo siguiente:	Mal	Mas o Menos	Bien	Muy Bien	Excelente	No Aplicable
1. La facílidad de hacer citas por telefono----	☐	☐	☐	☐	☐	☐
2. La facílidad de hacer citas en persona----	☐	☐	☐	☐	☐	☐
3. La cantidad de tiempo que espero entre el día preferido de su cita y el dia que le dieron su sita---	☐	☐	☐	☐	☐	☐
4. El tiempo que espero en la sala de espera----	☐	☐	☐	☐	☐	☐
5. La cantidad de tiempo que espero en el cuarto de examinación antes que entre el doctor----	☐	☐	☐	☐	☐	☐
6. Acceso al cúidado medíco en caso de emergencia	☐	☐	☐	☐	☐	☐
7. La facílidad de ver al doctor que ústed prefiere----	☐	☐	☐	☐	☐	☐
8. La facílidad de reciber·informacion medíca cúando usa el Telephone Advice System----	☐	☐	☐	☐	☐	☐

Conveniencia:

Como calífica lo siguiente:

	Mal	Mas o Menos	Bien	Muy Bien	Excelente	No Aplicable
1. La localídad del centro de salud que visito----	☐	☐	☐	☐	☐	☐
2. Las horas que atiende el centro de salúd que visito	☐	☐	☐	☐	☐	☐
3. El estacionamiento que hubo cúando ústed llego----	☐	☐	☐	☐	☐	☐
4. El servicio que le ofrecieron en la farmacia----	☐	☐	☐	☐	☐	☐
5. El recíbir su receta/medicamentos----	☐	☐	☐	☐	☐	☐
6. El obtener servicios del laboratorio cúando su doctor los orderna----	☐	☐	☐	☐	☐	☐
7. Obteniendo rayos-X cuando su doctor lo ordena----	☐	☐	☐	☐	☐	☐

Comunicación

Como clasifica ústed lo siguiente:	Mal	Mas o Menos	Bien	Muy Bien	Excelente	No Aplicable
1. La explicación de su doctor sobre su problema medíco--	❑	❑	❑	❑	❑	❑
2. La explicación de su doctor sobre procedimientos medícos o examenes de laboratorio--------------------	❑	❑	❑	❑	❑	❑
3. La explicación sobre el medícamento que le receto	❑	❑	❑	❑	❑	❑
4. La comunicación entre el doctor y el resto del personal--	❑	❑	❑	❑	❑	❑
5. El deseo de su doctor a escúcharle ------------------	❑	❑	❑	❑	❑	❑
6. La explicación de algún consentimiento--------------	❑	❑	❑	❑	❑	❑
7. La educación sobre las maneras de controlar su problema de salúd actúal----------------------------------	❑	❑	❑	❑	❑	❑
8. La educatión sobre maneras de evitar las enferme-dades---	❑	❑	❑	❑	❑	❑
9. La abilidád de ofrecer programas educacionales que promocíonan una vida mas saludable-----------	❑	❑	❑	❑	❑	❑
10.El apoyo/mensaje de usar los servicios prevenen-tivos (como el papanicolau, del prostate, etc)-------	❑	❑	❑	❑	❑	❑

Calídad del Cuidad de Salúd que Recibió

Como clasificá ústed los siguiente:						
1. La efícez del exámen médico que le hizo su doctor-	❑	❑	❑	❑	❑	❑
2. La cantídad de tiempo que el doctor le dio a usted--	❑	❑	❑	❑	❑	❑
3. La efícez del tratamiento medíco que recibió--------	❑	❑	❑	❑	❑	❑
4. El modo en que el doctor y las enfermeras trabaja-rón juntos para mejor servirle----------------------------	❑	❑	❑	❑	❑	❑
5 La calídad total del cúidado que recibió de su doctor	❑	❑	❑	❑	❑	❑
6.La calídad total del cúidado que recibió de las	❑	❑	❑	❑	❑	❑

Cuídado Personal

Como clasifica usted lo siguiente:						
1. La amabílidad y cortesia que recibió de su doctor--	❑	❑	❑	❑	❑	❑
2. La amabílidad y cortesia que recibió de enfermeras	❑	❑	❑	❑	❑	❑
3. La amabílidad y cortesia que recibió de recepción-istas---	❑	❑	❑	❑	❑	❑
4. El respeto que recibió de su doctor----------------------	❑	❑	❑	❑	❑	❑
5. El respeto que recibió de las enfermeras--------------	❑	❑	❑	❑	❑	❑
6. El respeto que recibió de la receptionista--------------	❑	❑	❑	❑	❑	❑
7. La atención personal que recibió de su doctor-------	❑	❑	❑	❑	❑	❑
8. La atención personal que recibió delas enfermeras-	❑	❑	❑	❑	❑	❑
9. La atención personal que recibió de la recepción-istas---	❑	❑	❑	❑	❑	❑
10. Llamada de cortesia cúando le hablan----------------	❑	❑	❑	❑	❑	❑

Friendly Hills Health Care Center Facility

Como clasifica usted lo siguiente:	Mal	Mas o Menos	Bien	Muy Bien	Excelente	No Aplicable
1. La apariencia exterior del Centro de Salúd	☐	☐	☐	☐	☐	☐
2. La apariencia de las señales en el exterior	☐	☐	☐	☐	☐	☐
3. La limpienza del area de recepción	☐	☐	☐	☐	☐	☐
4. La limpienza del area de tratamiento	☐	☐	☐	☐	☐	☐
5. La termperatura adecuada dentro del centro	☐	☐	☐	☐	☐	☐
6. Como de ordenado se ve el area de recepción	☐	☐	☐	☐	☐	☐
7. Como de ordenado se ve el area de recepcionista	☐	☐	☐	☐	☐	☐
8. Como de ordenado se ve el area de tratamiento	☐	☐	☐	☐	☐	☐
9. El nivel de ruido en la oficina	☐	☐	☐	☐	☐	☐
10. La calídad de aire (frescura) en el Centro de Salud	☐	☐	☐	☐	☐	☐

Informacion General

1. Fue esta su primera visita a Friendly Hills Health Care Center?   ☐ Si   ☐ No

2. Cuantas veces ha visto al doctor en el último año?

   ☐ Una   ☐ Dos   ☐ Tres veces o mas

3. Es ústed (el paciente):   ☐ Masculino   ☐ Femenino

4. Que édad tiene (el paciente)?:

   ☐ 36-45 años   ☐ 56-65 años

   ☐ menos de 6 años   ☐ 16-25 años   ☐ 46-55 años   ☐ 66-75 años

   ☐ 6-15 años   ☐ 26-35 años   ☐ sobre 75

5. Cuanto tiempo ha sido miembro de Friendly Hills HealthCare Network?

   ☐ Menos de 1 año   ☐ 1-2 años   ☐ 3-5 años   ☐ 6-10 años   ☐ 11 años o mas

6. Ústed planea seguir siendo miembro de Friendly Hills HealthCare Center? ☐ Si   ☐ No

7. Considerando todo, que satisfacción siente ústed con Friendly Hills Health Care Center?

   ☐ Completamenta satisfecho, no podría estar mejor   ☐ Un poco desatisfecho

   ☐ Muy satisfecho   ☐ Muy disatisfecho

   ☐ Un poco satisfecho   ☐ Completamente desatisfecho

     ☐ No estoy satisfecho ni desatisfecho

8. Ústed recomendaria el centro de Friendly HIlls Health Care Center aun familiar o una amistad?

   ☐ Si   ☐ No

Por favor ponga este questionario en la caja que dice "SURVEY COLLECTION BOX"

GRACIAS POR SU COOPERACION!

COMENTARIOS

_____

_____

_____

_____

_____

_____

_____

_____

_____

_____

_____

_____

Grácias por su cooperación!

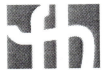

FRIENDLY HILLS HEALTHCARE NETWORK

"Calídad cúidado de salúd con enfasis en atención personal"

Principles of Continuous Quality Improvement: Presentation Slides

Courtesy of Friendly Hills HealthCare Network.

"Desired results in the organization are created not by the <u>mechanic</u>, but by the <u>gardener</u>. The gardener knows that life is within the seed."

- Stephen R. Covey

CONTINUOUS PROCESS IMPROVEMENT

F.O.C.U.S.- P.D.C.A.

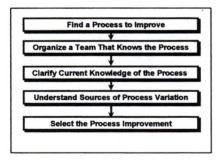

Find a Process to Improve

Organize a Team That Knows the Process

Clarify Current Knowledge of the Process

Understand Sources of Process Variation

Select the Process Improvement

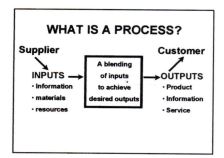

WHAT IS A PROCESS?

Supplier   Customer

INPUTS → | A blending of inputs to achieve desired outputs | → OUTPUTS

· Information   · Product
· materials   · Information
· resources   · Service

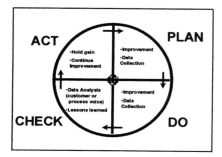

ACT   PLAN

· Hold gain   · Improvement
· Continue   · Data
Improvement   Collection

· Data Analysis   · Improvement
(customer or   · Data
process voice)   Collection
· Lessons learned

CHECK   DO

**FIND A PROCESS
TO IMPROVE**

· Who is the customer?
· What is the name of the process?
· What are the process boundaries?
· Clearly written opportunity statement?
· Who will benefit from the improvement?
· Tied to organization's priorities?

ORGANIZE A TEAM THAT KNOWS THE PROCESS

- How big is the team?
- People who work in the process?
- Does the team's knowledge of the process align with the boundaries in the opportunity statement?
- Roadmap to chart team progress?

_____
_____
_____
_____
_____
_____
_____
_____

CLARIFY CURRENT KNOWLEDGE OF THE PROCESS

- Document "as is" process flow? (vs. "ideal")
- Easy improvements in "C" of PDCA?
- Agreement on best process flowchart?
- Detailed enough to I.D. variation causes?

_____
_____
_____
_____
_____
_____
_____
_____

UNDERSTAND SOURCES OF PROCESS VARIATION

- I.D. Key Process Variables (KPVs) and Key Quality Characteristic (KQC) (specific, measurable & controllable)
- Clear data collection plan?
  - What data?...Who collects it?...How Long?
- KPV & KQC show special causes of variation in process?...How to resolve?

_____
_____
_____
_____
_____
_____
_____
_____

SELECT THE PROCESS IMPROVEMENT

- How is potential improvement selected?
- What data or other evidence supports the selected improvement?
- What criteria will be used to select the process improvement?

REQUEST FOR PERFORMANCE IMPROVEMENT TEAM

- Opportunity for Improvement
  - What process/system/outcome have you identified for an improvement team?
  - What data/information is available to substantiate the need for improvement?

- Scope of Performance Team
  - Opportunity Statement
  - Function - see CAMH *Special Update 3/97*
- Dimension of Performance
  - Doing the right thing
  - Doing the right thing well
    - Ava

CAUSE ANALYSIS

- Affinity diagramming
- Cause-and-effect diagramming
  - Ishikawa
  - Fishbone

AFFINITY DIAGRAMMING

- Identify an adverse outcome
  - Problem or process condition
- Generate potential causes - Post-Its
- Arrange Post-Its into related groups
- Create a heading for each group

GROUP TITLE/HEADING

- Best describes theme/focus of group
- Short - one to three words
- Place similar groups adjacent
- May combine groups - new title
- Team consensus essential

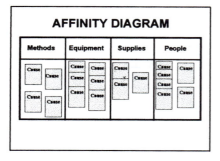

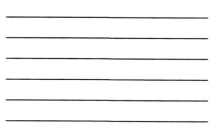

CAUSE-AND-EFFECT DIAGRAM

- Helps identify root causes
- Helps generate ideas
- Orderly arrangement of theories
- Helps to guide further inquiry
- "Head" = effect of causes
- Major headings in boxes

CAUSE-AND-EFFECT DIAGRAM

- Start with problem statement
- "Fish head" = problem effect
- Place major categories in boxes
- Refine categories
  - Ask "why?" five times
  - Specific enough to take action on

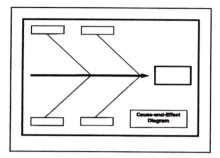

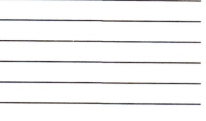

OPPORTUNITY STATEMENT DEFINITION

A written description of the specific process problem(s) the team will address first (or next) and how this was determined.

OPPORTUNITY STATEMENT ANSWERS 3 QUESTIONS

- What circumstances or process problem(s) , among several that may have been identified, have been selected to be addressed next?

- How was this selection made? What process and criteria were used to make the selection?

- What data or other evidence supports the selection?

OPPORTUNITY STATEMENT PURPOSES

- To clarify the task for the team and the steering committee and help keep both focused on the task
- To foster understanding and support for the decision to make this problem a priority vs. other problems in the process
- To document team activity for reporting purposes.

OPPORTUNITY STATEMENT EXAMPLE

"Timely Medical Record Availability"

IMPROVEMENT PLANNING

- **Brainstorm list of action steps to make the improvement**
  - Indicate who will be responsible for each step
  - Indicate start and end date(s) for each step
- **Complete a cost / benefit analysis**
  - Estimate hard and soft dollar costs and benefits

IMPROVEMENT PLANNING

- **Complete a force field analysis**
  - Indicate driving and resisting forces for change
- **Modify the plan to overcome resistors and enhance drivers**
- **Prepare and present written plan for approval before implementation**

CQI TEAM STRUCTURE

- Team Leader
- Recordkeeper
- Scribe
- Timekeeper
- Members
- Team Coach/ Facilitator/ Advisor

TEAM PRESENTATIONS - STORYBOARDS

- Baseline Data, Flow Chart, Cause Data, Opportunity Statement
- Improvement Plan for Approval
- Improvement Results Data & Next Steps
- Gain Sharing & Recognition

TEAM PRESENTATION - STORYBOARDS

Storyboards help teams effectively explain their work to people who may not be familiar with the CQI process. The aim is to summarize the team information from the entire FOCUS PDCA process on a single 4' by 4' board, using words, pictures and graphs.

TEAM PRESENTATION - STORYBOARDS

- Map the board in advance with labels for each section
- Update the board as the team progresses through the process. Use post-it notes.
- Prepare clean boards for group presentations and display.
- Keep detailed information in a team record binder for reference.

ROLE OF CQI COACH/ FACILITATOR / ADVISOR

- Help team select appropriate CQI tools
- Teach and train team on use of CQI tools & monitor use
- Keep teams on the FOCUS PDCA cycle

ROLE OF CQI COACH/ FACILITATOR / ADVISOR

- Observe group behaviors, skills and advise leader how to improve or handle problems
- Encourage
- Provide general assistance where needed

THE COACH / FACILITATOR / ADVISOR DOES NOT:

- Act as a team member or perform member roles
- Take sides
- Violate confidence
- Abandon the team

ROLE OF CQI TEAM LEADER

- Plan, prepare for and conduct team meetings or assign others
- Delegate assignments and responsibilities, then follow up
- Learn and apply CQI tools and FOCUS PDCA process
- Participate in discussions, give input
- Facilitate consensus discussions

_____

_____

_____

_____

_____

_____

ROLE OF CQI TEAM LEADER

- Resolve group dynamic problems quickly
- Develop group discussion skills of team members
- Make the team experience interesting and enjoyable
- Keep management partners informed, submit reports

_____

_____

_____

_____

_____

_____

THE TEAM LEADER DOES NOT:

- Make unilateral decisions
- Do all the work
- Show favoritism or discount others
- Lose sight of the objective or give up

_____

_____

_____

_____

_____

_____

4 ROLES OF LEADERS

- Modeling
  - Be the person others choose to follow
- Pathfinding
  - Scan the big picture (stakeholder needs)
  - Articulate mission / vision
  - Stay focused on the destination

4 ROLES OF LEADERS

- Aligning
  - People (focus on self)
  - Interpersonal - trust relationships
  - Managerial style, systems/processes, structures
  - Organizational mission / vision (compelling)

4 ROLES OF LEADERS

- Empowering
  - Create conditions of empowerment
  - Drive out fear to foster innovation - challenge the current state
  - Hold people responsible

CQI TEAM IMPLEMENTATION & REPORTING

- Project Recommendation
- Project Selection & Approval
- Team Charter
- Team Meeting Record
- Monthly Progress Reports
- Quarterly CQI Update

COST BENEFIT ANALYSIS

Hard Dollar - Direct outgo, income or savings of cash $

- Costs
  - Training manuals $500/yr.
  - Fax Machine $600
  - Print new forms $800
- Benefits
  - New enrollment $1000/yr.
  - -2 FTE $70K/yr.
  - -500 sq. ft. lease $5000/yr.

COST BENEFIT ANALYSIS

Soft Dollar - Deterioration, use of or savings of existing non-cash resources: labor, time, materials, equipment, work conditions, customer loyalty

- Costs
  - Stress out Joan on Monday
  - Deplete glove supply 1 yr.
  - Increase PC use 40% 2 years
- Benefits
  - Reduced pt. wait time 20%
  - Retain .5pts. per 1000/yr.
  - -5 hrs. work of Bill's time

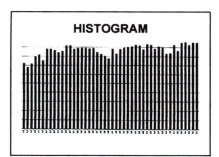

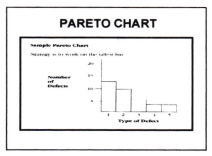

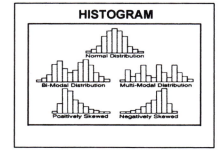

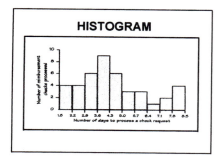

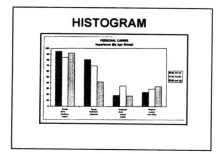

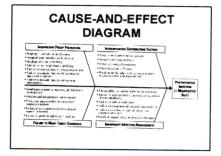

> Your actions speak so
> loudly that I can't hear what
> you say.

_____

_____

_____

_____

_____

_____

_____

Index

A